OCULAR PHOTOCOAGULATION
a stereoscopic atlas

OCULAR PHOTOCOAGULATION
a stereoscopic atlas

Francis A. L'Esperance, Jr., M.D.

Assistant Professor of Clinical Ophthalmology,
Columbia University College of Physicians and Surgeons,
New York, New York

with 562 illustrations and 112 stereoscopic views in full color on 16 View-Master reels and a View-Master compact viewer

The C. V. Mosby Company

Saint Louis 1975

Printed in the United States of America

Distributed in Great Britain by Henry Kimpton, London

Library of Congress Cataloging in Publication Data

L'Esperance, Francis A 1932-
Ocular photocoagulation.

Bibliography: p.
Includes index.
1. Light coagulation—Atlases. 2. Eye—Diseases and defects—Atlases. I. Title. [DNLM: 1. Light coagulation—Atlases. 2. Eye diseases—Therapy—Atlases. WW17 E77o]
RE992.P5L47 617.7′063′1 75-33111
ISBN 0-8016-2824-5

GW/U/B 9 8 7 6 5 4 3 2 1

To my wife, **ELLEN**

and **Franny**
Linda
Laura

Preface

Ocular photocoagulation was originally employed clinically in the spring of 1949 by Gerd Meyer-Schwickerath. Because of increased clinical experience and perfection of the various photocoagulation instruments since that time, indications for this method of therapy have become numerous. The xenon-arc photocoagulation instrument was the workhorse of photocoagulation therapy for nearly 15 years and was highly effective for various types of structural and vascular ocular abnormalities.

The discovery of laser action in 1960 provided the scientific community with a source of extremely precise, monochromatic light energy having predictable absorption potentials in various ocular tissues and the capability of producing a minute focus of high photon density. The ruby laser and later the argon, krypton, and frequency-doubled neodymium YAG laser have been used clinically, with each monochromatic wavelength used selectively to photocoagulate more effectively tissues that preferentially absorbed that wavelength.

The entire spectrum of ocular abnormalities, especially chorioretinal diseases, has been subjected to photocoagulation therapy for modification, control, or cure. In an effort to utilize the most advantageous and beneficial photocoagulation approach to a particular disease, clinicians have more critically analyzed many ophthalmic diseases and have learned more about the natural history, characteristics, and pathophysiology of these abnormalities.

The present work was undertaken in an effort to summarize and evaluate the response of various ophthalmic defects to photocoagulation. The book is designed to emphasize the important diagnostic and ophthalmoscopic aspects of chorioretinal diseases and is intended for use by the practicing ophthalmologist. With diagrams and stereoscopic photographs of photocoagulated defects, the book is also a comprehensive guide to the photocoagulation specialist for the proper and conservative therapy of these diseases. The effectiveness and the clinical experience (experimental or proved usefulness) of each photocoagulation approach have been indicated for each disease state. This monograph relates my personal experiences and convictions, although they have been tempered by the influence of many great clinicians.

The illustrations and diagrams are original, although several are reproduced from my previous publications. Except in those instances noted in the text, the photographs and color stereoscopic representations are taken from clinical examinations in my laboratory or office.

I am greatly indebted to the John A. Hartford Foundation for their generous support since 1966. Their financial assistance made possible the design, construction, and clinical evaluation of the first argon laser photocoagulation system. More recently, they have assisted my program to investigate, and normalize with argon laser photocoagulation, the pathologic hemodynamics of various chorioretinal diseases. I deeply appreciate their financial support during this time.

I was very fortunate to have the assistance of Arthur Vassiliadis, Senior Research Scientist at the Stanford Research Institute in Menlo Park, Calif., who wrote Chapter 2, which is concerned with the physical characteristics of lasers and which provides an understandable basis for photocoagulation therapy.

I wish to thank my associate, William A. James, Jr., for his constructive criticisms and suggestions during the preparation of the manuscript and for editing portions of it.

I wish to acknowledge the inestimable help I have had from Robert McGuffin, photographer for the John A. Hartford Laser Laboratory at the Edward S. Harkness Eye Institute. His skill as a photographer is outstanding, and he was unfaltering during the extremely arduous task of assembling the stereoscopic slides and representative prints. His unfailing cooperation has helped indispensably in the completion of this task.

Gloria Spevacek and Nancy Walsh of the Medical Illustration Department at the Veterans Administration Hospital in the Bronx, N.Y., were invaluable for their artistic help; they rendered all of the diagrams and drawings with painstaking care. I am grateful to Arnall Patz, Morton F. Goldberg, and Robert M. Ellsworth for their photographs of various diseases.

I am also indebted to Nan Gray, Diana Schleifer, Ada D'Amore, and especially to Rosemarie Verry, who typed the manuscript with meticulous care.

Francis A. L'Esperance, Jr.

Contents

Part III COMPLICATIONS OF OCULAR PHOTOCOAGULATION

Part IV DIAGNOSTIC AND FUTURE THERAPEUTIC INSTRUMENTATION

OCULAR PHOTOCOAGULATION
a stereoscopic atlas

Part I

INTRODUCTION

Chapter 1

History of photocoagulation

Plato's *Phaedo* contains a passage in which Socrates admonishes that one must take care not to look directly at the sun during an eclipse but to view the sun's reflection in water or some other such medium. The effect of solar radiation was well known to the ancients, and references continued into the Middle Ages, when the first description of a central scotoma following a solar burn of the retina was reported by Theophilus Bonetus (1620-1689). Descriptions of the ophthalmoscopic appearance of solar burns became widespread after the ophthalmoscope came into use, and many ophthalmologists collected cases following solar eclipses (Cords, 1912; Blessing, 1912; and Birch-Hirschfeld, 1912).

Accordingly, experimentation of the effect of light on the retina was carried out by a series of investigators, including Czerny (1867), Deutschmann (1882), and Widmark (1893). These investigators used either the effects of the sun or the carbon arc to produce a lesion in the retina. Early experimentation of the effect of radiation damage on the human retina was carried out by Maggiore (1927), who focused sunlight on two eyes scheduled for enucleation; these eyes were studied histologically and were found to show marked hyperemia and edema of the retinal structures. Móran-Salas performed numerous experimental procedures on human and rabbit eyes during the late 1940's to utilize light coagulation therapeutically. He failed to publish his results until after Meyer-Schwickerath, who was working concurrently, published his first clinical experiences with light photocoagulation in 1949. Móran-Salas then published his findings in 1950, corroborating the previous publications of Meyer-Schwickerath.

Since the eclipse of the sun on July 10, 1945, Meyer-Schwickerath had worked with various methods of instrumentation that he felt could produce a therapeutic photocoagulation burn. Sunlight was used for some time, but this method proved impractical because of the length of time needed for therapeutic coagulation; the intricate optical systems required; and the dependence on weather conditions, time of day, and time of year. Between 1949 and 1956 a Beck arc was modified to be used as a photocoagulation source but had the disadvantages of having a short photocoagulation span and producing gases saturated with soot and carbon particles. In 1956 the high-pressure xenon lamp was used as a photocoagulation source, and the xenon-arc photocoagulation instrument, pioneered by Meyer-Schwickerath, was made commercially available by Zeiss.

In 1960 Maiman produced the optical maser (or laser, as it was eventually called), using a ruby crystal to produce a 200μsec pulse of intense red light energy. This monochromatic light had a wavelength of 694.3 nm and provided the ophthalmologic world with an intense, pure beam of light that could produce extremely small burns of varying intensities. In 1961 Zaret began experimentation with ruby laser photocoagulation in animals, and both Campbell and Zweng treated human patients the following year. The ruby laser was found to be highly effective in producing an adhesive chorioretinitis but was not useful in the treatment of vascular diseases.

The use of the argon ion laser in the treatment of ophthalmic vascular disease was first considered in our laboratory in early 1965, and histopathologic studies with animals and the design and development of multiple photocoagulation systems to deliver the argon laser beam to the human eye were undertaken there from 1966 to 1968. At the Edward S. Harkness Eye Institute in the Columbia-Presbyterian Medical Center, on February 14, 1968, we conducted the first photocoagulation trial using argon laser radiation on a human. During the following year over 500 cases of various ophthalmic diseases were treated in our laboratory with our newly designed direct, indirect, and slit lamp biomicroscopic argon laser photocoagulation delivery systems.

In May 1969 Little, Zweng, and Peabody (1970) began their clinical argon laser photocoagulation studies (as did Patz, Okun, and others) with instrumentation that incorporated modifications of our original design. Commercial argon laser photocoagulation systems became available in 1971, 6 years after the inception of the argon laser project; presently, over 700 argon laser photocoagulators have been distributed to various parts of the world.

In 1971 our laboratory conducted clinical trials concerning the photocoagulation potential of the krypton (1972) and the frequency-doubled neodymium (1971) yttrium-aluminum-garnet (YAG) lasers in a series of patients. Although the laser radiations from these particular sources were more highly absorbed by the pigments of the eye, the technologic difficulties in producing the laser beam militated against their immediate use for therapeutic photocoagulation.

In 1971 the carbon dioxide laser was used by Beckmann and his associates to produce keratectomies and sclerectomies in animals. Extensive research is still being done on these procedures.

In 1973 Krasnov reported the treatment of the trabecular meshwork by a Q-switched ruby laser in patients with glaucoma to make this area more permeable to the outflow of aqueous fluid. His success was limited, but a new dimension of laser therapy in ophthalmology was introduced.

At the time of this writing, the helium-cadmium, helium-neon, xenon, and a host of other lasers have not been used therapeutically in ophthalmology. The introduction of dye lasers with the capability of producing laser wavelengths in any portion of the visible spectrum holds great promise for the laser beam's being tailored to a particular disease process. These newer laser systems, hopefully, will be utilized in the future to increase our armamentarium against ocular disease.

Chapter 2

Photocoagulation source technology and ocular effects

Arthur Vassiliadis, Ph.D.

The purpose of this chapter is to present a summary of the interactions and mechanisms involved in the application of laser radiation to photocoagulation of the eye. A review of some fundamentals of optical radiation is presented, followed by a discussion of material systems and how they interact with radiation fields. Characteristics of sources of radiation are discussed; the fundamentals of laser operation are summarized; and the properties of two lasers important to photocoagulation are enumerated.

Interactions of radiation of various wavelengths with biologic material is discussed, and the application of laser radiation to the eye is analyzed. Experimental evidence indicating the relationship of photocoagulation to simple thermal damage associated with denaturation of proteins is discussed.

Finally, photocoagulation of the retina is discussed in terms of a thermal model, and a number of considerations important to qualitative photocoagulation are presented.

RADIATION AND MATTER

Background

The turn of this century marked the beginning of the modern theories of matter and radiation and the end of the classical period.

In 1900 Planck presented the first modern theory with his explanation of black body radiation. A black body is, by definition, one that absorbs all the radiation that it receives. Very general reasoning based on thermodynamics indicates that the radiation emitted by a black body must be a function of temperature only and that the spectral distribution of the intensity of the radiation is derivable from the basic laws governing interaction between matter and radiation. The distribution thus derived from the classical theory, however, is in serious disagreement with experimental evidence (Fig. 2-1).

Planck took the bold step of postulating that matter consisted of material oscillators that could give up or absorb energy in discrete or quantized amounts only, rather than in a continuous manner. He also showed that the individual lumps of energy, called quanta, must be of the form

$$E = nh\nu$$

where n is any integer, ν is the frequency of oscillation, and h is a proportionality constant, now known as Planck's constant. With this assumption he derived an expression for the

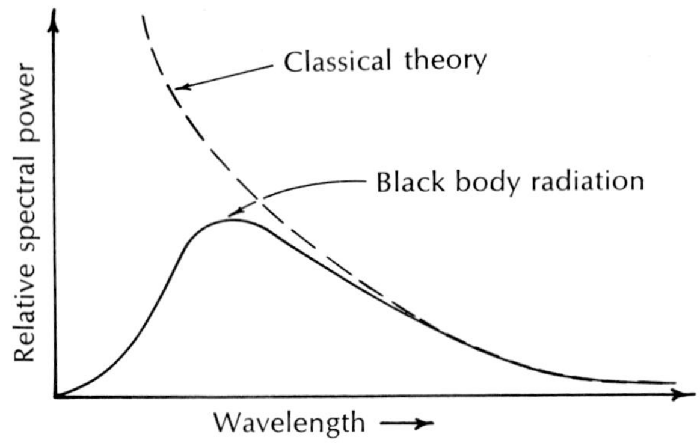

Fig. 2-1. Spectral distribution of a black body.

spectral distribution of a black body that agreed with experimental evidence. The success of the derivation of the radiation law did not immediately lead to acceptance of Planck's hypothesis; however, additional experimental facts and analyses confirmed this quantum nature.

Quantization of radiation photons

In 1905 Einstein took an even bolder step by hypothesizing that light radiation itself consists of a beam of quanta called photons, whose energy is $h\nu$ and whose velocity is c (velocity of light in a vacuum). He then showed how this hypothesis explains a number of phenomena, including the photoelectric effect, which could not be explained classically.

Thus, according to Einstein's theory, the minimal amount of radiation energy that can enter into an interaction with matter is equal to the energy of a single photon. Although this "corpuscular" picture of light explains certain observations, the wave nature of light cannot be renounced, and, indeed, a dual nature must be maintained; one or the other aspect is manifest, depending on the phenomenon being investigated.

Quantization of material systems

The existence of discontinuities in the interaction of radiation and matter not only upset the classical theory of light but also gave insight to the knowledge of atoms and molecules.

One of the important features of emission and absorption spectra of light by matter is the existence of narrow spectral lines. These frequencies vary from atom to atom, the more complex atoms having more complex spectral characteristics. These observations are again in disagreement with the classical theory, which predicts emission of a continuous light spectrum and does not explain the stability of atoms.

In order to explain the experimental evidence, in 1913 Bohr postulated the quantization of the energy levels of atoms. According to Bohr, the atom cannot exchange energy with its environment in a continuous manner (as expected classically); it can exist only in a certain number of stationary or quantum states, each having a well-defined energy associated with it. Fig. 2-2 is a diagram depicting the energy level of a hypothetical atom. The atom can change in internal energy only by going through a transition from one state to another, whereupon the atom must either gain or lose energy by absorbing or emitting a photon, for example. Thus, an atom can go from a lower state (E_i) to a higher state (E_j) $(>E_i)$ provided that energy is conserved; that is, the atom absorbs a photon whose energy is given by:

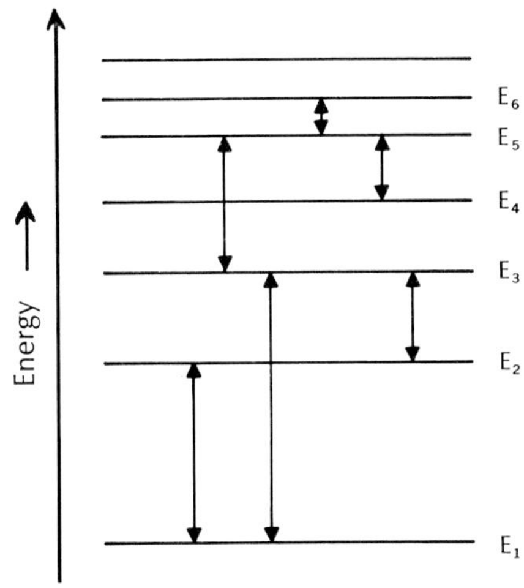

Fig. 2-2. Energy levels and transition of an atom.

$$h\nu = E_j - E_i$$

Similarly, employing the same relationship, an atom can emit a photon

$$h\nu = E_j - E_i$$

in going from the higher state to the lower state. The lowest energy state is called the ground state, and the atom in this state cannot radiate; it remains stable.

Simple atoms

An atom, as we have seen, has an innumerable number of levels. For simplicity, we are considering a hypothetical simple system where only two energy levels are possible. In this configuration the lower level, E_1, is the ground state, and the upper level, E_2, is the excited state (Fig. 2-3).

If an atom is in the ground state, E_1, and a radiation field containing photons of the appropriate wavelength is incident upon it, it can absorb a photon and go into the excited state. After some time the atom will spontaneously emit a photon of the same wavelength and return to the stable ground state. By considering the basic processes of emission and absorption of radiation at equilibrium, Einstein, in 1917, showed that an excited atom has an additional way of returning to the ground state. If the excited atom is in an external radiation field of the appropriate wavelength, the atom can be induced or stimulated into emitting a photon and returning to the ground state. Spontaneous emission is emitted randomly in any direction and bears no relation to an incident radiation field; whereas, as Einstein showed, the energy radiated by stimulated emission is in phase and coherent with the incident beam. As we will see in the next section, it is the stimulated emission of atoms or molecules that makes a laser possible.

Radiation sources

The radiation from natural and man-made sources (except lasers) typically is a combination of radiation from many lines, as well as a continuum approximation of the black body radiation profile, because most sources of light are a result of increasing the temperature of matter to a degree sufficient to cause it to radiate effectively in the spectral range of interest. From Fig. 2-1 it is apparent that the radiation is broad in spectral extent; that is, it contains all wavelengths of the spectrum.

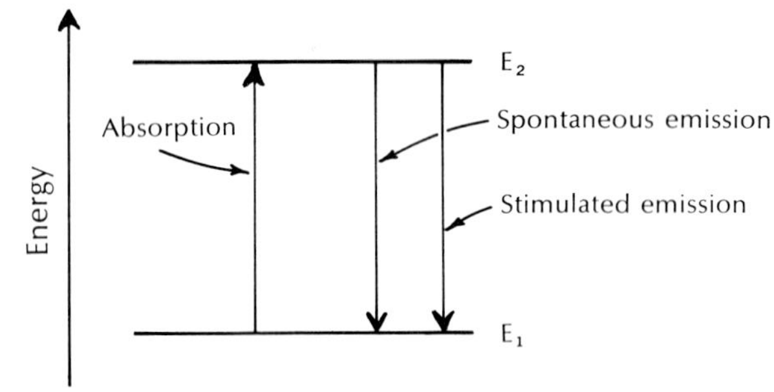

Energy of photon$=h\nu=E_2-E_1$

Fig. 2-3. Interaction of radiation and matter.

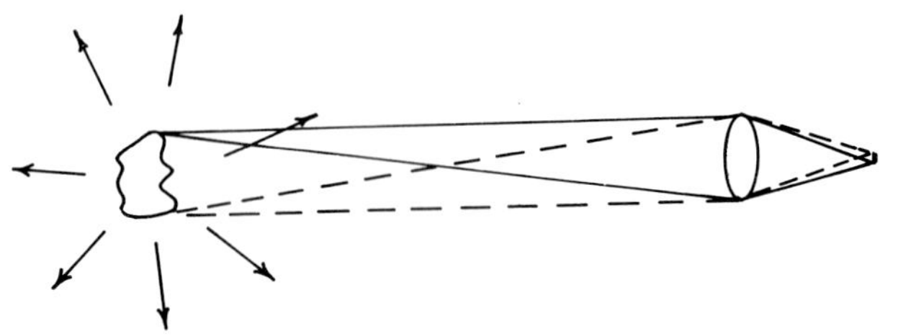

Fig. 2-4. Effect of concentrating radiation from a natural source.

More important, the light is radiated randomly in all directions, and the radiation source is finite. Thus, each part of the source is radiating independently from every other part. If one tries to focus the source in order to increase the intensity of radiation, the best that one can do is to image the source (Fig. 2-4). Indeed, there are fundamental reasons why the intensity of the image cannot be made greater than that of the source.

It is true that if one goes farther from the source, the image gets progressively smaller. However, in direct proportion, a progressively smaller fraction of the radiation from the source is being captured. Thus, the intensity of the image remains the same. The image size ultimately reaches the smallest possible diameter limited by diffraction effects.

Another way of looking at this phenomenon is to consider the angular subtent of the source. As the source recedes, the spherical waves that were generated by the various parts of the source come closer and become more and more indistinguishable. Eventually, the phase fronts of the various waves become one, and the wave is said to be spatially coherent. Thus, to focus down to a small spot, a light beam must have good spatial coherence.

LASERS

General considerations

In a quiescent state a collection of atoms or molecules will predominantly populate the lowest energy level, since this level is the only stable one. More accurately, the population of the levels depends on the temperature of the material. If the temperature is sufficiently high, significant numbers of molecules will be found in upper levels. The distribution of atoms in these levels is described by Boltzmann's distribution, that a higher energy level always has fewer atoms populating it than a lower level.

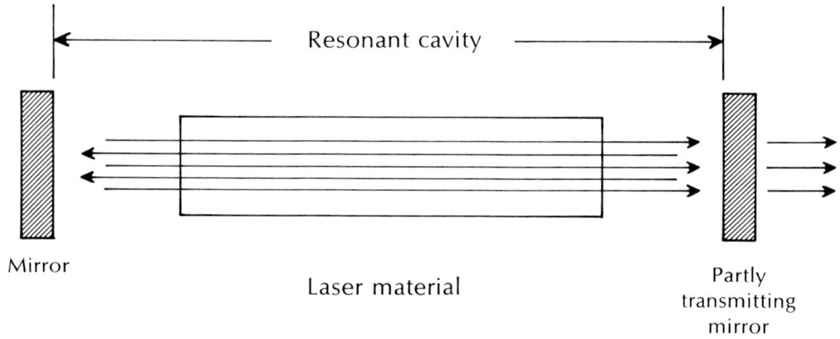

Fig. 2-5. Typical laser cavity, showing the laser material, the totally reflecting mirror, and the partly transmitting mirror that allows a portion of the resonating beam to escape from the cavity.

For transitions whose energy separation is equivalent to photons in the optical part of the spectrum, virtually all atoms or molecules are in the ground state. Thus, if a light beam of the correct wavelength is introduced into the medium, the beam will be attenuated because atoms will absorb photons of the beam and be excited to an upper level, from which they will, for the most part, spontaneously emit photons in random directions and return to the ground state.

If, however, by some stratagem we could achieve a condition where there were more atoms in an excited state than in a lower state or the ground state, then, if a beam of light were introduced, the beam would be amplified because the exicted atoms would be stimulated into emitting photons in phase and coherent with the exciting light beam.

The basic requirements for attaining laser operation are now apparent. First, a population inversion must be obtained; that is, more atoms must be placed in an upper or excited state than in a lower state. Second, a light beam of the correct wavelength must be introduced to stimulate the excited atom into emitting light coherent with the exciting light beam.

There are a number of methods that have been used to obtain population inversion; two of these methods are briefly described here. The method that is used to provide radiation of the proper wavelength is to place the laser medium in an optical cavity that acts as a resonator (Fig. 2-5). The resonant cavity consists of two mirrors carefully aligned to each other; the laser material is between them. One of the mirrors is made partially transmitting so that some of the radiation will be coupled out of the cavity.

Once population inversion has been achieved, the laser radiation buildup begins with some of the excited atoms in the medium emitting spontaneous radiation in various random directions. Some of the radiation, however, will hit one of the mirrors and return, passing through the medium. This radiation that is reentering is exactly the correct wavelength (since the material itself radiated it) and will therefore stimulate some of the atoms into emitting radiation, thus amplifying the beam. After the wave bounces back from the other mirror, it will be amplified as it passes through the medium again. As the intensity of this beam increases, the probability of stimulating additional atoms into emitting radiation increases. Thus a coherent beam is built up very quickly; stimulated emission becomes the dominant mechanism of deexcitation of the atoms; and one obtains laser action. Only waves propagating in directions closely parallel to the laser axis will be greatly amplified; consequently, the device emits a highly coherent beam because of the geometry of the cavity and the fact that stimulated emission is radiated in phase with the exciting beam. The laser beam will also be relatively monochromatic because the energy levels of the material are narrow and well defined.

Examples

Optically pumped pulsed laser

The first laser to be demonstrated was the ruby laser; it was demonstrated by Maiman in 1960. The ruby is a crystalline sapphire with a small percentage of chromium. The chromium ions are found to absorb strongly in the green-violet part of the spectrum and to fluoresce in the red part of the spectrum when flashed with white light.

A simplified energy level diagram for the ruby laser is shown in Fig. 2-6. The ruby laser has a large number of levels; in fact, there are whole bands of absorption. These bands explain the absorption of green, blue, and ultraviolet light.

The ruby is usually excited by being pulsed with a xenon flash lamp that emits radiation in all usable wavelengths. The chromium ions are thus excited and move to the upper energy states, where they nonradiatively lose some energy and pile up in a metastable level that has a relatively long lifetime (compared with the other transitory lifetimes). In this way a population inversion is obtained; that is, more ions are accumulated in this upper level than there are left in the ground state.

The ruby laser is termed a three-level system because the lower level of the laser transition is also the ground state (where the ions were initially). Thus there are only three levels: the ground state, the initial excited states grouped into one level, and the upper level of the laser transition, where the excited ions relax and accumulate.

The ruby laser is a pulsed laser; after population inversion is obtained, the laser emissions consist of a train of random pulses grouped together and lasting for times on the order of a millisecond. This mode of operation is termed long pulsed, and energy outputs of several hundred joules are obtained. In another mode of operation called Q switched, a single, very short pulse on the order of tens of nanoseconds is obtained with tens of joules output.

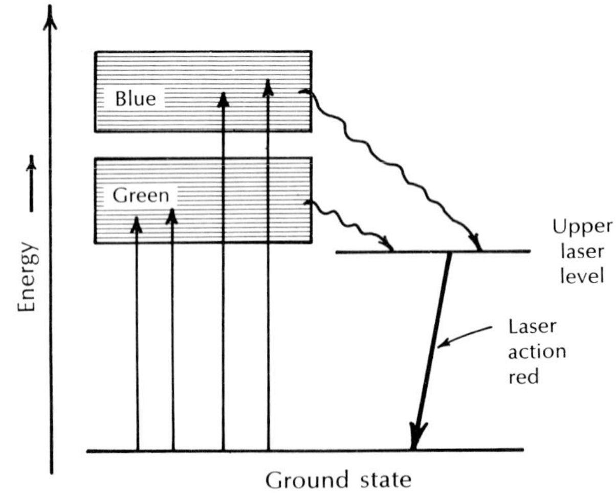

Fig. 2-6. Energy levels of the ruby laser.

Gas laser

Although there are numerous gas lasers that have been operated, I will only comment briefly on the argon ion laser. In the argon ion laser a high-current electrical arc discharge is started and maintained in an argon gas. The gas is then first ionized by energetic collisions with electrons. The singly ionized argon ion is then excited and moves to upper levels by additional collisions with electrons. A simplified schematic diagram of the energy levels of the argon ion laser is shown in Fig. 2-7.

In the argon ion laser some of the upper energy levels have somewhat longer lifetimes than others; ions can thus accumulate at these levels. Some energy levels below these have very short lifetimes and are virtually empty. Thus, laser action can take place in these unpopulated levels above the ground state; the argon ion laser can therefore be considered to operate as a four-level system: the ground state is the first level; the ions are excited and move to the high-excitation states, which may be grouped as one level (second level); the ions then accumulate at the upper laser states (third level) and emit radiation through laser action to the lower laser states, which comprise the fourth level. From the fourth level the ions quickly return to the ground state, from which they can begin the cycle again. This closed cycle makes possible the operation of the argon ion laser in a continuous mode; that is, laser radiation is emitted continuously.

The argon ion laser can lase over several lines simultaneously; these lines are all located in the blue-green part of the spectrum. Several watts of continuous power output can be obtained from an argon ion laser.

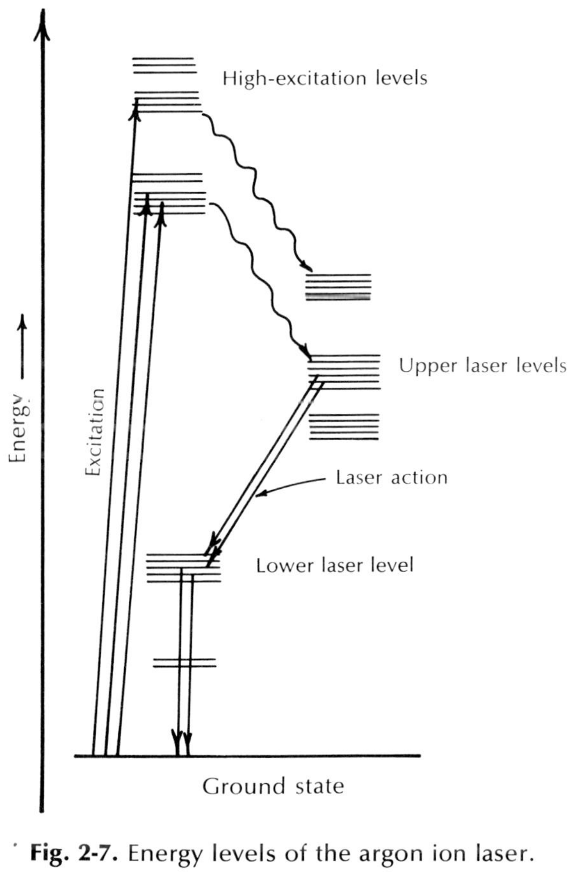

Fig. 2-7. Energy levels of the argon ion laser.

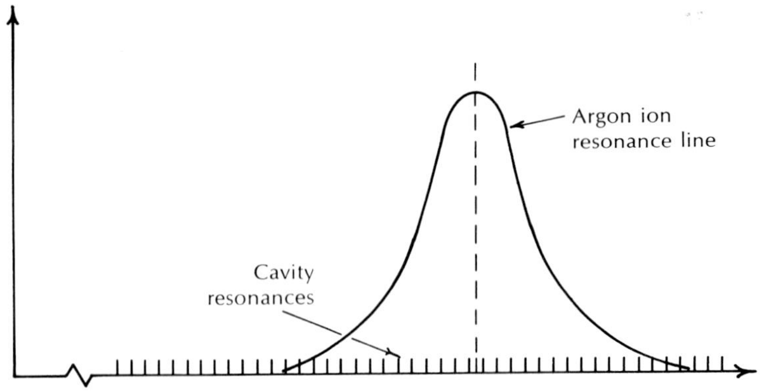

Fig. 2-8. Laser cavity resonances of a typical argon ion laser.

Other laser characteristics

The energy levels of atoms have been discussed here as very sharp and distinct levels. In fact, although they are sharp, they have a measurable width, and the line associated with transition is broadened because of a number of effects. The dominant mechanism in an argon ion laser is caused by the Doppler effect. Because the ions are moving randomly in all directions, when an ion emits a photon, its wavelength will be somewhat shifted, depending on whether the ion is moving toward or away from the direction in which it emits. This broadened line is shown schematically in Fig. 2-8. The gaussian, or bell-shaped, curve represents the resonance associated with one of the argon ion resonances, and it is only on the order of 0.001 nm in width spectrally.

In addition to this resonance of the laser medium, there are other resonances associated with the laser cavity and the light waves that are traveling back and forth in the cavity. The traveling waves, in transversing back and forth, set up standing waves that have resonances in the same way that a piano wire that is struck has resonances. This type of resonance is associated with the number of half wavelengths that are set up in the length of the cavity and refers to longitudinal modes. Because the wavelength of light is so short (about 0.5×10^{-4}cm), while cavity lengths are long, there are many combinations of half wavelengths that can fit within the line width. For example, a typical cavity length may be 1 m in length; then there can be about 4×10^6 half wavelengths in the cavity. Within the argon ion resonance line, there can be about 20 modes that can lase simultaneously, depending on the length of the cavity, as schematically shown in Fig. 2-8. All of these modes are, of course, equally effective for photocoagulation.

One final aspect of lasers needs to be mentioned briefly: the variation of intensity across the beam of the laser. The profile of the intensity of the beam will depend on the laser cavity and what are called transverse modes. Some lasers can, by proper restriction, be forced to lase in the simplest transverse mode that has a profile of a bell-shaped distribution.

In argon laser photocoagulators the lasers are operated so that a number of the low-order modes are operating simultaneously. The intensity is therefore relatively uniform across the beam.

In photocoagulation, multimode operation is of no consequence unless it is excessive. If a laser has too many higher-order modes, then the divergence of the beam is too large, and it cannot be focused to as small a spot as might be desired. This, however, is not a problem with the argon ion laser.

PHOTOCOAGULATION

Interaction of radiation with biologic material

We have seen that even a simple atom has numerous possible energy levels, and consequently the possible transitions are innumerable. In the optical part of the spectrum these transitions are associated with changes in electron orbits of the atom. When molecules are considered, the situation is much more complicated because of the vibrational, bending, and rotational energy levels that are possible. Thus, there are a large number of possible transitions, even in a simple molecule. For photons of high energy, such as those in the short ultraviolet and x-ray region, interactions will usually dissociate or ionize the molecule. In the visible region interactions predominantly involve electron orbit changes; whereas for photons in the infrared and longer wavelengths, interactions will usually involve complex vibrational, bending, and rotational changes. Once a molecule has reached an excited state, there are a number of different ways that the energy may be converted. They fall into three major categories:

1. Some or all of the energy may be reradiated in the form of resonant scattering, Rayleigh and Raman scattering; or it may be reradiated at appreciably longer wavelengths in the form of fluorescence or phosphorescence.
2. All or some of the energy will be converted into heat.
3. All or some of the energy can be used to provide free energy of activation to a chemical reaction.

Molecules involved in biologic systems are extremely complex and can maintain vital activity only in very specific configurations and ambient conditions. Thus, depending on the wavelength of the photons, widely different interactions are observed. Photons in the ultraviolet region are so energetic that interaction with biologic systems leads to disruption or alteration of DNA and RNA into abiotic forms, and cell death follows. Photons in the visible part of the spectrum lead to two forms of interaction. First, the photons can provide energy for photochemical reactions, such as photosynthesis and those that take place in the visual process. Second, the energy of the photons that are absorbed is degraded into heat, and since temperature is a very critical parameter in the normal operation of a living cell, a small increase in temperature can lead to thermal damage. Similarly, photons in the infrared or longer wavelengths are usually involved in thermal-type interactions with biologic material.

The type of damage caused in photocoagulation is thermal in nature. This damage is associated with the denaturation of proteins or the inactivation of enzymes. The temperature rise is required for this type of damage is only in the range of 10° to 30° C for the retinal damage associated with minimal to heavy clinical exposures.

Application to the eye

Characteristics of the eye

For interactions in the fundus of the eye, it is important to select wavelengths that are transmitted well by the ocular media and that at the same time are effectively absorbed by the target material so that good interactions can be obtained at the target site with minimal effects to other media.

To this end Fig. 2-9 shows the transmission characteristics of the ocular media and the absorption characteristics of the pigment epithelium and choroid in terms of incident radiation. The curves are based on in vitro measurements of human eyes. Light in the visible and near-infrared parts of the spectrum is transmitted very well by the ocular media. Thus, radiation whose wavelengths fall in this range will reach the retina with very little

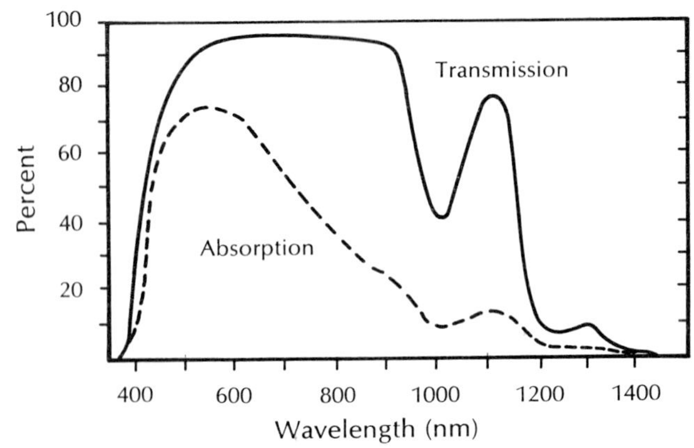

Fig. 2-9. Ocular transmission and absorption of the pigment epithelium and choroid.

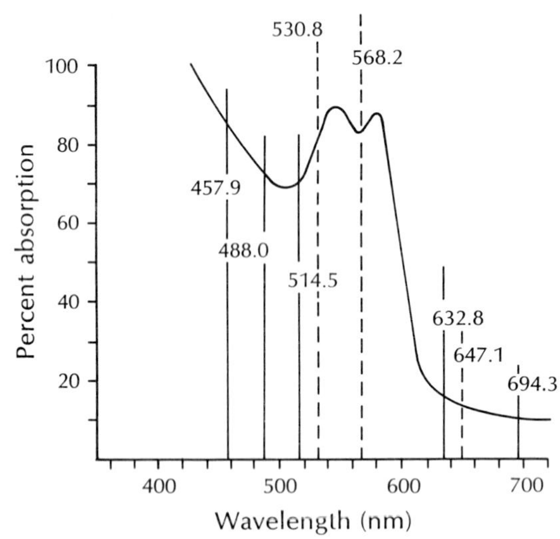

Fig. 2-10. Percent of energy absorbed per wavelength by a 100μ film of oxygenated blood: argon laser (457.9, 488.0, and 514.5 nm), krypton laser (530.8, 568.2, and 647.1 nm), helium-neon laser (632.8 nm), and ruby laser (694.3 nm).

loss to the ocular media. Wavelengths in the infrared region, however, are highly absorbed because of the water content in the media; radiation in the infrared region would not be useful for retinal interactions.

Fig. 2-9 also shows the absorption characteristics of the melanin granules responsible for the major part of the absorption in the pigment epithelium and choroid. This absorption falls off more rapidly as the wavelength is increased. The most effective part of the spectrum for heating the pigment epithelium is the blue-yellow part of the visible spectrum. The falloff of the curve on the short wavelength end is caused by the decrease in transmission characteristics of the ocular media, rather than by a decrease in absorption by the melanin granules.

Another important material with which interaction is desired is hemoglobin. Fig. 2-10 shows the absorption characteristics of hemoglobin in a 100-micron (μ) thickness of blood. The shorter wavelengths, particularly the blue-yellow part of the spectrum, are far more effective than the red and near-infrared wavelengths. Thus, red lasers, such as ruby, which emits radiation at 694 nm, is virtually totally unabsorbed by hemoglobin. If one wants to interact with blood vessels, one must use wavelengths that are shorter than 550 nm.

Because the argon ion laser usually emits several wavelengths in the blue-green part of the spectrum, all the wavelengths of this laser are located in a relatively narrow part of the spectrum that is almost optimally located for effective interactions with both the pigment epithelium and hemoglobin. Calculations show that in interactions with the pigment epithelium and choroid, the argon ion laser, in terms of power entering the eye, is 2.2 to 3.5 times more effective than the xenon-arc, depending on the pigmentation of the individual. Thus, appreciably less power need be used to generate the same effect. Similarly, calculations show that the argon ion laser is at least five times more effective than the xenon-arc as far as absorption by hemoglobin is concerned. Experimental evidence in rhesus monkeys has shown that vessels can be occluded with the argon ion laser beam by a power 10 times less than that used with xenon-arc radiation. The wavelengths of the argon ion laser appear to be extremely effective for photocoagulation of both the pigment epithelium and the choroid and for interactions with blood vessels.

Thermal interactions

Interactions of laser beams and the retina have been studied by a number of investigators. It has been shown that at the power levels used for interactions of minimal damage and for clinical applications, very little of the energy is absorbed by the photopigments of the eye. The majority of the energy that reaches the fundus is absorbed by the pigment epithelium and choroid. The resulting interaction results in thermal damage of the tissues in the fundus of the eye.

Because of its high density of melanin granules, the pigment epithelium is the place where the highest absorption per unit volume takes place. The highest temperature rise in the back of the eye will thus take place near or inside the pigment epithelium layer. Because of the geometry of the absorbing layers and because thermal conduction can take place away from the interaction region, the size of the interaction area plays a very important role as far as temperature rise and decay of the exposed site are concerned.

The temperature rise in the pigment epithelium, calculated on the basis of a simple thermal conduction model, is shown in Fig. 2-11 as a function of time for the same power density incident at the retina. In small spot sizes the temperature quickly rises and reaches a constant value. This temperature is the point of equilibrium where the heat being introduced into the interaction region is equal to the heat being conducted away to the surrounding tissues. In larger spot sizes it takes longer for equilibrium to be reached; more important, a higher temperature is reached (even though the power density is the same) because the thermal conduction of heat from a small spot size is more effective than that from a large spot size. In a small spot size we have a small absorbing area; as the heat is absorbed and the temperature begins to rise, there will be thermal relaxation or conduction of heat away from the site. In a small area the center part of the absorbing area, which is the part that gets the hottest, can cool in virtually all directions, so that the cooling of a small spot is fairly effective (Fig. 2-12). In contrast, in a large spot all the central area begins to heat up simultaneously, so that the center part of the region cannot cool as effectively because its immediate neighbors are also heating up. Thus, in a large area it takes less photon absorption per unit area to generate a certain temperature than in a small area (Fig. 2-13).

Since in photocoagulation the goal is to generate the same temperature rise at the

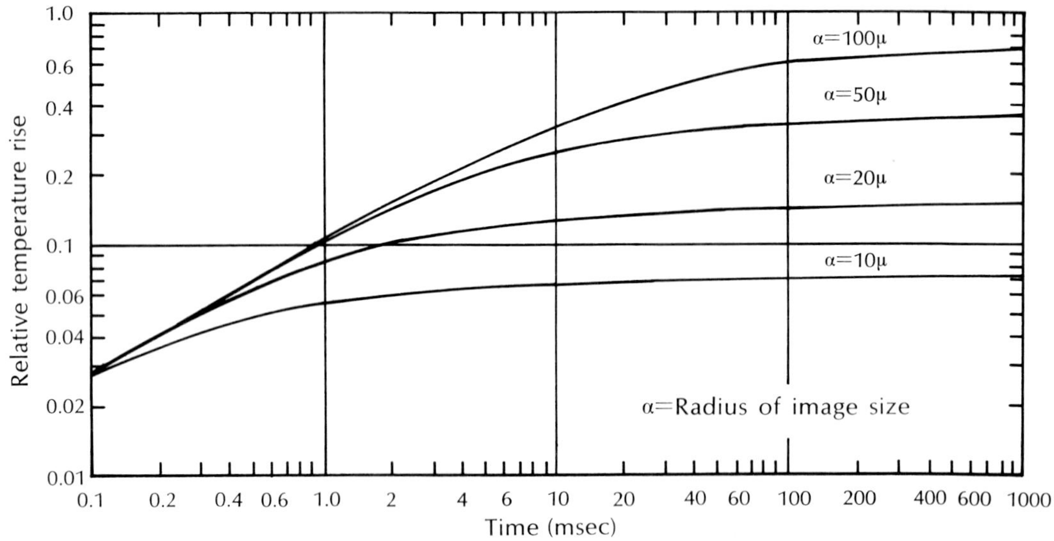

Fig. 2-11. Temperature rise at the center of the pigment epithelium as a function of time.

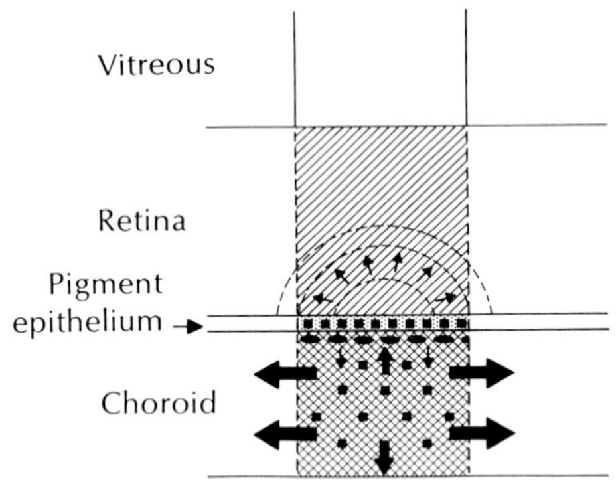

Fig. 2-12. Thermal dissipation of a threshold retinal laser dose in a small impact area. The central portion of the lesion cools more quickly because of easier conduction to the surrounding tissue.

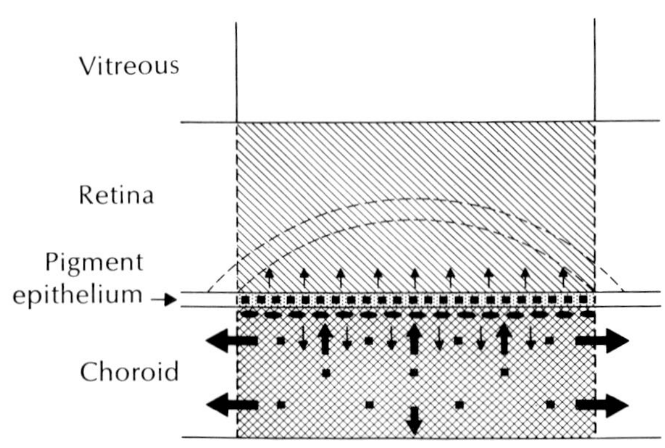

Fig. 2-13. Thermal dissipation of a threshold laser dose in a large impact area. The difficulty of cooling the central region of the lesion is caused by inadequate thermal conduction to the surrounding tissues.

center of any lesion, the power density used must be correspondingly reduced as the spot size is increased. This requirement is demonstrated in Fig. 2-14, which shows the total beam power theoretically required to cause the same temperature rise in each spot size as a function of exposure time.

At very short exposure times the power requirement varies in a way that is proportional to the area. Thus, if the spot size is increased by a factor of two, the area correspondingly increases by a factor of four, and four times as much power will be required to reach the same temperature. In this time regime the heating of the tissues takes place in a short time in comparison with the thermal relaxation time; that is, no cooling because of conduction takes place. However, at long exposures, which is the regime where most clinical argon laser exposures are made, the situation is totally different. This is seen, for example, in the region in Fig. 2-14 where the curves have leveled off. Here, we see that if the spot size is increased by a factor of two, the power required increases only by a factor of two, *not* a factor of four, because the smaller spot is more efficiently cooled by conduction than the larger spot. Thus, whenever the spot size is adjusted, the power must always be correspondingly adjusted.

Actual experimental data of retinal damage are shown in Fig. 2-15. These data were taken on threshold retinal damage in rhesus monkeys. Each point represents a large number of exposures that have been averaged. Although the curves should have leveled off, as theoretically predicted by simple thermal models, the curves continuously decrease as a function of exposure time. This factor is related to the fact that the damage is caused by protein denaturation or inactivation of enzymes. Therefore, because there is a rate relationship associated with these processes, the length of time at which tissues are kept at a certain temperature is important. Thus, there is no unique critical temperature; for a longer interaction one can generate the same effect by using a slightly lower temperature and therefore a slightly lower power in the laser.

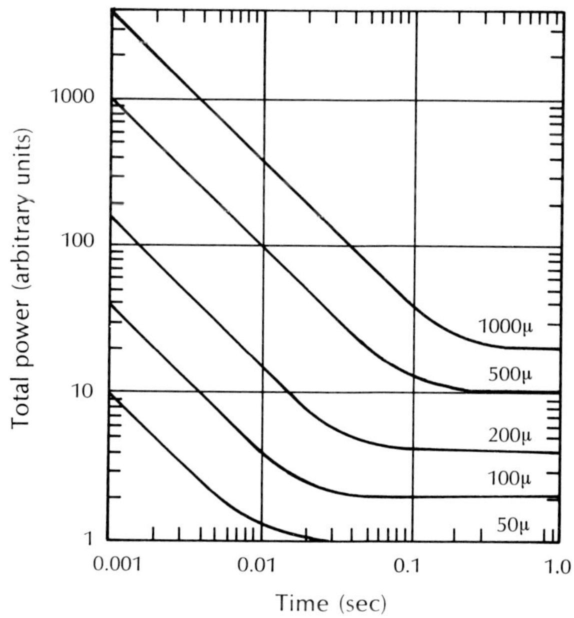

Fig. 2-14. Power required for an equal temperature rise in coagulations of various sizes.

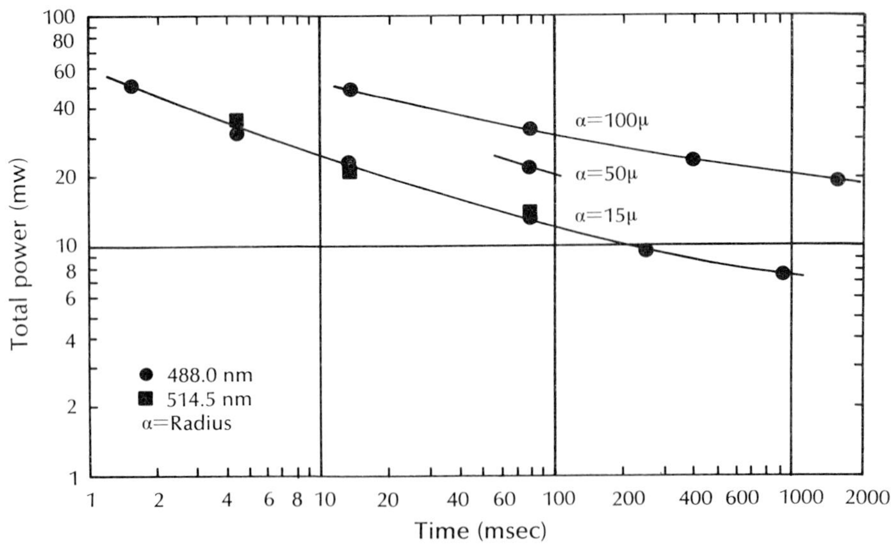

Fig. 2-15. Threshold retinal damage in rhesus monkey by argon ion laser photocoagulation.

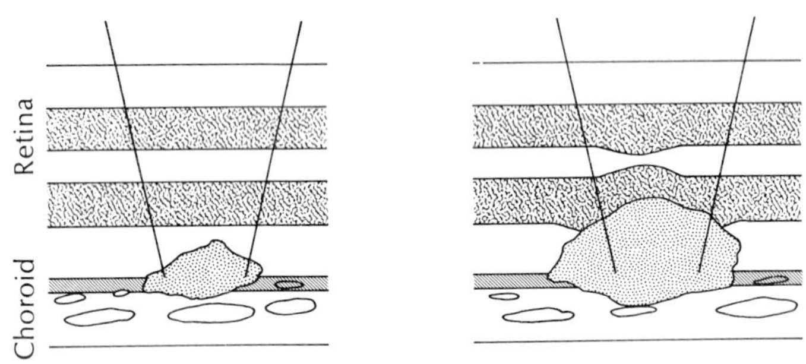

Fig. 2-16. Increase in coagulation's diameter and depth that occurs when either the exposure time or power level is increased while the spot size is retained.

Other considerations

There are numerous other considerations that must receive attention in the development of effective photocoagulation techniques.

In all applications of photocoagulation in the fundus, it is important to obtain a good estimate of the clarity of the optical media, including a careful examination for lenticular changes and hemoglobin in the vitreous.

In all applications one is interested in interaction with a certain area; one must therefore be careful to observe and estimate the amount of pigmentation in the area, because the temperature rise will depend on the fraction of the beam that is absorbed by the target. Even in a normal eye the pigmentation varies from one location to another, so that different power levels must be used.

As the power is increased beyond the point where one is getting a minimal effect, the lesion size will tend to increase beyond the size of the spot size. Thus, if one sets the spot size at 50μ, one generates a lesion of this size at a minimal interaction level. If, however, the power is increased, the area of the lesion will increase correspondingly.

The response of the tissues from minimal to very heavy photocoagulation results from a small increase in temperature. Accordingly, it takes a small power increase to go from a minimal effect to a strong effect. Thus, increases in power level should be made in small increments.

In changing the spot size, as has been shown, one should make a corresponding change in power level. If one decreases the spot size by a factor of two (thereby quadrupling the power density), one should always decrease the power level by a factor of three. If one increases the spot size by a factor of two, for safety the power should be increased by a factor of 1.5. Subsequent adjustments can then be made for proper effect.

Depending on the disease entity, the kind of interaction that is desired for effective treatment is different. If a minimal extent of damage away from the pigment epithelium is desired (in other words, longitudinal damage is to be kept to a minimum), as with central serous choroidopathy, for example, small spot sizes and very short exposure times should be used. On the other hand, if damage is required deep into the choroid or into the retina (as with choroidal neovascularization or the neovascular response of histoplasmosis), larger spot sizes and long exposure times should be used (Fig. 2-16).

Chapter 3

Technical considerations for ocular photocoagulation

PHOTOCOAGULATION INSTRUMENTATION AND BEAM CHARACTERISTICS

Physical differences between xenon-arc and laser radiation

The characteristics of electromagnetic radiation produced by each type of photocoagulator must be considered if one is to comprehend the potential effect that these radiations may have on ocular structures. The effect on the retina and other tissues basically depends on: (1) the magnitude of the intensity of the radiation energy; (2) the length of time that this energy is applied to an absorbent substance; and (3) to some extent, the diameter and area of the coagulation spot.

The intensity of radiation incident on the retina with the xenon-arc or laser system varies with and depends on three factors.

1. The aperture of the ocular system (the ratio between the size of the pupil and the focal length of the eye). Clinically, the intensity of radiation on the retina is increased when the pupil is widely dilated and the eye is hypermetropic; conversely, the intensity of radiation on the retina is reduced when the pupil is poorly dilated or the eye is myopic, despite the use of a correcting contact lens.

2. The absorption of light energy by the ocular media. The various photocoagulation sources (Fig. 3-1) available for ocular photocoagulation must have most of their emissions concentrated in the visible portion of the spectrum (Fig. 3-2). The absorption potentials of the transparent structures from the cornea posterior to the retina have been recorded for many of the clinical and experimental photocoagulation systems (Fig. 3-3). These observations are of paramount importance, since electromagnetic radiation, both xenon-arc and laser, produces effects only in sites at which it is absorbed. Certain tissues absorb only a particular wavelength, but the intensity of this wavelength may be sufficient to cause irreparable damage. The polychromatic radiation from the xenon-arc source is likely to affect all portions of the retina and choroid; with slightly longer exposures it will create some degree of coagulation of all layers (Fig. 3-4). On the other hand, the monochromatic light from the laser sources affects only several tissues in the choroid and retina, primarily those containing the melanin, xanthophyll, and hemoglobin pigments. The spectrally pure monochromatic beam from various lasers affects the pigment epithelium in most cases and various other cellular areas of the retina, depending on the particular wavelength emitted

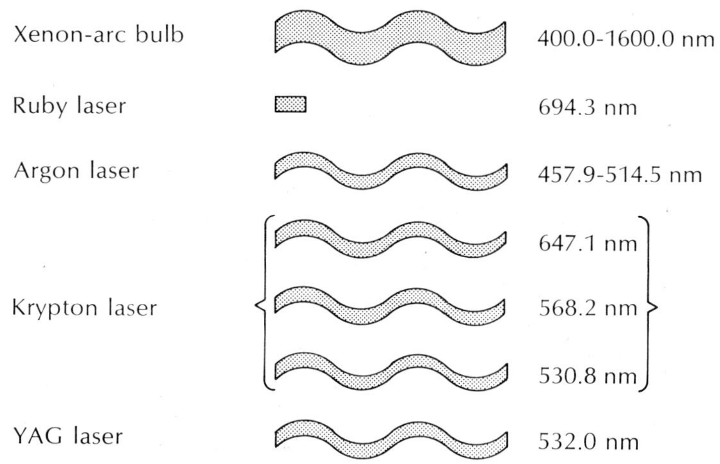

Fig. 3-1. Light sources available for photocoagulation and their representative wavelength emissions.

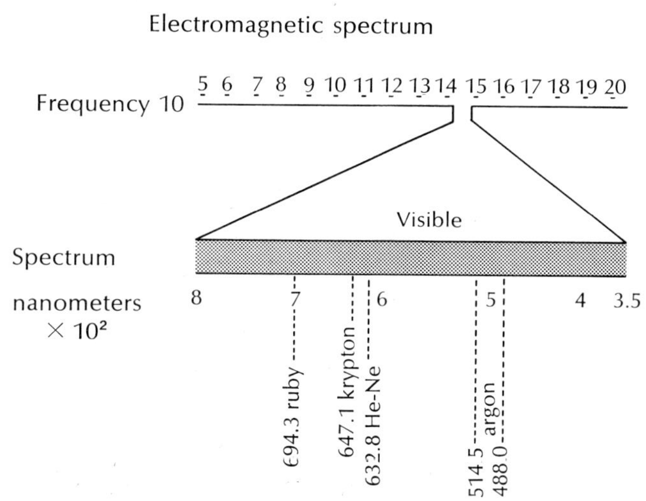

Fig. 3-2. Relationship of laser photocoagulation sources to the visible spectrum and the overall electromagnetic spectrum.

by the laser (Fig. 3-5). The ocular media transmit 95% of the radiations between 400 and 900 nm but absorb rather highly between 300 and 400 nm and beyond 900 nm (Fig. 3-6).

3. The spectral distribution and density of the radiations from the light source. Every light source emits energy as electromagnetic waves, but these radiations may be more concentrated at one wavelength than at another. The typical 1-w argon ion laser emits 9 wavelengths between 457.9 nm and 528.7 nm, but more than two thirds of the power of the total beam is concentrated at the 514.5 nm (pea green) and 488.0 nm (blue) wavelengths (Fig. 3-7). It may be difficult to determine the concentration of the individual wavelengths from the overall intensity of radiation, since the percentage of one particular wavelength varies with the overall power. For instance, radiation from an argon ion laser at low power is primarily blue (488.0 nm), whereas higher-power radiation is primarily pea green (514.5 nm).

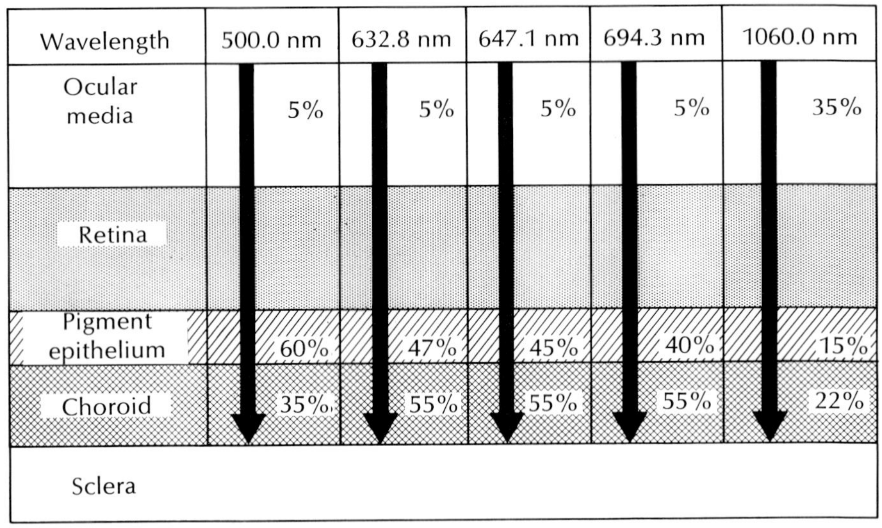

Fig. 3-3. Maximum amount of laser energy that would be absorbed by various posterior ocular layers from laser beams as they struck those individual layers: argon (500 nm), helium-neon (632.8 nm), krypton (647.1 nm), ruby (694.3 nm), and neodymium (1060.0 nm) laser beam radiations.

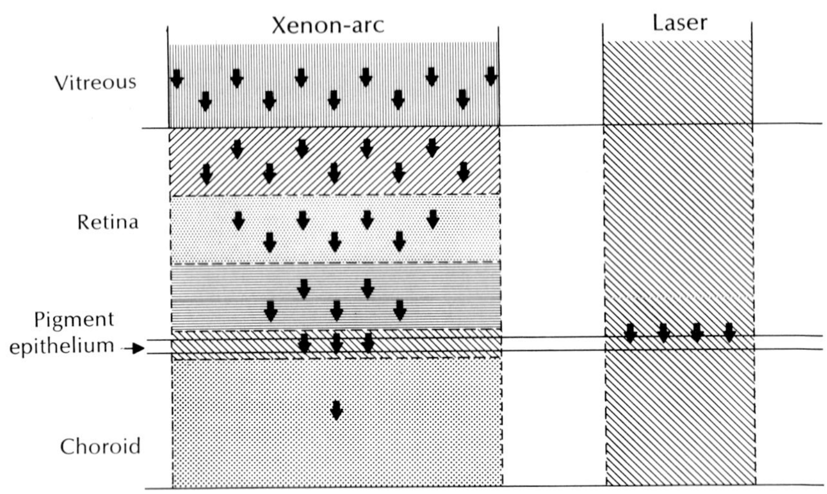

Fig. 3-4. Choroidal and retinal potential for absorption of polychromatic radiation (xenon-arc), and pigment epithelial absorption of laser (argon and ruby) radiation.

The output of continuous-wave sources, such as the xenon-arc and argon laser instruments, is considered in terms of power; watts or milliwatts are used as the unit of measurement. If a power meter is allowed to measure the output of a continuous-wave photocoagulation source for 1 sec, it will record the number of joules emitted during that 1-sec interval. Since 1 w is equal to 1 joule emitted over a period of 1 sec, the number of joules recorded by the power meter can then be converted directly to watts (joules per second). Regardless of the length of the photocoagulation exposure, the increment of the beam utilized is a portion of the beam being produced continuously at a particular rate of a certain number of joules per second (or watts).

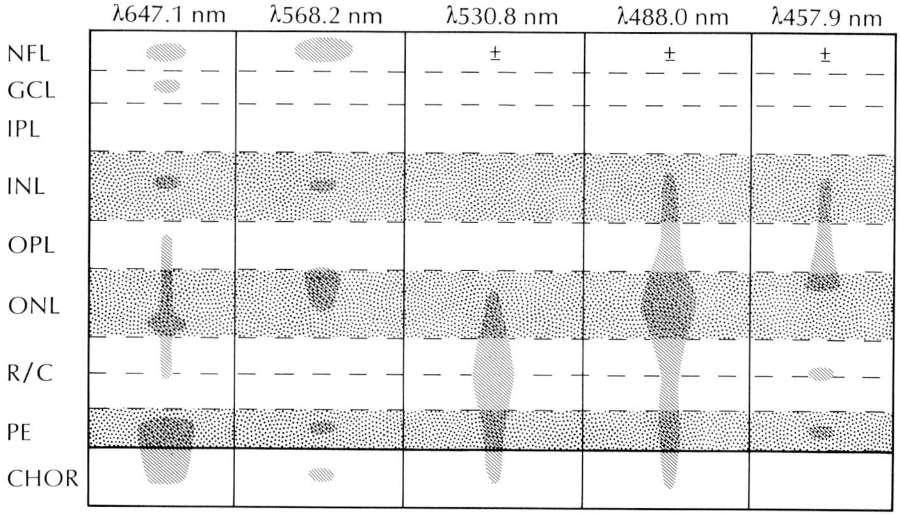

Fig. 3-5. Chorioretinal zones of maximal absorption and damage from laser photocoagulation of various wavelengths: krypton (647.1, 568.2, and 530.8 nm) and argon (488.0 and 457.9 nm) laser radiations.

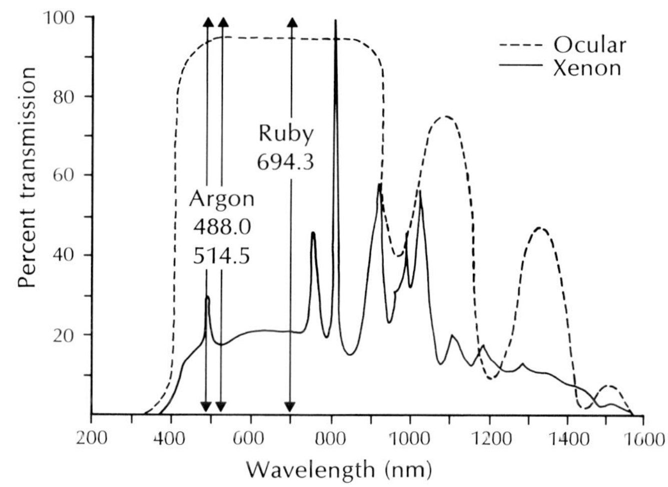

Fig. 3-6. Xenon-arc and laser energy distributions in comparison with the ocular refractive media transmittance.

Output wavelength (nanometers)	528.7	514.5	501.7	496.5	488.0	476.5	472.7	465.8	457.9
Output power (watts)	0.005	0.24	0.09	0.12	0.42	0.095	0.005	0.005	0.02

Fig. 3-7. Output power distribution of a typical 1-w argon laser.

The ruby laser and any pulsed photocoagulation system must be measured on a slightly different basis. Since most pulsed lasers (such as the long-pulsed ruby laser and the Q-switched ruby laser) cannot be operated continuously for a 1-sec period, their energy is simply recorded by the recording meter along with the inherent length of each laser pulse. The pulse length is then divided into 1 sec, and the resulting factor is multiplied by the energy in a single pulse from the laser source (expressed in joules). The energy output of the pulse laser can then be expressed in terms of joules per second. Occasionally, pulsed laser systems are considered in terms of their energy output (joules) in an individual pulse, provided that the pulse length is well known.

With an argon laser or xenon-arc photocoagulation system, a 0.5-sec exposure at a 2-w power level does not deliver 2 w of power; rather it delivers 1 joule of energy to the eye. If the exposure were maintained for 1 sec at the 2-w power emission level, the energy delivered to the eye would then be 2 joules over a 1-sec exposure interval, or 2 w of power (Fig. 3-8).

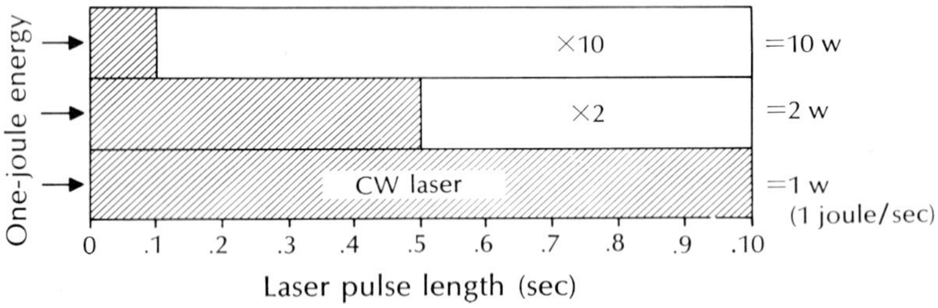

Fig. 3-8. Relationship of energy (joules) and power (watts). One watt is equal to 1 joule of energy delivered over a 1-sec interval.

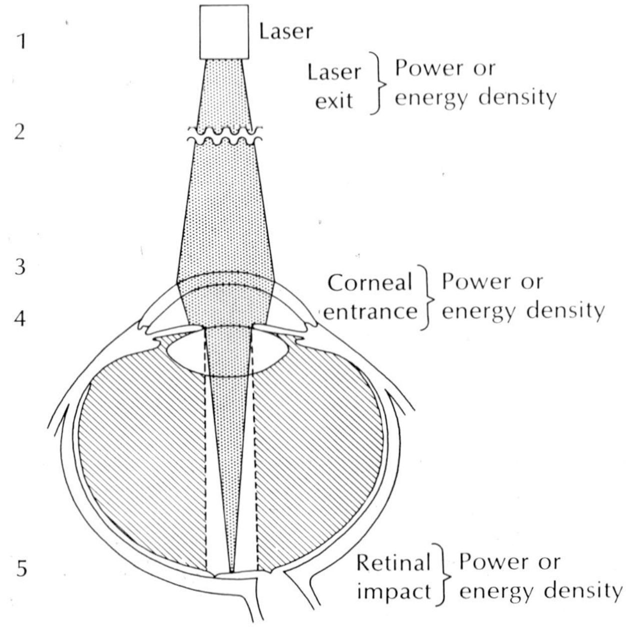

Fig. 3-9. Laser exit, corneal entrance, and retinal impact energy or power density as calculated at these areas. Power and energy density are expressed in terms of watts or joules per square centimeter.

Whether we are dealing with a pulsed (energy) or a continuous-wave (power) photocoagulation system, the power or energy should be considered in terms of the area of the beam as it exits from the laser of the photocoagulation system or as it impinges on the cornea, the retina, or other ocular tissue. The number of watts or joules per square millimeter or square centimeter can be calculated and is known as the laser exit, corneal entrance, or retinal impact power or energy density (Fig. 3-9). Consideration of the power or energy density as the photocagulation beam impinges on an ocular tissue is most important when one is comparing or determining the photcoagulation effect on that particular area.

Xenon-arc radiation

The xenon-arc photocoagulator produces radiation that has spectral qualities similar to sunlight and power capabilities many times that emitted by the sun. The element xenon is made to glow by high-intensity current, and the resulting white light is an unequal mixture of all wavelengths from 400 to 1,100 nm. The spectral energy distribution of the xenon arc after it passes through the optical system of the light coagulator is illustrated in Fig. 3-6. A comparison of the energy distribution with the transparency curve of the ocular media shows that most of the radiation energy is transmitted with little absorption, particularly in the visible and shorter infrared range that is most effective for tissue coagulation at the absorption site. Longer infrared radiations (from 930.0 to 1,030.0 nm) are still present, however, and are partially absorbed by the refracting media. This partial absorption creates a potential hazard that must be considered in xenon-arc photocoagulation. These longer infrared radiations are effective in the penetration and coagulation of intraocular tumors, telangiectatic and saccular vascular abnormalities, and other thick abnormal tissue masses.

The actual creation of an exudative choroiditis for chorioretinal adhesions depends on the accumulative effect (time factor) of a certain intensity of radiation of 1 or more wavelengths. The coagulation produced by the xenon-arc source tends to involve a greater amount of chorioretinal tissue, because of the polychromaticity and larger spot size, than

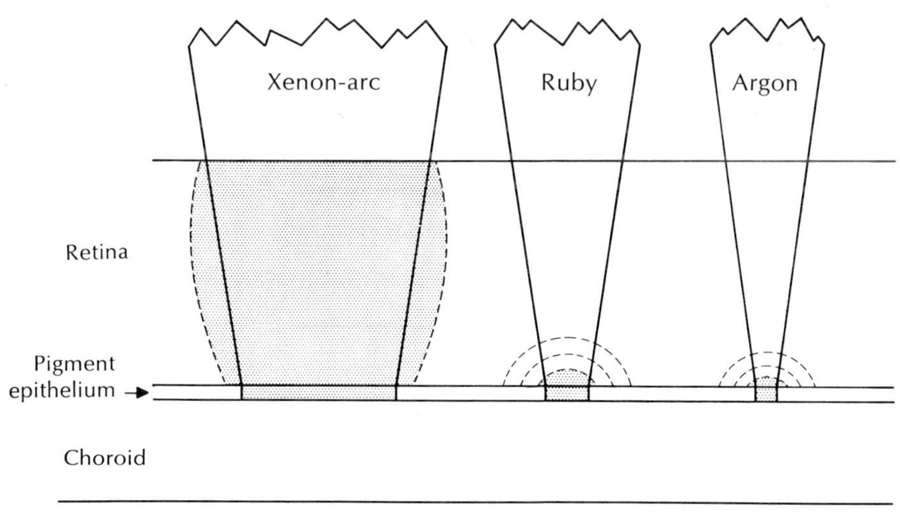

Fig. 3-10. Beam coagulation characteristics of the xenon-arc, ruby laser, and argon laser photocoagulation systems. The larger and more widespread retinal xenon-arc coagulations are compared with the small ruby laser coagulations and the extremely small argon laser coagulations.

do the ruby and argon laser coagulations, which are confined primarily to the pigment epithelial layer (Fig. 3-10). The minimal coagulation size afforded by the xenon-arc source is between 150μ and 200μ, as compared with 80μ for the ruby laser and 50μ for the commercial argon laser photocoagulation devices. Melanin absorption characteristics show that energy from the xenon-arc, ruby laser, and argon laser sources is absorbed almost completely and converted to heat energy. The pigment epithelium and choroidal pigment are the sites of maximal heat production, but there are conduction losses to adjacent tissues. The choroidal vessels are affected directly in proportion to the amount of choroidal pigment present and inversely with the rate and magnitude of choroidal blood flow, which carries away some of the heat produced. Each area of the fundus should be evaluated with these factors in mind, and the initial treatment performed at a low-energy or low-power output.

Laser radiation

The argon ion or ruby laser produces a light output that has great inherent power capabilities and is extremely directional, essentially coherent, and, above all, monochromatic. The laser's energy can be considered as a small packet delivered in a sufficient quantity to produce an effective coagulation.

Laser radiation is highly directional, and this aspect assumes importance when one considers that a well-constructed laser beam will be deviated from a single direction of propagation only by the effects of diffraction from the aperture of the emitting surface; thus, sources with an angular spread of several milliradians are readily obtainable. This minimal divergence is particularly possible with continuous-wave lasers, such as the argon laser photocoagulation source, which produces a beam of much higher collimation than the ruby or other crystal lasers (Fig. 3-11). This extremely small deviation from an essentially parallel light beam allows the radiant energy to be focused to a very small spot on the retina with greater concentration of energy than would be possible with any incandescent light source (Fig. 3-12). The most highly collimated incandescent beam cannot approach the collimation afforded by the most rudimentary laser; therefore, almost any laser is capable of producing a coagulation spot size many times smaller than the smallest spot created by the xenon-arc instrument. In addition, the monochromatic nature of the output beam of the lasers used for photocoagulation avoids chromatic aberration and the multiple foci (blue, red, yellow, and so on) that are inherent with xenon-arc photocoagulation (Fig. 3-13). The monochromaticity and exceptional collimation of the laser beams permit the

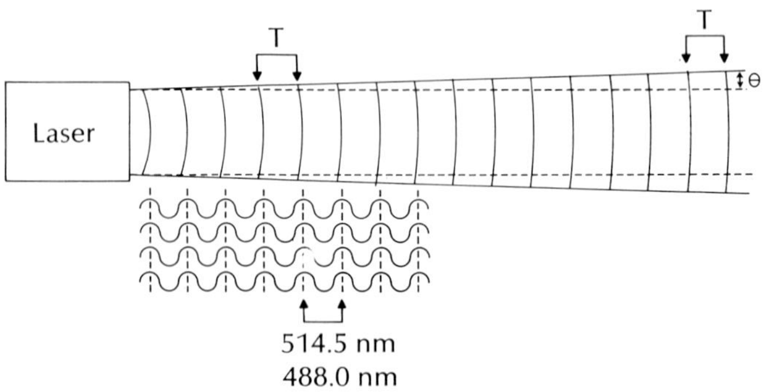

Fig. 3-11. Minimal beam divergence (angle Θ) and temporal and spatial coherence of the beam of a typical continuous-wave argon laser system.

creation of an extremely small coagulum in any ocular tissue. This coagulum is many times smaller than one obtainable by the xenon-arc source.

In addition to the differences in their degrees of collimation and in wavelength emissions, the coagulation characteristics of the ruby and argon laser photocoagulation systems are different in other ways. The argon ion laser is used at a relatively slow exposure interval (from 0.01 to several-sec exposures), which produces a slow coagulum that affects primarily the pigment epithelium and occasionally the deep vascular plexus and nuclear layers (Fig. 3-14). The ruby laser, on the other hand, produces its tissue effect in a matter of 200μsec to 500μsec. Its impact can be explosive: a vapor vacuole is formed; coagulation is primarily at the pigment epithelial level; and there is a slightly larger overall tissue effect. One must take these factors into consideration, along with the absorption capabilities of the target tissue, when selecting the proper incandescent or laser source for photocoagulation.

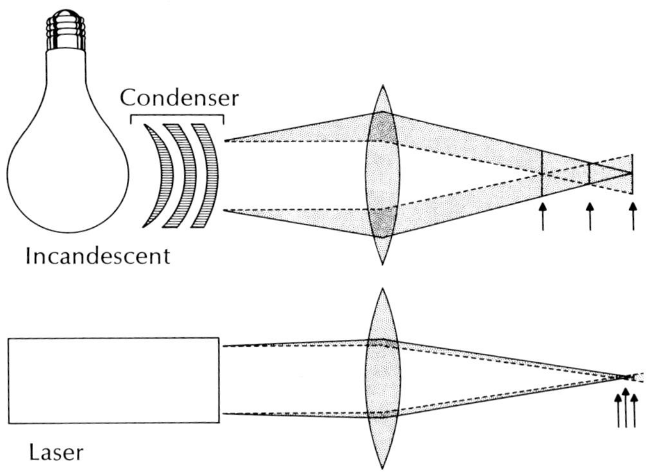

Fig. 3-12. Precise focusing potential of a laser beam because of the high collimation and lack of divergence inherent in laser systems.

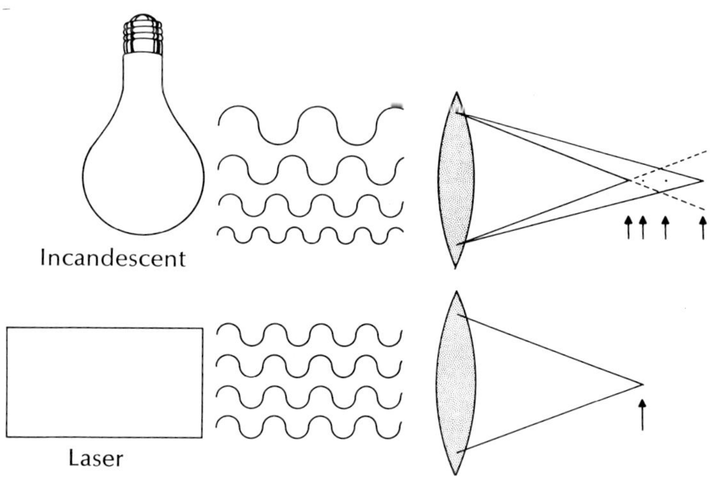

Fig. 3-13. Precise focusing potential of a laser beam because of the lack of chromatic aberration inherent in laser (argon or ruby) photocoagulation systems.

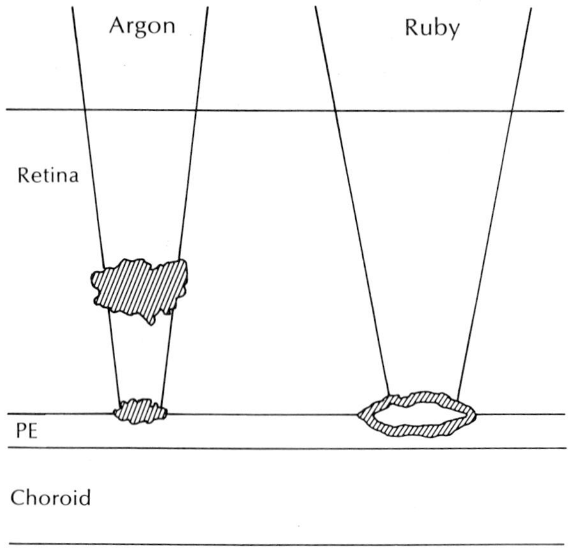

Fig. 3-14. Characteristics of an argon laser beam with controlled coagulation of the pigment epithelium **(PE)** and nuclear and vascular elements in the region of the deep vascular plexus, and typical coagulation with a vapor vacuole in the region of the pigment epithelium at the site of a ruby laser beam impact.

Table 1. Currently available argon laser photocoagulators*

Argon laser photocoagulators	Type laser	Cooling	Power (mw)	Retinal spot size (μ)
Britt Electronic Products Corp.	Pulsed 3,000/sec	Air	Variable to 1,500	40, 100, 200, and 700
Coherent Radiation	Continuous wave	Water	Variable to more than 2,000	50, 100, 200, 500, 1,000, and 2,000
Medical Instrument Research Associates (MIRA)	Continuous wave	Water	Variable to 550 at 488.0 nm, 650 at 514.5 nm	50, 100, 150, 250, and 500 with microscope variable to 1,000
Optics Technology, Inc. (OTI)	Continuous wave	Water or air	Variable to more than 2,000	50, 100, 200, and variable to 1,000

*Data compiled from advertisements from respective companies.

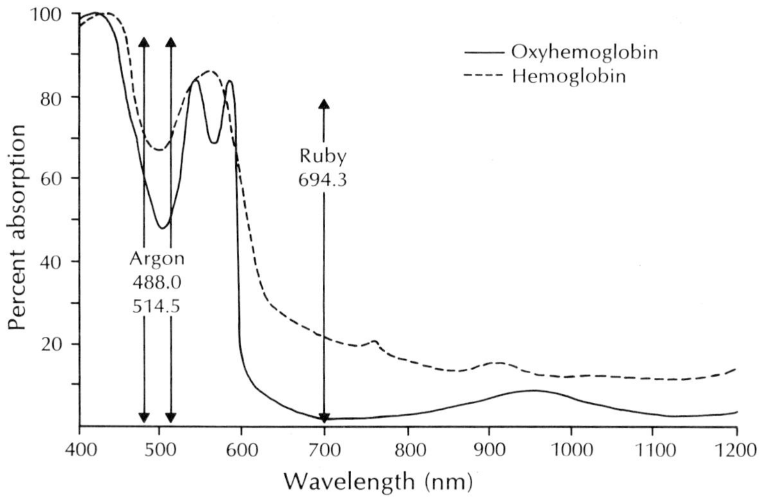

Fig. 3-15. Percent of energy absorbed per wavelength for reduced hemoglobin (veins) and oxyhemoglobin (arteries). Venous systems must be photocoagulated with lower energies and greater caution because of higher absorption of argon laser radiation and greater resultant heat production.

Exposure time (sec)	Delivery systems	Slit lamp	Input power
0.02, 0.05, 0.1, 0.2, and continuous	Slit lamp via articulating arm	Zeiss	230 v single-phase model
0.01, 0.02, 0.05, 0.1, 0.2, 0.5, 1, 2, 5, and continuous	Slit lamp and direct-viewing ophthalmoscope via articulating arm	Zeiss and AO (modified)	208 v three-phase model
0.05, 0.1, 0.2, 0.3, 0.5, 0.8, 1.0, and 2.5	Slit lamp and binocular indirect-viewing ophthalmoscope via articulating arm	Zeiss modified	208 v three-phase model
Selectable range of 0.01, 0.02, 0.05, 0.1, 0.2, 0.5, 1, 2, 5, and continuous	Slit lamp and direct-viewing ophthalmoscope via fiber optics cable	Haag-Streit, Zeiss, AO, Gambs, Rodenstock, and Mentor (no modifications)	230 v single-phase (air-cooled) and 208 v three-phase (water-cooled) models

In particular, the argon ion laser produces a coherent monochromatic blue-green beam of light energy that has the following unique features of ophthalmologic importance:

1. Argon laser radiation is five times more effectively absorbed by hemoglobin and vascular structures than is xenon-arc radiation.
2. The transverse electromagnetic mode (TEM_{00}) argon beam can be focused to a theoretical spot size at least 40% smaller than that produced by the ruby laser.
3. The argon ion laser can produce a greater continuous-wave (CW) power density at the retina than can any other light source.
4. The blue-green beam has greater inherent energy per photon than does any other laser source considered for photocoagulation.
5. The argon ion laser produces radiation that is more highly absorbed per incident photon at the pigment epithelium than does any other existing photocoagulation system available commercially.
6. The argon ion laser produces radiation that is more highly collimated and directional than any other commercial photocoagulation beam. Argon laser radiation appears to be absorbed selectively at the pigment epithelium and at areas of hemoglobin concentration, as well as slightly at the nuclear layers and outer segments of the rods and cones.
7. The argon ion laser produces radiation that is 7 to 8 times more effectively absorbed by oxyhemoglobin and reduced hemoglobin than is ruby laser radiation. Arterial systems have oxyhemoglobin primarily, whereas venous vessels are a mixture of reduced hemoglobin (primarily) and oxyhemoglobin (Fig. 3-15).
8. Argon laser radiation creates no detectable adverse effects, other than thermal ones, on the ocular tissues, plasma proteins, or blood constituents. Nonlinear and acoustic effects have not been demonstrated during widespread investigations.

Table 1 compares more precisely the various features of the four argon laser photocoagulation systems now commercially available and used throughout the world. Further information can be obtained from individual manufacturers.

GRADATION OF ARGON LASER PHOTOCOAGULATION LESIONS

Argon laser photocoagulations can be graded on a simple system ranging from *Grades 1 to 4* for coagulations of chorioretinal layers or ocular tissues other than the retinal vasculature (Figs. 3-16 and 3-17) and *Grades I to IV* for coagulations of vascular tissue (Figs. 3-18 and 3-19). Characterization of the coagulations is important for determining the proper end result when one is coagulating a particular abnormality. When appropriate, reference is made to these gradations throughout this text.

Chorioretinal coagulations

GRADE 1 Barely visible, blanching of pigment epithelium
GRADE 2 Hazy, mucoid, translucent, foggy
GRADE 3 Opaque, dusky, gray, dirty white, off-white
GRADE 4 Dense, chalk colored, hard-boiled egg white

Vascular coagulations

GRADE I Slight constriction of coagulated vessel
GRADE II Complete constriction and spasm of coagulated vessel
GRADE III Complete constriction and surrounding paravascular coagulum
GRADE IV Complete constriction, coagulum, and charring of coagulated vessel

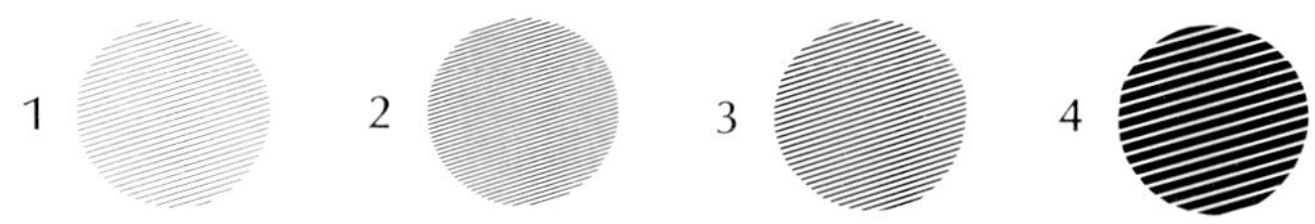

Fig. 3-16. Density of the coagulum in relation to the various chorioretinal coagulation gradations (Grades 1 to 4).

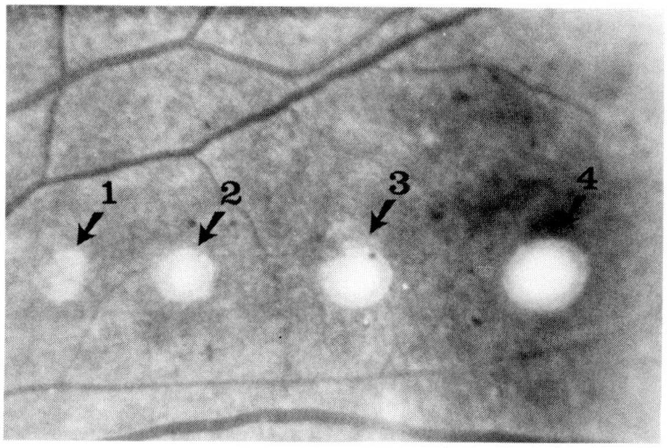

Fig. 3-17. Typical chorioretinal coagulation gradations (Grades 1 to 4).

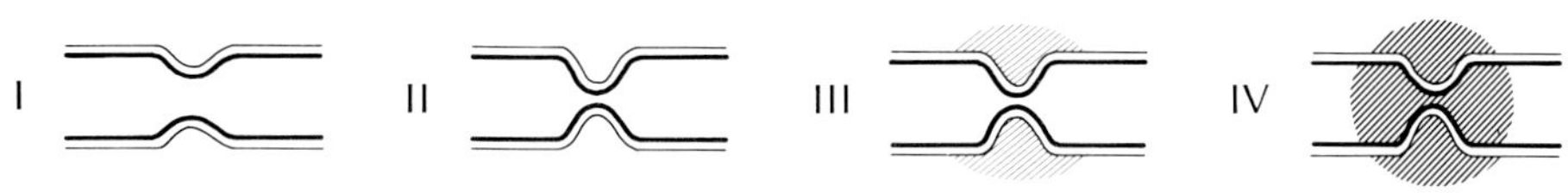

Fig. 3-18. Blood vessel and surrounding tissue with various degrees of vascular coagulation (Grades I to IV).

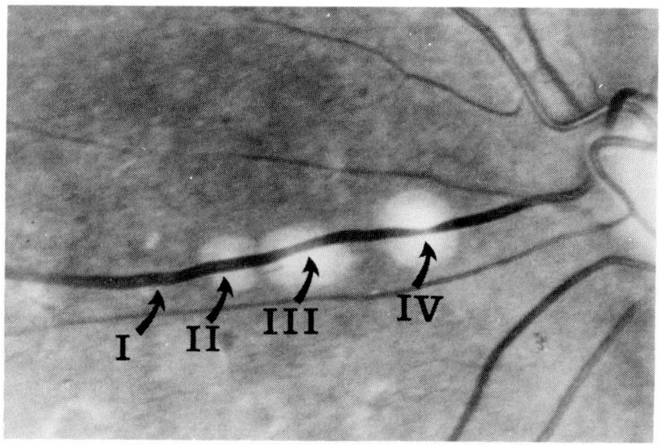

Fig. 3-19. Gradations of vascular coagulations (Grades I to IV).

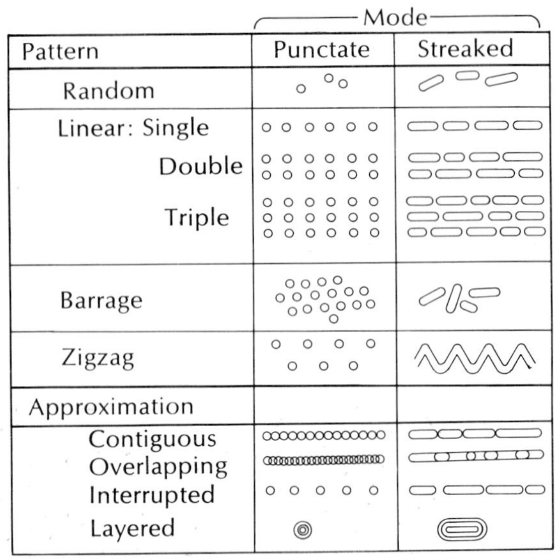

Fig. 3-20. Coagulation configurations, including the mode, pattern, and approximation of the ocular coagulations.

COAGULATION CONFIGURATIONS

One can describe a coagulation by defining its nature according to three categories: mode, pattern, and approximation (Fig. 3-20). The *mode* is concerned with delivery of the coagulation in a punctate, discrete, and solitary fashion or in a streaked, painted, and elongated manner. The *pattern* of the coagulation impacts is characterized as random; as single, double, or triple linear types; or as barrage or zigzag configurations. The *approximation* of one coagulation to another is further designated as contiguous, overlapping, interrupted, or layered.

PHOTOCOAGULATION PARAMETERS

Throughout this atlas all diagrams have been constructed in a manner that should be easily understood from a photocoagulation standpoint. The SEP at the side denotes the spot size (S), exposure interval (E), and power level (P) usually required with argon laser photocoagulation for the desired result for a particular disease under average conditions with clear media. When applicable, xenon-arc and ruby laser photocoagulation parameters are discussed in each section.

MAINTENANCE OF POWER DENSITY

One of the most important concepts in photocoagulation is maintenance of the power density of the coagulating beam when it is directed on the diseased tissue. Usually, the coagulation spot size can be predetermined for a particular lesion; the power setting and exposure interval are then carefully adjusted for production of the proper coagulation. When the proper coagulation energy (power intensity × exposure interval) has been determined, this dosage should be maintained while any changes in the exposure interval are being considered. It is quite advantageous in the performance of therapeutic photocoagulation to maintain the power density at the proper level. The energy transmitted to the retina can be considered in terms of energy per unit area or, with continuous-wave lasers such as the argon ion laser, more appropriately as the power per unit area, or power density. If the spot size does not vary, the product of the exposure interval and the input power or power density should be kept approximately constant. This relationship is fairly linear and rather simple to maintain. However, if the spot size changes, the energy input must be decreased or increased with the decrease or increase in the diameter of the spot size (see Fig. 14-13).

ALTERATIONS IN PHOTOCOAGULATION INTENSITY, SECONDARY TO REFRACTIVE MEDIA OPACIFICATIONS

The approximate values for power density (SEP) expressed in each of the chapters are related to and dependent on ideal conditions. These conditions include an emmetropic eye that has a normally clear cornea, anterior chamber, lens, and vitreous humor. Any opacification of any of these parts of the ocular media can lead to reflection, scatter, or absorption of the argon laser beam; the effective energy impinging on the retinal surface would thus be decreased. Table 2 emphasizes the approximate energy increase necessary with the various degrees of opacification of the individual tissues. This table can serve only as a rough guide; the appropriate power level must always be determined by increasing the power setting from a weak level to the ideal photocoagulation intensity for a particular disease. If the power increase necessary for a coagulation response far exceeds these listed values, one should search for other conditions or problems that are responsible for the ineffectiveness of the photocoagulation beam.

Table 2. Power increases necessary for various degrees of opacification

Area of opacification	Percentage of power increase required
Cornea	
1+ epithelial edema	5
2+ epithelial edema	15
1+ stromal haze	10
2+ stromal haze	35
1+ endothelial disruption	5
2+ endothelial disruption	25
Aqueous	
1+ flare	10
2+ flare	30
1+ cells	15
2+ cells	35
Lens	
1+ nuclear sclerosis	10
2+ nuclear sclerosis	25
3+ nuclear sclerosis	45
1+ cortical opacities	10 to 30
2+ cortical opacities	10 to 40
1+ posterior subcapsular opacities	15
2+ posterior subcapsular opacities	40
Vitreous	
1+ vitreous haze	15
2+ vitreous haze	35

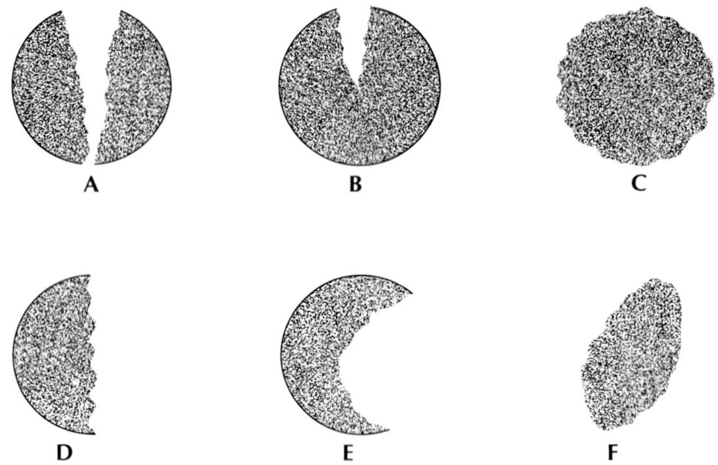

Fig. 3-21. Attenuation or distortion of the appearance of the attenuated argon laser photocoagulation target beam on the retina. **A,** A large cortical lenticular wedge interfering with the laser beam; **B,** a short cortical lenticular spoke; **C,** a hazy, indistinct retinal image caused by ocular media haze; **D,** disappearance of a portion of the retinal target beam spot because of impingement of the beam on the border of the iris; **E,** loss of a portion of the argon laser beam image on the retina because of a large lenticular or vitreous opacity; **F,** distortion and elongation of the retinal target spot because of lenticular astigmatism.

ATTENUATED RETINAL BEAM IMAGE

It is most important that one consider the appearance of the attenuated argon laser photocoagulation target beam on the retina when determining whether the total energy impinging on the cornea is being properly transmitted to the chorioretinal structures. The focus of the argon laser beam should appear as a circular spot of uniform intensity. Lenticular, corneal, or vitreal opacities can block portions of the incoming beam, producing a shadow in the circular spot area (Fig. 3-21). Cortical lenticular opacities can block out a wedge of the beam, and vitreous opacities can prevent a larger, more irregular portion of the beam from striking the retina. If the opacification is diffuse, such as that encountered with nuclear cataracts or vitreous cellular debris, the attenuated argon laser focus spot may be hazy and ill defined. Occasionally, a poorly delimited circular spot on the retina will indicate improper focusing of the argon laser beam. Large areas of the beam can be blocked if the incoming laser beam impinges on the borders of the iris, thereby producing an eclipselike loss in the circular spot on the retina. In cases of high lenticular astigmatism the beam may be elongated, rather than circular, as it is projected on the retinal surface. To obviate these problems, the argon laser circular spot on the posterior structures of the eye should be evaluated carefully before photocoagulation.

LOCALIZATION OF THE FOVEA

The dimensions of the anatomical regions of the posterior pole (macula, fovea, foveola, and centrally located umbo) should be known. Fig. 3-22 illustrates the radii of the various anatomical regions as compared with the radius of the optic disc (750μ). Knowledge of these dimensions permits the more precise evaluation of chorioretinal abnormalities in relation to their anatomic placement. It is sometimes extremely difficult to find the fovea before and during photocoagulation because of the presence of marked retinal edema,

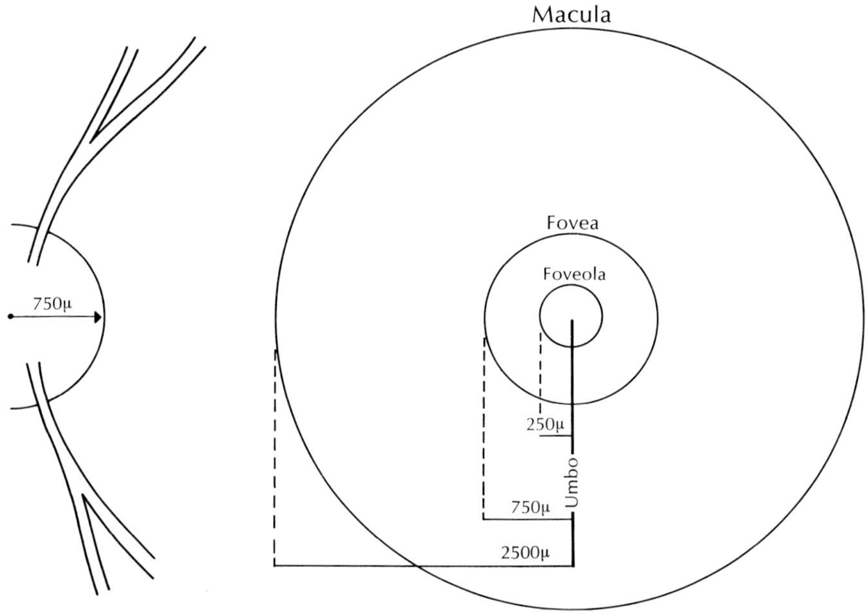

Fig. 3-22. Anatomical regions of the posterior retina and their respective dimensions.

cystic changes, hemorrhages, or other disorganizing factors. It is most important that this region be located, so that the proper therapeutic approach to a disease may be determined and precise therapeutic photocoagulation impacts rendered. The following sequence has proved useful for the exact location of the fovea.

Prephotocoagulation evaluation

Following indirect ophthalmoscopy and contact lens biomicroscopy, it may be difficult for the patient to fixate on a target light or pointer accurately with his fovea because of retinal exhaustion resulting from the bright examination sources. The patient can be asked to look directly at the very small beam from the slit lamp during the initial examination; this procedure will usually demonstrate the foveal region somewhat accurately. If the fovea cannot be accurately located, it is advisable to proceed to the next step.

With his pupils dilated, the patient is asked to sit in a darkened room for approximately 20 min, until his retinal sensitivity is partially reactivated. He is then asked to sit before the biomicroscope and locate the very small spot of light from the slit lamp. The intensity of the light should be minimal, sufficient only for allowing the patient to fixate with his foveal region. This procedure may, however, be extremely difficult when advanced degenerative, edematous, or hemorrhagic conditions of the macular region are present. Once this estimation has been completed, the patient is moved to the photography room so that a permanent record can be made of the presumed fixation point.

With the illumination at its lowest value, the patient is asked to locate the fixation pointer within the fundus camera (Fig. 3-23). The patient is directed to look at the end of the pointer, and some determination is made concerning the accuracy and overall ability with which the patient follows the pointer as it is moved in various directions. While the patient is fixating on the end of the pointer, a Polaroid or Kodachrome 35-mm picture is taken. This photograph is used for foveal reference at the time of photocoagulation.

Any photography, indirect ophthalmoscopy, or examination using the bright light

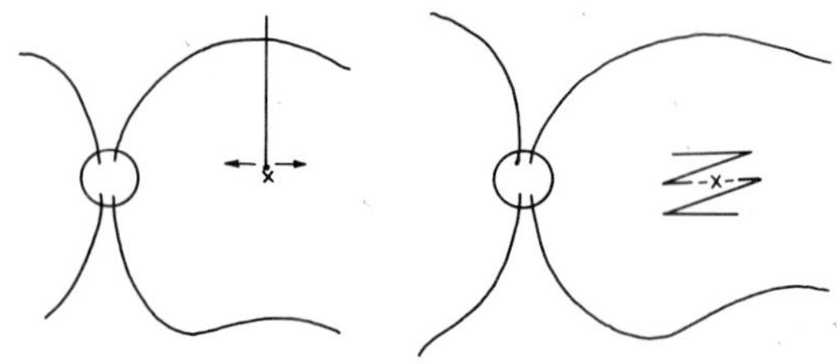

Fig. 3-23. Method of foveal localization with the fundus camera pointer during photography before photocoagulation and with extinction of the low-powered blue argon laser beam during foveal scanning at the time of photocoagulation.

source on the biomicroscope will exhaust the retina sufficiently to cause an erroneous localization of the fovea, particularly in those patients with damaged maculas. Therefore, localization of the fovea should always be done with reduced illumination and before any of the previously mentioned examinations involving a bright illumination beam.

Foveal localization during photocoagulation (scanning and extinction technique)

Particularly with those patients whose macula has been damaged, resulting in a decrease in macular function, the foveal region should be carefully located before indirect ophthalmoscopy or bright light biomicroscopy is done. The patient is seated before the photocoagulator slit lamp, and the contact lens is inserted on the patient's cornea. Under markedly reduced illumination, a very small spot is projected into the patient's eye, and the patient is asked to fixate on this small spot of white light. The geographic location of the fixation point, with regard to surrounding exudates, retinal folds, hemorrhages, or blood vessels, is then determined and documented by a small drawing, which is compared with the drawings and photographs made during the prephotocoagulation examination. If the fixation regions are identical, it can be assumed that the patient is using this particular retinal area for fixation and for his maximal visual function. His fixation point and his foveal region may not be the same, since his fovea may have been damaged sufficiently to cause him to fixate eccentrically in some other perifoveal or macular area.

When the fixation point has been determined, the attenuated target or marker argon laser beam can be used to locate the anatomic foveal region; a *100μ* diameter spot at a power of *25 mw* or less is placed in the macular region near the suspected foveal area. With the least dense attenuator filter in position and a rather bright, readily visible spot on the fundus, the very low-powered beam is brought across the suspected foveal region in a scanning, raster-type motion until the deep blue argon beam diminishes markedly in brightness because of its absorption by the xanthophyll pigment in the fovea (Fig. 3-23). This decrease in reflected intensity is quite noticeable, particularly if the argon beam is maintained at a very low power intensity, so that it contains energy predominantly composed of the 488.0-nm blue wavelength. If the power intensity is increased, the less highly absorbed 514.5-nm green wavelength appears in the beam, and the decrease in reflected intensity is not so pronounced. The argon laser beam is composed mainly of the blue wavelength (488.0 nm) at powers below 50 mw; percentages of the green wavelength (514.5 nm) are increasingly higher as the overall power is increased. Therefore, the power

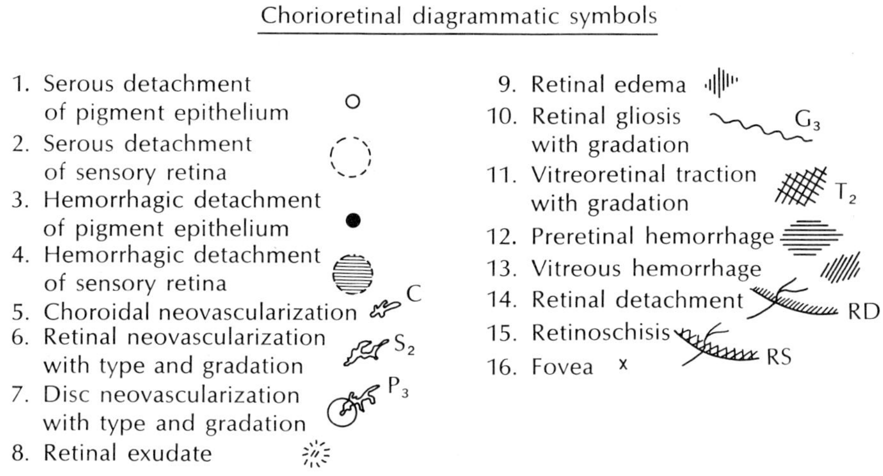

Fig. 3-24. Chorioretinal diagrammatic symbols of various chorioretinal peripheral and macular diseases.

should always be at an extremely low level when localization of the fovea is done with the blue argon laser beam by the scanning and extinction technique.

The fovea, fixation point, and surrounding localizing structures (such as blood vessels or hemorrhages) should be drawn on a chart, and these areas should be avoided during the photocoagulation procedure. It is most important to avoid an eccentric fixation area outside the foveal region, since destruction of this zone during the photocoagulation process could lead to a marked decrease in the visual level. The careful determination of the eccentric fixation point and the fovea by the slit lamp and the scanning-extinction technique using the blue argon laser beam, before photocoagulation, can be most helpful.

REPRESENTATION OF CHORIORETINAL DISEASE BY SYMBOLS

Although stereoscopic color fundus photography (with and without magnification) is extremely useful in the documentation and analysis of macular and posterior chorioretinal disease, an accurate drawing of the pathologic process can be most useful, particularly in the constructive analysis of the forthcoming photocoagulation approach. My colleagues and I have attempted to draw all posterior chorioretinal lesions with great care so that we can document the particular morphologic problems that we encounter. In this way we can accurately evaluate patches of edema, serous accumulations between portions of the retina, hemorrhagic activity, and various separations, splitting, and other derangements of chorioretinal function (Fig. 3-24).

It is also advantageous if structural defects can be represented by a simple pen or pencil drawing rather than multicolored diagrams (Fig. 3-25). The former approach is satisfactory, much quicker, and less laborious than the use of shading and polychromatic representations. The drawings can be copied by any black-and-white copying machine and sent to the referring doctor or attached to the hospital chart, along with a small list indicating the various symbols and their meanings.

A separate sheet, designed specifically for macular and posterior chorioretinal drawings, is most useful (Fig. 3-26). This chart can be used for drawings of the posterior polar region of either eye, showing the inverted image observed during indirect ophthalmoscopy or the erect image as seen during direct biomicroscopy. Small dots radiating from the

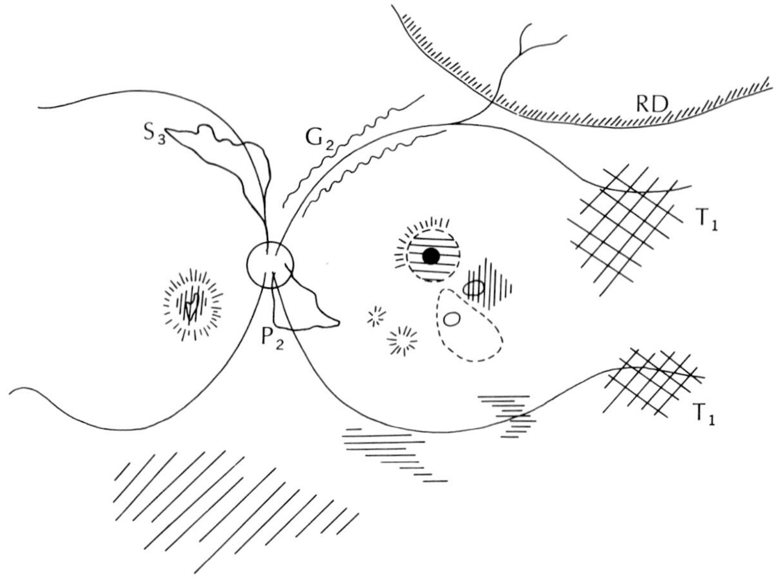

Fig. 3-25. Typical schematic representation of chorioretinal diagrammatic symbols illustrating various disease states.

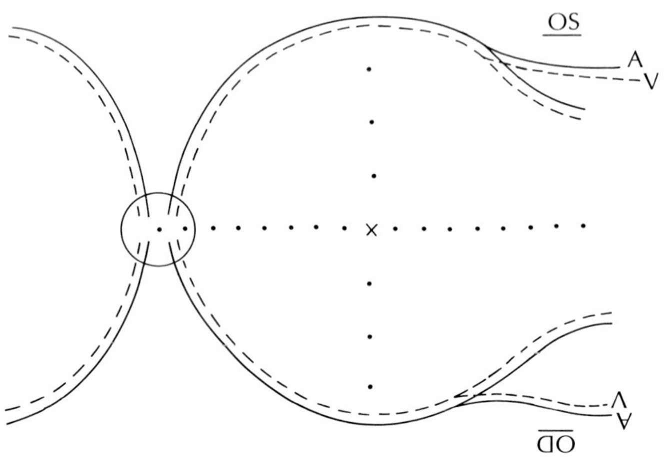

Fig. 3-26. Drawing sheet used to diagram macular disease in either eye. Dots radiate from the umbo horizontally at 500μ intervals and vertically at 1,000μ intervals, providing for proper placement of the diagrammatic symbols.

foveola horizontally at 500μ intervals and vertically at 1,000μ intervals describe accurately the extent and position of the lesions. The symbols are drawn as accurately as possible and have been selected in such a way that the deeper lesions are represented by less complicated symbols; the more superficial retinal diseases are represented by additional diagrams drawn over the previous symbols.

Chapter 4

Clinical considerations

THERAPEUTIC RATIONALE FOR PHOTOCOAGULATION

The goal of photocoagulation therapy is to maintain the hemodynamics and the fluid dynamics of the macular region in the healthy state. Alterations in the normal adhesiveness of the pigment epithelium to Bruch's membrane can lead to serous detachments of the pigment epithelium. The normal approximation of the pigment epithelium to Bruch's membrane may be restored by cauterization of serous detachments of the pigment epithelium before the process becomes more widespread or deteriorates with the growth of neovascularization.

Degeneration of the pigment epithelium allows the fluid from the choriocapillaris and Bruch's membrane region to filter freely inward through the pigment layer beneath the sensory retina. These areas of defective pigment epithelium can be cauterized and transformed into a thin layer of scar tissue, thereby preventing further leakage influx of the serous fluid beneath and into the sensory retina. More serious breakdown from the degeneration of Bruch's membrane or the pigment epithelium, with rupture and bleeding beneath the pigment epithelium and sensory retina, can be ameliorated by prompt and accurate photocoagulation of the defects.

The breakdown, deterioration, instability, and permeability defects of the retinal vessels can also be treated effectively by proper photocoagulation techniques. The increase in fluid transport through the usually nonpermeable retinal vessels in disease states such as diabetes, hypertension, Leber's disease, and Coats' disease can lead to rapid and irreparable damage and scarring of the macular and paramacular regions. The leaking blood vessels can be obliterated, and the hemodynamic pressures, as well as the nutrient and metabolic transport systems in the macular region, can be returned to a more normal condition. The selective photocoagulation of defective retinal vessels in various occlusive diseases can also be beneficial when these particular vessels are leaking actively into the sensory retina and the subretinal space.

In summary, in cases of anatomic barrier breakdown, photocoagulation is utilized to destroy the offending tissue elements or retinal vessel in an effort to seal the abnormal area and prevent leakage from a retinal or choroidal vascular system into the sensitive sensory retina.

The breakdown and deterioration of the cellular elements of the retina can have an extremely destructive effect on the visual function of the macular region. The hypoxia and subsequent accumulation of intraretinal fluid secondary to an arterial occlusion of one of the nutrient arteries to the macular region can be devastating and is usually not responsive to any photocoagulation therapy. Similarly, toxic and structural changes in the macular region resulting from the topical application of epinephrine or other medications have not been treated successfully by photocoagulation. In the case of the Irvine-Gass syndrome or macular changes secondary to vitreitis and peripheral uveitis, the structural changes secondary to the accumulation of fluid from the retinal vasculature in the extracellular spaces of the macular retina have a damaging effect on retinal function.

In these cases early photocoagulation techniques have attempted to decrease the extracellular fluid by providing egress routes by way of the retinal veins or Bruch's membrane–pigment epithelial–choriocapillaris layers. The purpose of photocoagulation is to increase the permeability in areas that would otherwise be nonpermeable (Bruch's membrane–pigment epithelial–choriocapillaris region or the retinal veins) in an effort to provide a transport route away from the zones of fluid accumulation that are causing the ultimate deterioration and scarring of the macula.

The proliferation of neovascular tissue is probably a result of localized hypoxia in the region of Bruch's membrane–pigment epithelium junction (choroidal or subretinal neovascularization) or the retinal vessels (retinal neovascularization) near the internal limiting membrane. It would seem obvious that these blood vessels are proliferating in response to some biochemical stimulus, and neovascularization seems to be an appropriate defense and reparative mechanism of the body. However, the ingrowth of neovascularization and its supportive glial tissue, as well as the attendant leakage from these vessels into the surrounding retinal spaces, the transport of heavy lipoproteinaceous material through the neovascular walls into the retina, the resulting hemorrhages, and the dynamic changes occurring from the interposition of the fibrovascular sheet, can irreparably damage the macular retina.

In these cases the purpose of photocoagulation is the total obliteration of the neovascularization to prevent further deterioration of the involved regions.

INITIAL EXAMINATIONS

A complete ocular examination should contain an extensive evaluation of the following items in the approximate order that they are listed:

1. *History of chief complaints.* Time of onset of symptoms, suddenness of onset of symptoms, portion of visual field first affected and nature of progression of the visual field change, medications taken for the ocular problem and how they affected the course of the disease, results of any ocular or systemic laboratory tests, general health status of the patient with regard to any systemic diseases that might affect the eyes and the particular medications the patient takes for these conditions, and a complete evaluation of the family history of the patient with regard to other ocular problems.
2. *Refraction.* Complete refraction, with examination at distance and at reading distance; use of low-vision aids and magnifiers where applicable.
3. *Anterior segment.* Cornea: haze, maculas, leucomas, pterygii, epithelial or endothelial defects, pigment accumulations on the posterior cornea, or other keratic precipitates. Anterior chamber: presence of flare, cells, hyphema, hypopyon, lens debris, or pigment flecks. Iris: abnormal configurations, growths, neovascularization, anterior or posterior synechias. Lens: cataract type, if present; exfoliation; pigment flecks on lens surface.
4. *Applanation tonometry.* Should be performed on all patients.

5. *Central and peripheral visual field examinations.* Campimetry and perimetry to be carefully performed on all diseased eyes so that the status and progress of the disease can be well documented.
6. *Macular retinal function tests.* Amsler grid examination to be performed on all patients, particularly those with macular disease. Macular stress evaluation to be conducted with white, red, and blue lighting sources.

When evaluation of these items has been completed, the patient's pupils are dilated with a solution of equal mixtures of proparacaine hydrochloride 0.5% (Ophthaine), phenylephrine (Neo-Synephrine) hydrochloride 10%, and cyclopentolate (Cyclogyl) hydrochloride 2%. The topical use of an anesthetic decreases the burning and stinging that is commonly found with the use of an ordinary mixture of phenylephrine and cyclopentolate. The topical use of an anesthetic in this manner has not affected the epithelial integrity in any way.

7. *Indirect ophthalmoscopy.* Ophthalmoscopy utilizing the indirect method and the 20-diopter (3× magnification of retinal image) and the 30-diopter (2× magnification) to be conducted in an extremely careful and meticulous manner. (Indirect ophthalmoscopy with magnifying loupes has also been helpful for certain portions of the macular and paramacular regions.) Defects to be drawn carefully and accurately on the macular or peripheral chorioretinal chart provided for that purpose; vitreous membranes, diffuse hemorrhages, blood clots, pigment, collagen condensations, and areas of fibrin accumulation to be documented; a complete, accurate drawing of the chorioretinal lesions and surrounding retinal landmarks to be included in the representative drawing.
8. *Contact or precorneal lens biomicroscopy.* Should be performed to determine the presence and extent of microscopic defects in the macular and posterior polar regions; pertinent findings to be recorded on the macular chart.
9. *Fundus color photography.* Should be done stereoscopically, if possible, with the 45°, 30°, and magnified images. Also possibility of Polaroid fixation pictures to be taken after about 20 min, when the patient's eyes have adapted to the dark.
10. *Fluorescein angiography.* Should be performed on all patients with posterior choroidal or retinal defects, particularly those with macular disease. Black-and-white (or color) fluorescein angiography to be done stereoscopically, if possible.

A compilation of all of these factors is extremely important for a total analysis and evaluation of the patient before photocoagulation.

PREPHOTOCOAGULATION PROCEDURES

When photocoagulation has been designated as the treatment of choice, the patient is brought to the photocoagulation theater; if an interval has elapsed since the initial examination, the patient undergoes a repeated examination of his visual acuity, anterior segments, and intraocular pressure values. The patient's pupils are then dilated with a mixture of phenylephrine 10% and cyclopentolate 2%; a small amount of proparacaine 0.5% is usually added to this mixture, as noted previously.

Patient information and permission forms

While the patient's pupils are dilating, the patient and accompanying relatives are given several typewritten sheets describing the condition to be treated, the reason and purpose of treatment, the photocoagulation procedure, expected results, and possible complications. This description includes several paragraphs concerning the aftercare and

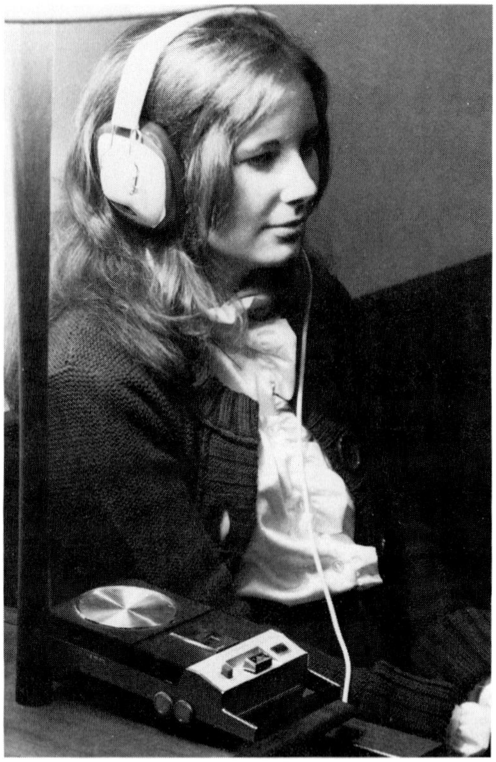

Fig. 4-1. Tape recorder and headphones used to explain the methods and purposes of the photocoagulation treatment to the patient and accompanying relatives.

possible discomfort that might be experienced by the patient. In addition, the patient and his relatives are asked to listen to a 15-min tape recording of the same material. All individuals wear headphones so that the recorded message will not bother other patients in the waiting room, and they are allowed to listen to the tape as many times as they wish (Fig. 4-1). The written and taped explanations of the methods and purposes of the photocoagulation treatment have proved to be of great assistance in increasing the patient's sense of well-being and understanding of the photocoagulation process; it has also been extremely helpful in eliminating many patient-to-physician telephone calls and questions. After he listens to the explanatory tape and reads the typewritten sheets, the patient is asked if he has any further questions concerning either the purpose or method of treatment or anything else in connection with the forthcoming photocoagulation session. If he has none, he is asked to sign a permission sheet similar to that shown in Fig. 4-2, which is used specifically for patients undergoing photocoagulation therapy. The patient is also asked to sign the ordinary operative procedure permission sheet that is required at the Columbia-Presbyterian Medical Center. The purpose and scope of the permission sheets should be explained in detail to the patient after he has read the explanatory sheet and heard the tape, because the patient usually has a few questions concerning the purpose of the permission sheet.

Corneal evaluation

After his pupils have been dilated, the patient is brought to the photocoagulation suite and reexamined thoroughly with the biomicroscope. The anterior segment is evaluated

PHOTOCOAGULATION CONSENT FORM

Patient's name______________________________ Date____________

Address:______________________________

____

Description of procedure to be undertaken:

Argon Laser
Xenon-Arc
Ruby Laser

Photocoagulation of the__________eye for__________

____

____

____

I have fully explained to the patient the nature and purpose of the procedure described above and such risks as are involved in its performance.

____________________ M.D.

____

Witness

Permission is hereby given for the administration of any anesthetic and the performance of any ophthalmic operation that may be advisable to facilitate the above procedure. I have been fully informed of the risks and possible consequences involved in the performance of the procedure described, have listened to the recorded explanatory tape or have read the identical typed explanatory sheet, have been advised that unforseen results may occur, and, nevertheless, hereby authorize ________________ to perform the procedure upon me and hereby release and forever discharge him, The Presbyterian Hospital in the City of New York, and Columbia University from liability for any injury which may result directly or indirectly from the performance of the procedure.

____

Patient signature

Fig. 4-2. Typical permission form used specifically for patients undergoing photocoagulation.

with regard to opacities in the tear film, such as mascara, flecks of dust, face powder, grease, or mucous films, that would scatter the photocoagulation beam. If any of these are found, they are washed from the cul-de-sac with a gentle lavage of isotonic saline or Ringer's solution.

The cornea is examined for defects in the epithelium, embedded foreign bodies, small disruptions of Bowman's membrane, stromal haze, stromal maculas or leucomas, or other stromal opacities that could conceivably scatter, deflect, or absorb the incoming laser beam. The endothelium is also carefully searched for any increase in guttata, pigment deposition, breaks, doubling or rolling of Descemet's membrane, or any accumulations of red or white cells or other keratic precipitates on the posterior surface of the cornea. Any of these defects will decrease the effectiveness of the argon laser beam as it traverses the tear film and cornea and could introduce several complications that are discussed in subsequent sections.

Anterior chamber evaluation

The anterior chamber is examined for the presence of cells, protein accumulation (flare), blood, pigment flecks, or other unusual particles in the aqueous fluid. An increase in protein concentration or red or white blood cells in the anterior chamber can decrease the effectiveness of laser photocoagulation as well as the effective visualization of the posterior segment. Photocoagulation should be deferred until the hyphema or concentration of the blood elements in the anterior chamber has decreased by natural absorption. An increase in the protein concentration should be evaluated, and the possible topical use of steroid or cycloplegic drops, or both, should be considered.

Iris evaluation

The pupil should be dilated to a minimal diameter of 4 mm for adequate photocoagulation of the chorioretinal layers. Most pupils will dilate to 6 or 7 mm in diameter, and this pupillary aperture allows excellent visualization of most areas of the retina. Rubeosis iridis or any synechias of the iris to the lens structure should be noted by a small drawing so that the proper photocoagulation approach can be determined.

Lenticular examination

The lens of the eye is one of the most important elements in the refractive media to be examined before photocoagulation. Wedgelike cortical opacities can effectively decrease the impact power of the laser beam by occluding a segment of the beam as it passes through the cataractous lens. Nuclear sclerotic lenses tend to scatter and absorb the argon laser beam at the cortical-nuclear junction. In addition, nuclear cataracts can refract the beam in various directions, depending on the density of the cortical and nuclear lenticular layers, so that a distinct focus cannot be obtained. Posterior subcapsular cataracts can diminish the effectiveness of photocoagulation therapy tremendously, sometimes negating the procedure altogether. Anterior and posterior polar cataracts present a difficult problem if the pupil cannot be dilated, but this problem usually can be circumvented if the argon laser beam is channeled eccentrically through the outer portion of the pupillary space; it thereby avoids the central opacifications. All of these cataract types must be analyzed thoroughly for the most appropriate photocoagulation approach to be planned.

Vitreous examination

The vitreous should be inspected by indirect and direct ophthalmoscopy for obvious opacities, such as blood clots, pigment accumulations, or collagen condensations and membranes, that could decrease the effectiveness of the photocoagulation beam. Diffuse vitreous blood can be effectively penetrated by the argon laser beam if there is sufficient clarity to permit visualization of the retinal lesion by direct ophthalmoscopy. If the retinal defect cannot be seen clearly by direct ophthalmoscopy, photocoagulation should be deferred because of the possibility of vitreous contraction secondary to excessive absorption of the laser beam by the erythrocytes in the vitreous cavity. Pigment flecks and glial or collagen proliferation or condensations should be mapped precisely and avoided during the photocoagulation procedure. Absorption of light energy by pigment flecks or clumps will create a localized coagulum in the vitreous humor. Inadvertent photocoagulation of glial proliferations or collagen condensations could lead to further vitreous contraction and traction stress on the retinal surface. Photocoagulation can be directed around the clots of blood, but solid preretinal or vitreal accumulations of blood or partially organized clots should not be photocoagulated under any conditions, because of the localized traction, glial proliferation, and intense heat that could be produced at those particular sites. Syneresis cavities should be located in the vitreous, if possible, since these interruptions in the continuity of the vitreous gel can lead to dispersion and scatter of the laser beam.

Retinal examination

At the time of photocoagulation the retina should be carefully examined to determine whether any changes from the initial examination have taken place. Areas of hemorrhagic activity, edema or exudate formation, retinoschisis, or serous accumulations beneath the sensory retina or pigment epithelium must be scrutinized so that the photocoagulation approach can be changed if necessary. An increase in sensory retinal edema or serous accumulations beneath the sensory retina can involve a marked increase in the photocoagulation energy required for adequate coagulation of underlying neovascularization on the surface of the pigment epithelium. Hemorrhages into serous detachments of the sensory retina or pigment epithelium can increase the uptake of the argon laser photocoagulation beam and lead to severe scarring secondary to the excessive production of heat in these

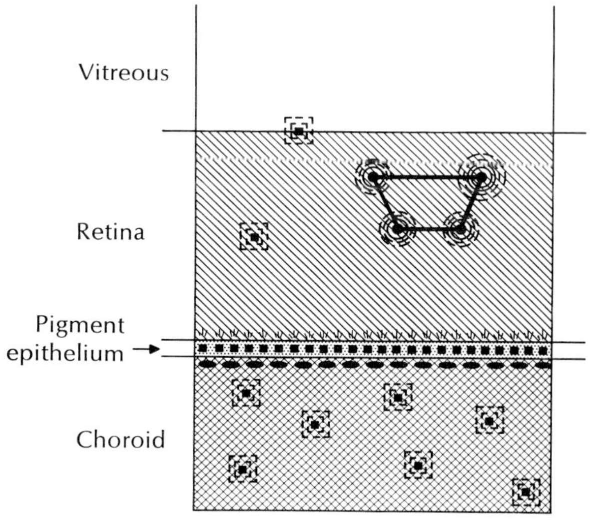

Fig. 4-3. Potential photon absorption sites that must be documented and evaluated before photocoagulation: retinal and preretinal pigment or hemorrhages, retinal or preretinal shunting or neovascular systems, pigment epithelial hypertrophy, choroidal hyperpigmentation, and areas of preretinal or vitreal blood.

layers. Large, blot, deep retinal hemorrhages, zones of pigment proliferation or macroaneurysm formation, or regions of retinal atrophy or pigment epithelial hypertrophy should be carefully evaluated with regard to the correct photocoagulation approach under the existing circumstances (Fig. 4-3).

Selection of ocular anesthesia

The reliability, stability, and cooperativeness of the patient must be determined and the retrobulbar administration of an anesthetic considered. Although argon laser photocoagulation is essentially painless, unless longer exposures and higher powers are used, the bright light from the photocoagulation beam and the general aura of the procedure can sometimes be quite disturbing to the patient. In these circumstances a retrobulbar injection has been shown to be most effective in reducing the extraocular excursions and eliminating the photophobia and discomfort.

It is advisable to give a retrobulbar injection of 3 ml of a 2% solution of lidocaine (Xylocaine) hydrochloride with hyaluronidase (Wydase) (and without epinephrine) in addition to anesthetic drops, such as proparacaine, to provide adequate akinesia and anesthesia for the following patients:

1. Unreliable, senile, apprehensive patients
2. Uncooperative or photophobic patients, or patients with marked Bell's phenomena
3. All patients with perifoveal and macular lesions
4. Most patients with neovascularization extending from the optic disc or the vascular arcades (focal treatment)
5. Most patients undergoing panretinal photocoagulation procedures
6. Most patients undergoing iridotomies
7. All patients who will undergo iridocyclitic membrane discissions
8. All patients with iris cysts
9. Most patients with choroidal neovascularization
10. Most patients with moderately hazy ocular media
11. All patients when exposure time exceeds 0.5 sec regularly
12. Most patients when the power density is necessarily high
13. Most patients when the length of the treatment session is expected to exceed 30 min

Occasionally, injection of anesthetic near the horizontal and vertical recti muscles is necessary in addition to the retrobulbar injection for complete immobilization and stabilization of the globe. If the surgeon momentarily considers the possibility of using a retrobulbar or recti muscle injection, a general rule is that he probably should employ it. Because the most reliable patients can lose their composure for a fraction of a second, causing devastating results, it is better to be conservative; this way, a steady, easily treatable eye is obtained.

If a topical anesthetic is used alone and the patient complains of discomfort, several steps can be taken to reduce the pain:

1. Stop all photocoagulation treatment for a period of at least 15 to 20 sec, and then continue at one half the previous photocoagulation rate.
2. Reduce the exposure interval by one half and adjust the power appropriately to obtain the same power density and desired reaction.
3. Reduce the diameter of the spot size by approximately 20% and adjust the power accordingly.
4. If the maximal pain or discomfort is related to the 12, 3, 6, or 9 o'clock meridian,

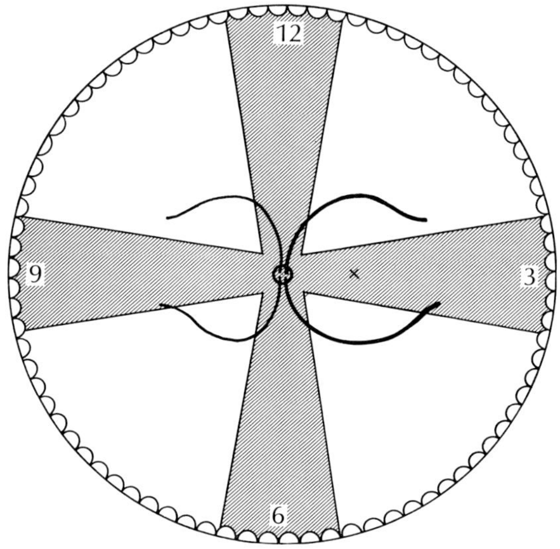

Fig. 4-4. Zones of possible pain or discomfort (shaded areas) during the photocoagulation procedure.

treat another region of the retina and return intermittently to the painful area for a few exposures at a time (Fig. 4-4).

5. If the pain continues despite these steps, give a retrobulbar anesthetic (2 to 3 ml of 2% lidocaine without epinephrine).

Pain during argon laser photcoagulation is caused by one or more factors:

1. *Retinal area.* The retinal area most sensitive to photocoagulations of any exposure or power is in the midperiphery at the 12, 3, 6, or 9 o'clock meridian, possibly because the sclera and certain other coats of the eye are thinner and have less thermal diffusion and because of the concentration of neural elements in those regions.
2. *Rapidity of photocoagulation exposures.* If the exposure rate is faster than 1 coagulation per sec, pain is likely to develop after the twelfth or fifteenth exposure. This process appears to be a summation of subliminal pain that then becomes manifest.
3. *Diameter of the coagulation size.* There is a greater chance of pain with a larger spot size because of the greater heat generated at the center of the larger coagulum. Spot sizes of 300μ or less rarely give discomfort.
4. *Power level.* There is a greater chance of discomfort with higher powers because of the greater degree of heat production and the depth and extent to which the coagulum is produced. Power levels less than 500 mw rarely give pain.
5. *Exposure interval.* There is a greater chance of pain with longer exposures, again because of the depth and extent of the coagulation, as well as the buildup of heat energy. Exposures of 0.05 sec or less seldom produce discomfort.

Patient preparation

The patient is seated on the chair in the argon laser slit lamp photocoagulator, and the photocoagulation tray (Fig. 4-5) is inspected to ensure that the various components are present. This tray contains the following items: a Goldmann three-mirror contact lens, a Goldmann fundus contact lens, Goniosol solution, a plano low-vacuum contact lens, a diagonal low-vacuum contact lens, an anterior segment lavage contact lens, a low-vacuum

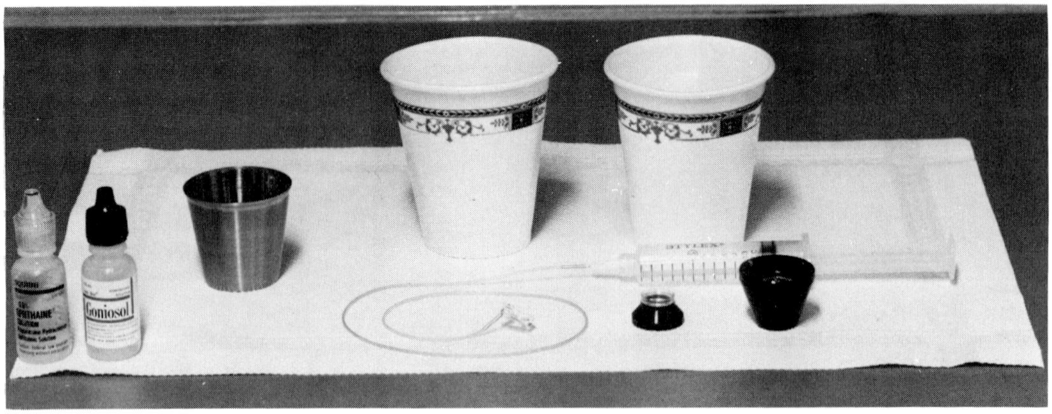

Fig. 4-5. Tray containing items possibly required during photocoagulation.

anterior segment magnification contact lens, a lukewarm water bath containing several drops of detergent, two lukewarm water rinsing baths, paper tissue wipes, a large barrier surgical sheet, towel clips for the barrier sheet, Instant Glucose jelly, proparacaine drops, and an ammonia smelling salts ampule. It is useful to have all of the contact lenses that might possibly be required available on the photocoagulation tray. The inclusion of Instant Glucose* is important, since many of the patients are diabetic and could experience early hypoglycemic shock. If nondiabetic patients feel faint, the breakage of an ammonia smelling salts ampule has proved most useful.

A plano low-vacuum contact lens is applied to the cornea of the eye. Gentle suction is then created with a syringe filled with Ringer's solution to hold the low-vacuum contact lens onto the surface of the cornea. The posterior segment regions are then examined as outlined previously.

A three-mirror Goldmann lens or similarly mirrored contact lens can also be used, if desired, with a drop of 0.5% methylcellulose between the contact lens and the anterior surface of the cornea. A restraining strap is usually placed around the back of the patient's head to hold him more securely into the chin and headrest supports of the biomicroscope. The contact lens must be held firmly against the eye during the photocoagulation procedure by the surgeon, and this procedure can become tiring. An elbow support is recommended so that the surgeon's arm can be relaxed when hand-held corneal mirrored lenses that do not have self-retaining flanges are being used.

Selection of technical parameters

The spot size is next selected for the particular condition requiring photocoagulation; ranges are between 50μ and $2,000\mu$. The exposure time is then determined and set on the photocoagulation instrument. Finally, the minimal power setting is established for the particular retinal or anterior segment problem. The photocoagulation power is then increased in increments of 25 mw until the desired coagulation effect is produced. A small joy stick, located on the biomicroscope, allows the beam to be accurately placed or moved during the photocoagulation sequence. In most cases an average power density should be maintained in the treatment area for the proper coagulation of the various abnormal elements. (The concept of an adequate power density for photocoagulation and the

*Diabetes Association of Cleveland, 10205 Carnegie Ave., Cleveland, Ohio 44106.

maintenance of this power density during the procedure are emphasized in subsequent chapters dealing with specific disease states.)

PHOTOCOAGULATION TREATMENT RECORD

The argon laser photocoagulation treatment record (Fig. 4-6) should contain spaces for the patient's name, diagnosis of his disease, hospital record number, dates, the treating doctor, the condition of the optical media, and the name of the individual who is compiling the data. Categories depicting the type of photocoagulation technique may also be tabulated on the record sheet, and a small section for notations on complications may be provided.

The record sheet consists of seven sections vertically arranged according to the area of the fundus to which the photocoagulation treatment has been directed. These sections are: disc, macula, paramacula area, peripapillary area, vascular arcades, midperiphery, and periphery. Seven horizontal categories for each of the retinal areas include: location of the area of the primary photocoagulation treatment, technique used in that particular area, diameter of the spot size in microns, exposure time in seconds, power designated in milliwatts, the number of exposures for that particular area, and the number of hemorrhages encountered in that region. Each section has tabulations sufficient for 14 individual photocoagulation attempts. In this way the information concerning all parameters of photocoagulation to any area of the retina is documented in a complete manner so that the total or fractionated energy input to an eye can be computed without difficulty. At the bottom of this treatment record, it can be noted if the patient is to return after a certain interval for a specific type of diagnostic evaluation or therapy. In addition, the designation of the degree of discomfort during the photocoagulation procedure can be noted.

Because argon laser photocoagulation is a precise technique, it should be employed in a qualitative and quantitative manner for all types of chorioretinal diseases; it is mandatory that such a record sheet be kept so that the patient's response to photocoagulation, as well as his reparative and healing potential, can be evaluated critically. This type of record also allows the surgeon to reassess his treatment approach to a particular disease so that he can make more constructive recommendations for that patient or other patients in the future.

A summary data sheet should also be completed after each photocoagulation session in order to record the response of the eye to treatment and to quantitate the overall amount of laser energy employed (Fig. 4-7).

PATIENT CARE AFTER TREATMENT

The following directions are summarized on a photocopied sheet and given to the patient after any type of photocoagulation. The patient is urged to follow these instructions for a minimal period of 3 weeks after treatment.

1. Keep your head up and move slowly. Do not move suddenly or bend over to tie your shoes or pick up objects. If it is absolutely necessary to grasp low objects, try to bend your knees only, keeping your back straight and your head up, and hold onto a table or chair for support.

This particular section is provided to prevent the patient from increasing the venous pressure in his head, neck, and eyes by bending at the waist. As they bend over to pick up a low-lying object, patients have a tendency to hold their breath and to increase the venous pressure even further.

2. Do not strain at anything. Do not lift any objects heavier than 10 lbs. Do not carry luggage. Do not hold your breath for any reason. Do not strain during bowel movements, and try to avoid constipation (take mineral oil, milk of magnesia, Colace, or the like, regularly). Do not

PATIENT ____ Rx NO.____ NO. ____ DATE ____

DX ____ DR. ____

EYE ____ OPTICAL MEDIA ____ DATA BY ____

TECHNIQUES: 1. FOCAL 4. PRP

2. FEEDER 5. C Rx

3. FROND 6. CEP

NO. ____ OTHER COMPLICATIONS ____

VISIT NO. ____

TIME ____

AREA	L M H	TECHN	SPOT SIZE μ	EXP. TIME (sec.)	POWER (mW)	NO. EXP.	HEM.	TECHN	SPOT SIZE μ	EXP. TIME (sec.)	POWER (mW)	NO. EXP.	HEM.
1. DISC													
2. MACULA													
A/B 1,2,3,4 H													
3. PARAMACULA													
4. PERIPAPILLARY AREA													
5. ARCADES													
6. MIDPERIPHERY													
7. PERIPHERY													

RETURN ____ DAY(S) ____ WEEK(S) ____ MONTH(S)

DISCOMFORT DURING Rx ____

FOR ____

Fig. 4-6. Typical treatment record used at the time of argon laser photocoagulation.

SUMMARY DATA SHEET
ARGON LASER PHOTOCOAGULATION

PATIENT NAME ______________________________ AGE __________

D_X ______________________________ GRADE __________

COMMENTS ______________________________

PRE–EXPOSURE		EXPOSURE		POSTEXPOSURE			DR.	SUMMARY
DATE	VA	DATE(S)	EYE(S)	DATE	VA	RETINA		

Fig. 4-7. Summary data sheet used to document the amount of laser energy employed and the ocular response after each photocoagulation session.

engage in any strenuous activities (athletics, sexual intercourse, gardening, or the like) for at least 3 weeks after photocoagulation unless advised otherwise. Avoid tight collars and chokers.

This paragraph emphasizes the role of Valsalva's maneuver, which can increase the venous pressure markedly in the region of the eyes. If the patient can learn to move slowly without holding his breath, a mild form of exercise can be conducted; walking and other mild activities are encouraged. Swimming should not be done during this period, but simple bathing in pools and lakes is permissible.

3. You may have some discomfort around your treated eye. Darvon or similar compounds are sufficient to relieve the pain in most cases; aspirin or related compounds should not be used. Do not be concerned if the lids of the treated eye are black and blue; this condition is caused by the occasionally required injection of an anesthetic and will disappear in a few weeks. The eye may be bloodshot; this condition is another common occurrence following photocoagulation. It is also common for the vision in the treated eye to be somewhat blurry and blotchy for 2 to 3 weeks or longer after treatment. Nearly always, but not invariably, vision will return to the pretreatment level.

This section is provided to allay any feelings of great concern caused by the presence of ecchymosis of the lids or subconjunctival hemorrhages. The knowledge that the central vision may be more blurred for a period of several weeks because of nearby coagulations is also reassuring to the patient when that particular problem occurs. It is advisable to have the patient refrain from taking the aspirin compounds, because of their anticoagulant effect, and to use medications other than the salicylates.

All of the following directions should be observed indefinitely:

4. Sleep with the head of your bed raised 15° to 20°. Put two pillows or a foam rubber wedge under your present pillow, or raise the head of your bed by placing bricks under the headpost supports. This maneuver will decrease the blood vessel pressure in your eyes.

This maneuver appears to be an important one for patients with hemorrhagic retinopathy, especially following photocoagulation, because venous pressure increases greatly when one is lying in a horizontal position. Decreasing this pressure (by elevating the head 20°) may decrease the possibility of hemorrhages, either from the choroid or from the retina, following any type of photocoagulation intervention.

5. Control coughing and sneezing with cough syrup or other medications. Try not to stifle a sneeze, since this action raises the blood pressure in your eyes to high levels. Do not blow your nose vigorously. Do not rub your eyes, since rubbing them may disrupt the blood vessels inside the eyes.

The momentary elevation of pressure in the retinal vessels to extremely high levels during the act of coughing, sneezing, or rubbing the eyes can prove to be disastrous for patients with hemorrhagic retinopathy or following photocoagulation. Cough syrups and other medications should be prescribed by the local physician, since several of these medications contain ingredients that are contraindicated with certain systemic problems that the patient may have.

6. Do not use nose drops, sprays, inhalators, or other medications that contain ephedrine or epinephrine, since these drugs tend to raise the blood pressure in the body and, therefore, in the blood vessels in the eye. Ask your physician about these medications.

The medications should be well monitored by a patient's internist, who should be advised of the goals of photocoagulation and of the restrictions imposed.

7. Avoid altitudes over 8,000 feet. Commercial aircraft cabins are pressurized below this altitude.

Altitudes over 8,000 feet may induce retinal hypoxia and lead to distension of the retinal or choroidal vessels and possibly other changes in the retinal vasculature that could be detrimental to the patient for an indeterminate period following photocoagulation. These changes of altitude are usually restricted only in cases where the individual cannot acclimate slowly but is subjected to higher altitudes and lower oxygen concentrations abruptly.

Chapter 5

Disease response

Photocoagulation of the choroid, retina, and anterior segment structures can be produced by the absorption of light energy from any of the three (argon laser, ruby laser, or xenon-arc) photocoagulation systems. All systems deliver light energy in the visible or infrared region of the spectrum, and the ultimate chorioretinal effect is determined by the total amount of light energy absorbed and converted to heat. The major physical difference between the laser and the xenon-arc systems is the type of radiation developed by each method.

ARGON ION LASER

The argon ion laser produces light energy consisting of six wavelengths in the blue-green portion of the visible spectrum. The 488.0-nm blue wavelength and the 514.5-nm pea green wavelength are the predominant wavelengths and make up approximately 90% of the argon laser beam. The argon laser beam is produced continuously from the electrical excitation of argon gas ions in a specially designed discharge tube, and segments of this continuous beam are used for the various exposures and bursts of light energy that are delivered to the retina. The ocular tissue effect depends on the amount of argon laser energy channeled through the refractive media to the choroid and retina or to the anterior segment structure, as well as on the tissue upon which the argon laser beam impinges. The retina itself absorbs little energy from the argon laser beam; the vitreous, lens, and cornea similarly are very slightly involved in the absorption process. However, the pigment epithelium (with its pigment granules), the xanthophyll pigment, and the hemoglobin pigment all absorb the argon radiation highly, resulting in marked conversion to heat. The nidi of heat production, therefore, are located and radiate from the pigment epithelium, the deep and superficial vascular plexus, the retinal vessels, the nerve fiber layer area (xanthophyll), and any defects or abnormalities containing these particular pigments. The damage is totally thermal in nature, and a coagulum is formed from denaturation of the involved protein. The healing process takes place by glial tissue repair; scarring and atrophy of the retina and the underlying choroid subsequently occur.

RUBY LASER

The ruby laser beam delivers light energy at one wavelength (694.3 nm) in the deep red region of the visible spectrum. The effect on an ocular tissue is determined by the specific tissue absorption for that wavelength only and by the instantaneous (0.0005 sec) intensity of the beam. This energy is not effective with blood vessels and blood-filled structures because of the lack of absorption by the hemoglobin pigment. The ruby laser beam is scattered, transmitted, and reflected by erythrocytes; the lack of absorption fails to produce a coagulum, although vascular injury can take place. The ruby laser beam is highly absorbed by pigment granules in the pigment epithelium, and the ruby laser energy has been found effective in producing a coagulum at this level, as well as in exciting an exudative chorioretinitis, which leads to the eventual production of an adhesive chorioretinitis. The coagulative effect is generated mainly from the pigment epithelial region, and the coagulum will extend into the inner retina and the choroidal region.

XENON-ARC SOURCE

The xenon-arc high-pressure bulb delivers radiation from all portions of the visible and near-infrared spectrum. This broad-spectral energy output is presented to the ocular tissues, and nearly all ocular structures can be coagulated by the absorption of sufficient amounts of light energy from one or more of the impinging wavelengths. Xenon-arc radiation can be absorbed by any tissue, although it is absorbed primarily at the pigment epithelium, whereas laser radiation is generally absorbed only by pigmented tissues. The xenon-arc emanations are continually produced by the nonlaser high-pressure xenon-arc bulb, and portions of the light output are shuttered into the eye at various exposures. The output power of the xenon-arc instrument, as well as of the laser instruments, can be varied to produce various gradations and severities of the ocular coagulum. These factors and the highly specialized manner of production of light energy by each particular system contribute to the diverse reaction of various ocular lesions to xenon-arc and laser radiation.

Peripheral chorioretinal diseases

PERIPHERAL RETINAL STRUCTURAL ABNORMALITIES

Retinal tears

Argon laser and xenon-arc photocoagulation

The period of treatment of retinal breaks is similar with argon laser and xenon-arc photocoagulation, and the chorioretinal adhesions produced are nearly identical. The manner by which the desired effect is accomplished with the two methods is quite similar. As the light energy from either the argon laser or xenon-arc source is delivered to the retina, the white retinal edema is an indication of the severity of treatment and the extent of the barrage. Retinal tears are seen in sharp contrast to the treated area. The light beam may be applied in a continuous fashion along the edges of the tear, or solitary impacts may be used in a similarly effective manner. Concentric secondary barrages are usually laid down peripheral to the primary treatment area, since the initial application stands out vividly. Detached areas of retina near a retinal tear may absorb sufficient energy to be coagulated directly, without necessarily exciting an underlying choroidal response. Coagulation near the operculum of a retinal tear may occasionally cause further vitreous shrinkage, elevation of the operculum, and extension of the retinal tear. Vitreous strands, flaky opacities, pigment specks, and other debris are always considered a dangerous sign in argon laser or xenon-arc photocoagulation, since they may absorb sufficient quantities of the various wavelengths of radiation available to cause localized coagulation or vitreous shrinkage.

Ruby laser photocoagulation

Therapeutic ruby laser photocoagulation immediately produces a barely perceptible spot of pigment dispersion and chorioretinal edema. The most demonstrable part of the impact may be only a slight jarring of the retinal tissue. If an intraretinal water vapor bubble forms, the retina may be bowed slightly toward the observer, creating a shiny reflection in the internal limiting membrane and the anterior wall of the bubble. Usually, some pigment granules are swept to the edge of the impact area, leaving the target area slightly less pigmented. These particular changes are usually the only indication of treatment, and it is sometimes difficult to determine the extent and degree of coagulation. Clear demarcation of the retinal tear or detachment does not occur with treatment, and it is only by carefully surveying and comparing the adjacent fundus areas that one can recognize former coagulation sites. The process of ruby laser photocoagulation differs from the longer exposures of the continuously operating sources, such as the argon laser and xenon-arc photocoagulation systems, because it assumes more of an instantaneous tacking process. Individual bursts of energy are placed precisely around the retinal tear to surround it effectively. Macular and posteriorly placed breaks can be coagulated accurately by either the argon laser or the ruby laser method, and there is minimal destruction of surrounding tissue because of the small size of the laser-created lesions. Impact sites are not intentionally overlapped, since the double accumulation of energy in the overlapped areas may cause disruption of the choroidal vessels. With the ruby laser, retinal blood vessels may be included within the target area, since they are relatively unaffected at the lower intensities (they reflect, transmit, or scatter most of the light). The retinal vessels are also sufficiently distant from the absorbent layer of the pigment epithelium to withstand the small temperature rise that occurs. With argon laser or xenon-arc photocoagulation, immediate and delayed necrosis of the retinal vessel wall can occur when vessels near a retinal tear are overtreated. Higher-energy ruby laser impacts can also shear a retinal vessel at the time of impact.

Higher-energy ruby laser impacts create a more easily recognizable reaction. Choroidal blanching, retinal swelling, and bubble formation are all more pronounced, and pigment granules may be arranged in mosaic patterns. Retinal edema and clouding appear much more quickly than with lower-energy coagulations, usually within several minutes. Intraretinal vapor bubbles are larger and last longer, absorbing completely in 20 min.

Retinal degenerations

Laser and xenon-arc photocoagulation

Lattice and pigmentary retinal degenerations occurring in the preequatorial region of the retina are treated effectively, when indicated, by argon laser, ruby laser or xenon-arc photocoagulation. Because of the relative decrease in the size of the pupil at this angle and the large degree of spraying and scattering of radiation, considerable amounts of energy must necessarily traverse the lens and anterior vitreous to create effective coagulations. With far-anterior lesions where scleral indentation is necessary, it may sometimes be preferable to employ transcleral cryocautery, especially if visualization of the degenerative site is difficult. Peripheral retinal degeneration, however, can usually be surrounded by coagulation sites; the results and limitations for photocoagulation for those degenerative lesions are similar to those mentioned for retinal tears.

Retinal detachments

Argon laser and xenon-arc photocoagulation

Laser or xenon-arc coagulation is a valuable adjunct to surgery during the postoperative period. Incompletely closed retinal tears, persistent, slightly elevated areas of retinal detachment, underdiathermized areas of choroid, meridional folds of retina, and retinal incarceration sites may all be treated by photocoagulation. However, photocoagulation by any method is capable of causing massive vitreous shrinkage, further elevation of retinal folds, and extension of retinal tears. To lessen the frequency of these complications, the vitreous structure should be assessed thoroughly and great care exercised in the extent of treatment.

The argon laser photocoagulation system is capable of coagulating any tissue that has a concentration of pigment granules or hemoglobin sufficient to absorb the beam, resulting in the creation of a coagulum. Atrophic areas and zones of fluid accumulation may not be coagulated as effectively, as observed with xenon-arc photocoagulation. Usually, sufficient pigment accumulation is present for adequate photocoagulation with the argon laser, and the ability of the argon laser to be used without contact with the globe and without anesthesia make it highly useful during the postoperative period.

The xenon-arc photocoagulator can coagulate any tissue capable of absorbing any portion of its radiations. Therefore, nonpigmented tissues, such as areas of choroidal atrophy, isolated retinal tissue, or fluids of a high protein content, can be coagulated much more easily by xenon-arc than by argon or ruby laser photocoagulation. Shallowly detached retinas and fluid-filled meridional folds over scleral buckles can be collapsed effectively by xenon-arc photocoagulation, resulting in contraction of the separated layers. The ability of the xenon-arc radiation to collapse thin chorioretinal separations by coagulation of the intervening space makes this method extremely valuable during the early stages of the postoperative interval.

The ruby laser, however, does not operate as efficiently as the xenon-arc or argon laser coagulator when the choroidal and retinal surfaces are slightly separated, because heat is generated only at areas of pigment concentration and usually not enough heat is dispersed to these layers to coagulate them. Nonpigmented areas and choroidal atrophy absorb only minute portions of the incident laser beam and are generally not affected by it. Therefore, the ruby laser can be used to create additional chorioretinal adhesions during the early postoperative period only if the chorioretinal surfaces are closely approximated. It is not suitable for treating shallow detachments or fluid-filled meridional folds. During the late postoperative period the ruby laser can be used to reinforce existing chorioretinal adhesions or to wall off areas of potential weakness.

One of the outstanding features of argon laser and ruby laser photocoagulation is the ability of these systems to create an adhesive chorioretinitis without any need for anesthesia or akinesia. This feature is most advantageous during the first 3 weeks of the postoperative period, when the globe may be easily ruptured in the areas of scleral diathermy, orbital vessels are dilated, and the eye is generally not suitable for external manipulation or retrobulbar injection. A speculum, focusing contact lens, and saline lavage, usually required for xenon-arc coagulation, are also unnecessary with laser photocoagulation. The laser therefore has a distinct value during this early postoperative period because the ocular structures need not be disturbed for the production of an effective adhesive chorioretinitis.

Retinoschisis

Laser and xenon-arc photocoagulation

Photocoagulation offers an effective treatment for retinoschisis under certain conditions; there are three main approaches.

Walling off smaller areas of retinoschisis is accomplished without difficulty with either laser or xenon-arc photocoagulation. The laser photocoagulators are preferable for this type of treatment because of the ease of application, smallness of coagulation sites, and relative sparing of normal retinal tissue. Usually, a double, interrupted barrage is laid down just posterior to the extent of retinal splitting along the entire extent of the bulla.

Photocoagulation treatments to the entire bulla of the retinoschisis have proved effective, especially with the more shallow bullas. The cystlike schisis area collapses over a period of several weeks, but the mechanism remains uncertain. Since ruby laser coagulation of the retinoschisis bleb is not as effective as argon laser or xenon-arc photocoagulation, it appears that some coagulation of the cyst fluid, rich in hyaluronic acid and mucopolysaccharides, takes place with the latter photocoagulation methods. Preferably, the argon laser or xenon-arc photocoagulation device is used when a large retinoschisis bleb is treated in this manner. A delimiting series of coagulations is usually applied to the normal retina near the edge of the retinoschisis area in conjunction with the bleb barrage.

The argon laser, ruby laser, or xenon-arc photocoagulator can be used, along with a preplaced encircling band, to reinforce diathermized areas. As noted previously, the argon laser and xenon-arc photocoagulation systems work better than the ruby laser when the inner layers of the retinoschisis are moderately elevated. When the schisis has been collapsed, the ruby laser can increase chorioretinal adhesions more effectively to create a delimiting row of coagulations. Generally, however, the argon laser is used in this situation because of the effectiveness of its wavelengths and because no specific kind of anesthesia or akinesia is needed.

PERIPHERAL RETINAL VASCULAR ABNORMALITIES

Argon laser and xenon-arc photocoagulation

Continuous-wave photocoagulation with either the argon laser or the xenon-arc source has been used effectively with retinal vascular lesions, including entities such as Eales' disease, Leber's disease, Coats' disease, proliferative sickle retinopathy, and retrolental fibroplasia. Treatments must be light, since a delicate balance exists between the therapeutic obliteration of the vessels and necrosis and rupture of the walls. The heat produced by the light energy at the vessel site is dispersed into the flow of blood and the adjacent retina and vitreous. Coagulation and scarring of the retinal tissue may constrict some smaller retinal vessels, and thrombosis of these vessels may occur. The absorption of large amounts of light energy, sufficient to cause clotting in the larger retinal vessels, is usually accompanied by subsequent vascular necrosis and scarring. It is important to note that argon laser and xenon-arc radiation is effective with most retinal vascular lesions because it can be focused on the defect and absorbed in sufficient quantities to produce a direct effect. Therefore, vitreal and preretinal neovascularization and the larger vascular abnormalities, more distant from the highly absorbent pigment epithelium, can be treated more successfully with argon laser and xenon-arc photocoagulation than with the ruby laser method.

Ruby laser photocoagulation

The vascular effect produced by the ruby laser is dependent on the proximity of the vessels to the pigment epithelium or melanocytes and on the flow rate and absorption characteristics of the enclosed hemoglobin. Ruby laser radiation can be effective with larger vascular lesions if pigment is interspersed intraretinally initially or as a result of repeated low-intensity laser bombardment to the vessel area. Coagulations at 2-week intervals can increase pigment proliferation greatly and shrink the surrounding retina. Some vessels and vascular abnormalities can become irregularly constricted and show disruption and pigment proliferation within their walls. Eventually, smaller vessels narrow sufficiently to allow restriction of the blood flow and occlusion. Generally, because of the low absorption of the ruby laser beam by vascular elements, it is preferable to use the argon laser or the xenon-arc modality for the obliteration of vascular abnormalities of the choroid or retina.

DIABETIC RETINOPATHY

Nonproliferative diabetic retinopathy

Argon laser and xenon-arc photocoagulation

Both the argon laser and xenon-arc photocoagulation systems are highly effective in the treatment of nonproliferative diabetic retinopathy. The treatment of this condition can be considered when the retinal vessels have passed through the stage of herniation and microaneurysm formation, and possibly rupture and hemorrhage, and are leaking grossly into the retinal tissue. The condition may take the form of moderately advanced diabetic maculopathy, as well as edema of the other portions of the posterior retinal area. Intraretinal microvascular abnormalities, such as large shunting channels, microaneurysms, and macroaneurysms, can be effectively obliterated with either of these photocoagulation systems; retinal edema and, possibly, exudate formation will subsequently be reduced. The areas of maximal leakage from the retinal vessels must be documented by fluorescein angiography, and the laser photocoagulation approach must be directed toward these areas of leakage.

If the vascular abnormalities are treated before exudate formation becomes prominent, there is an excellent chance that the vision can be maintained or improved; this chance is considerably better than that occurring when the disease runs its natural course. Macular defects are most satisfactorily treated with the small coagulations that are possible with the argon laser, whereas paramacular and other retinal areas can be treated effectively with either the argon laser or the xenon-arc photocoagulation system.

Ruby laser photocoagulation

In the paramacular and posterior polar areas, the ruby laser is still used in some instances to produce coagulations that are effective in stabilizing and improving early macular and retinal edema. Random coagulations and coagulations of the panretinal ablative type have proved useful in treating nonproliferative diabetic retinopathy but are probably less effective than those of the argon laser or xenon-arc devices.

Proliferative diabetic retinopathy

Argon laser photocoagulation

The proliferative phase of diabetic retinopathy can be divided into five categories, depending on the location and growth of the neovascularization. Argon laser photocoagulation is highly effective for focal treatment to surface, peripapillary, epipapillary, papillovitreal, and retinovitreal neovascularization. The photocoagulation is directed to the area of neovascularization, or indirect destruction of the peripheral retina during panretinal photocoagulation causes obliteration of the neovascularization. The high absorption of the argon laser beam by hemoglobin permits this photocoagulation system to be used advantageously for treating neovascularization extending from the optic disc or the retina into the vitreous body. In addition, the amount of energy necessary for coagulation of these abnormal vessels is much less than that expended by the xenon-arc source; hazards and possible subsequent complications are therefore minimized.

Xenon-arc photocoagulation

Xenon-arc photocoagulation is used effectively for treating surface neovascularization in any portion of the retina. The indirect approach used with panretinal photocoagulation can also be applied with xenon-arc impacts but cannot be used more peripherally in the fundus, because the xenon-arc beam cannot easily be reflected off the three-mirror lens. Most areas of surface or slightly elevated retinal neovascularization can be obliterated directly by xenon-arc photocoagulation due to the blue portion of the polychromatic beam and indirectly by the shriveling and scarring produced on retinal structures near the abnormal vessels.

Ruby laser photocoagulation

Ruby laser photocoagulation has a limited effect on proliferative diabetic retinopathy unless the procedure is employed in the very early stages of the disease and with the panretinal photocoagulation technique. The latter technique of destruction of retinal tissues appears to have an indirect effect on decreasing the stimulus for neovascularization and has proved successful in obliterating some types of surface retinal and vitreal neovascularization. Argon laser photocoagulation has proved preferable to ruby laser photocoagulation, however, for treating all categories of proliferative diabetic retinopathy.

PERIPHERAL CHORIORETINAL TUMORS

Retinoblastoma

Argon laser and xenon-arc photocoagulation

In the treatment of retinoblastoma, photocoagulation has assumed greater importance recently as a procedure used alone or as an adjunct to radiation and chemotherapy. Small tumors occupying less than 2 DD in the posterior pole can be destroyed by repeated photocoagulation treatments. Actual photocoagulation of the white tumor tissue by argon laser or xenon-arc radiation is not easily accomplished because of low absorption and considerable reflection. Pigment flecks in the tumor and choroidal pigment near the tumor tissue will absorb both types of radiation and secondarily affect the neoplastic cells. The main destructive course appears to be the interruption of the tumor's blood supply, which is vital to the tumor. In these cases argon laser and xenon-arc photocoagulation can both be moderately successful because of their effect on the blood supply. Further studies with higher laser outputs in these conditions are being conducted. If utilized, photocoagulation therapy probably should be in conjunction with cobalt plaque implantation or other types of localized radiation.

Ruby laser photocoagulation

Ruby laser photocoagulation is not effective for any type of chorioretinal tumor.

Malignant melanoma of the choroid

Argon laser and xenon-arc photocoagulation

Malignant melanomas less than 6 DD in size, confined to the posterior portion of the globe, and without an extensive secondary retinal detachment have been treated successfully by light coagulation in several series of patients. Argon laser or xenon-arc radiation is applied to the surrounding choroid and heavily over the tumor mass in a gradual, segmental manner, forming a coagulum to prevent metastasis of malignant cells. This treatment destroys the cells and blood vessels near the surface of the tumor mass; the resulting hemorrhage and gray coagulum veil usually prevent further treatment until they have cleared. Additional coagulations are performed over a period of months, until the tumor has been reduced to a slightly elevated, scarred mass. This type of photocoagulation therapy is experimental; it must be performed on relatively small melanomas, and it must not be excessive, because of the possible extensive necrosis and inflammatory reaction of the globe.

Angiomatosis retinae

Argon laser and xenon-arc photocoagulation

Either argon laser or xenon-arc photocoagulation is effective for large retinal angiomas. The latter source is preferred because of the infrared component of the radiation, which helps produce a greater penetration of the coagulum and affects the vascular tissue itself. The argon laser photocoagulation beam is also effective but has more of a capping effect; its penetration is limited in comparison with the xenon-arc source. The treatments are multiple and are spaced at 3- to 4-week intervals. Reduction of the tumor mass is gradual. Coagulations directed to the tumor mass itself are highly effective with either photocoagulation source and are the therapeutic technique of choice.

Macular diseases

MACULAR INTERRETINAL ABNORMALITIES

Macular serous detachment of the pigment epithelium or sensory retina

Argon laser photocoagulation is superior to xenon-arc and ruby laser photocoagulation for most macular diseases because of the small coagulation size that can be produced, as well as the high absorption by both melanin and hemoglobin. Because of these features, defects in the pigment epithelial layer, abnormally permeable retinal vessels, and areas of choroidal or retinal neovascularization can be obliterated with less effect on surrounding healthy tissue. In particular, serous detachments of the pigment epithelium can be located by fluorescein angiography and treated lightly with the argon laser; the results are flattening and correction of the detachment in a high percentage of cases. Similarly, choroidal leakage through the pigment epithelium beneath the sensory retina can also be corrected by cauterizing the abnormal leakage area in the pigment epithelium. Serous accumulations beneath the sensory retina from abnormal retinal vasculature, although less common, can also be improved by selective argon laser photocoagulation.

Hemorrhagic detachment of the pigment epithelium or sensory retina

Argon laser photocoagulation of hemorrhagic detachments of the pigment epithelium can be quite beneficial, particularly when located a small distance away from the fovea. Accumulations of neovascularization are usually found on the surface of the detached pigment epithelium or beneath it, and proper, intense photocoagulation of the hemorrhagic detachment usually prevents the occurrence of repeated hemorrhages into the area beneath the pigment epithelium or beneath the sensory retina. Subretinal hemorrhages are much less effectively treated, since the source of the hemorrhage is usually covered by the blood and treatment must be postponed until the hemorrhage beneath the sensory retina has been absorbed. The use of fluorescein angiography is imperative for detecting the small serous leakage zones and areas of degeneration or frank neovascularization. Argon laser photocoagulation can be highly effective for stabilizing these macular degenerative diseases and, particularly, the macular problems that are secondary to the development of choroidal neovascularization. In all such cases it is important to treat these abnormalities as soon as they are recognized ophthalmoscopically or by fluorescein angiography.

MACULAR INTRARETINAL ABNORMALITIES

Branch retinal vein occlusion

Branch retinal vein occlusion can be treated by three distinct photocoagulation techniques with any of the three photocoagulation systems (argon laser, ruby laser, or xenon-arc). The para-arteriolar, barrier, and barrage techniques have been found to be moderately effective for this disease process. The photocoagulation approaches are designed to reduce the arteriolar pressure head in the region of the occluded vein, and particularly in the paramacular zone. The para-arteriolar crimping technique is most innocuous and appears to decrease the arteriolar pressure by a moderate amount. The barrier technique around the macular region reduces the inflow to the macular zone enough to allow compensation of that area, and the barrage technique produces a greater degree of destruction of the pathologic, occluded region. All techniques attempt to preserve the macular function and reduce the edema, microcystic changes, and hemorrhagic activity in the macular and paramacular areas. In addition, it is conceivable that photocoagulation allows the trapped intraretinal fluid to escape into the choroid, but this theory has not been established. Photocoagulation can therefore be extremely useful if the natural compensation course is ineffective and the condition is worsening. Photocoagulation should not be used immediately when a branch vein occlusion has been recognized; it should be postponed for 3 to 6 months, and then employed only when it is obvious that the macular region is undergoing rapid deterioration.

Central retinal vein occlusion

The treatment of central retinal vein occlusion is experimental at the present time, but in several short series of patients panretinal photocoagulation to the posterior polar region has been beneficial in stabilizing the course of eyes that have sustained central retinal vein occlusion. These particular patients have not developed neovascular glaucoma over a very short follow-up period, and the microcystic changes and edema of the macular region have decreased following the panretinal photocoagulation application. Photocoagulation should not be employed at the onset of this disease state; it should be considered only after several months and in a situation where it is obvious that the macular condition is undergoing decompensation and degeneration.

MISCELLANEOUS MACULAR DISEASES

Macular hole or cyst

A macular cyst should not be treated by photocoagulation, and a macular hole should be watched carefully for rolling of the edges; there is also the possibility that a macular hole, if penetrating, may extend to a retinal detachment. Walling off the macular hole by argon laser or ruby laser photocoagulation is indicated if it is obvious that the macular area is undergoing contraction and detachment of that region.

Preretinal fibrosis

The use of photocoagulation for preretinal fibrosis is entirely experimental. Photocoagulation attempts have been directed toward the region of increased fluid accumulation, as observed with fluorescein angiography. At the present time photocoagulation is not recommended as a primary therapeutic method.

Toxoplasmic retinochoroiditis

Any photocoagulation system can be used to treat the border of the inactive (or occasionally active) toxoplasmosis scar. The rationale of such treatment appears to be the obliteration of resident dormant organisms, or hyperallergic or antigenic tissue. It has been debated whether this prophylactic treatment will reduce the average reactivation rate of these old chorioretinitic areas, but it is the impression of some investigators that this type of therapy can be considered, particularly if reactivation of the lesion is frequent.

Toxocara canis infestation

Photocoagulation of the posterior polar granuloma, primarily with the argon laser or xenon-arc source, has been undertaken experimentally. The granulomas appear to have decreased in size, and there has been little secondary reactivation of the uveitis or vitreous clouding.

Pigment epitheliopathy

The basic cause for most pigment epitheliopathies is not known. These elusive diseases include acute multifocal placoid pigment epitheliopathy, as well as helicoid and geographic or serpiginous chorioretinitis. The first disease mentioned is self-limiting and should not be subjected to photocoagulation, but consideration has been given to creating a "fire wall" between the foveal region and the tongues of affected pigment epithelium that have a tendency to extend toward the macular area in the latter condition. The serpiginous type of chorioretinitis reactivates at intervals and can extend into the foveal region, resulting in considerable destruction. Therefore, properly directed photocoagulation for this disease has been considered experimentally.

Anterior segment abnormalities

IRIS DEFECTS

Photocoreoplasty

Argon laser or xenon-arc photocoagulation has been effective in repositioning an eccentric pupil that is congenital or secondary to surgery or trauma. The photocoagulation technique is simple if the patient is aphakic; it must be more delicately applied, usually with the argon laser, if the lens is still present. The repositioning of the iris structure is usually considered for optical reasons rather than for cosmetic reasons.

Photomydriasis

The procedure called photomydriasis has been used to dilate pupils of individuals receiving intensive miotic therapy for glaucoma in an effort to increase the light transmitted to the retina. Certain patients are debilitated by the extreme miosis or by the underlying nuclear sclerosis or cataractous opacification of the lens; in many patients this procedure will increase the visual field and acuity.

Photoiridotomy

In certain situations, particularly iris bombé or incipient angle-closure glaucoma, it is advisable to perform an iridectomy or iridotomy. Argon laser photocoagulation has been used to perform photoiridotomies on phakic and aphakic eyes without operative interven-

Text continued on p. 68.

Table 3. Results of treatment of various ocular abnormalities by argon laser, ruby laser, and xenon-arc photocoagulation

	Argon laser	Xenon-arc	Ruby laser
Energy production	Source: electrically pumped gaseous discharge tube Maximum power density: 250.0+ watts/sq cm at cornea (approximately) Duration: 0.01 sec—continuous Repetition rate: instantaneous	Source: high-pressure xenon-arc bulb Maximum power density: 7.8+ joules/sq cm/sec at cornea (approximately) Duration: 0.1 sec—continuous Repetition rate: instantaneous	Source: ruby crystal pumped by xenon flash Maximum power density: 0.14+ joules/sq cm/0.0002 sec at cornea (approximately) Duration: 0.0002 sec Repetition rate: 1 to 5 sec
Energy characteristics	Directional, coherent, monochromatic beams at 6 wavelengths between 457.9 nm and 514.5 nm, predominantly 488.0 nm and 514.5 nm; 95% transmission by ocular media	Visible and infrared radiation (400 to 1,100 nm); 95% transmission by ocular media (400 to 900 nm), ⅔ transmission (900 to 1,100 nm)	Directional, coherent, monochromatic beam at 694.3 nm; 95% transmission by ocular media
Tissue reaction	Absorption primarily at pigmented areas, such as melanin, xanthophyll, and hemoglobin; heat production and coagulum formed, resulting in eventual pigment and glial proliferation	Coagulation with sufficient absorption of any wavelength (400 to 1,100 nm); edema, exudation, pigment proliferation, gliosis, and atrophy	Absorption primarily at pigmented areas, with production of heat; late result similar to light coagulation
Anesthesia	Topical anesthesia required; occasionally retrobulbar akinesia and anesthesia necessary	Occasionally preoperative sedation, retrobulbar and lid akinesia and anesthesia; topical anesthesia necessary	None required
Ancillary equipment	Low-vacuum or three-mirror contact lens for retinal photocoagulation; occasionally, cooling contact lens for anterior segment therapy	Contact lens for correcting high ametropia, lid speculum, and constant saline corneal lavage; forceps manipulation of eye may be necessary	None required
Hospitalization and aftercare	None required	Monocular patch for 12 hours	None required
Hazards	No danger to operator; overall hazards to patient minimal due to minute total energy transmitted through refractive media	Accidental retinal burn of operator; overheating of anterior chamber, thermal cataract, vitreous hemorrhages, secondary retinal necrosis and tears, secondary exudative retinal detachment, and macular deterioration	Accidental retinal burn of operator more probable because of coherency and energy density of stray laser beam; similar ocular complications; less total energy transmitted through media

Therapeutic effectiveness			
Peripheral retinal structural abnormalities			
Retinal tears	Excellent*	Excellent	Excellent
Retinal degenerations	Excellent*	Excellent	Excellent
Retinal detachments	Excellent—requires absorbent pigment*	Excellent—effective with slightly elevated retinas, meridional folds, tears	Good—effective if retina attached
Retinoschisis	Good—use limited to delimiting bulla,* possibly barrage	Good—used to barrage* or delimit bulla; with encircling element*	Fair—to delimit bulla after bulla has been collapsed by surgery
Peripheral retinal vascular abnormalities			
Eales' disease	Excellent*	Excellent	Poor
Leber's disease	Excellent—especially for macular lesions*	Excellent	Poor
Coats' disease	Excellent	Excellent*	Poor
Proliferative sickle retinopathy	Excellent*	Excellent	Poor
Retrolental fibroplasia	Equivocal*	Equivocal	Poor
Diabetic retinopathy			
Nonproliferative	Excellent*	Excellent	Poor
Proliferative	Excellent—especially for epipapillary, peripapillary, papillovitreal, and retinovitreal neovascularization*	Excellent—especially for surface neovascularization*	Fair—ablation technique only
Peripheral chorioretinal tumors			
Retinoblastoma	Fair	Good*	
Malignant melanoma	Good—<6 DD	Good*—<6 DD	Poor
Angiomatosis retinae	Excellent	Excellent*	Poor
Macular serous abnormalities			Poor
Serous detachment of pigment epithelium	Excellent*	Excellent	Good
Central serous choroidopathy	Excellent*	Excellent	
Macular hemorrhagic abnormalities			Excellent
Hemorrhagic detachment of the pigment epithelium	Excellent—especially for perifoveal and macular area*	Excellent	Poor

*Preferred method of treatment.

Table 3. Results of treatment of various ocular abnormalities by argon laser, ruby laser, and xenon-arc photocoagulation—cont'd

	Argon laser	Xenon-arc	Ruby laser
Hemorrhagic detachment of the sensory retina	Good*	Good	Poor
Choroidal neovascularization and secondary exudative maculopathy	Excellent—especially for perifoveal and macular area*	Excellent	Poor
Macular intraretinal abnormalities			
Branch retinal vein occlusion	Excellent*	Excellent	Good—ablation technique only
Central retinal vein occlusion	Equivocal*	Equivocal	Equivocal
Miscellaneous macular diseases			
Macular hole, penetrating	Excellent*	Fair	Good
Preretinal fibrosis	Equivocal*	Equivocal	Equivocal
Toxoplasmic retinochoroiditis	Good(?)*	Good(?)	Good(?)
Toxocara canis infestation	Good(?)	Good(?)*	Poor
Pigment epitheliopathy	Good*	Good	Fair
Angioid streaks	Good*	Good*	Poor
Anterior segment photocoagulation			
Photocoreoplasty	Excellent—especially if lens is present*	Excellent	Poor
Iris cyst	Excellent*	Excellent	Poor
Photomydriasis	Excellent—especially if lens is present*	Good	Poor
Iridocyclitic membrane	Excellent*	Excellent	Poor
Photoiridotomy	Excellent—especially if lens is present*	Good	Good

Table 4. Photocoagulation effectiveness classification for various ocular diseases

Ocular disease	Classification
Peripheral retinal structural abnormalities	
Retinal tears	4d
Retinal degenerations	4d
Retinal detachments	4d
Retinoschisis	4d
Peripheral retinal vascular abnormalities	
Eales' disease	4d
Leber's disease	4d
Coats' disease	4d
Proliferative sickle retinopathy	4d
Retrolental fibroplasia	3a
Diabetic retinopathy	
Nonproliferative	4c
Proliferative	
Epipapillary neovascularization	3c
Peripapillary neovascularization	3c
Papillovitreal neovascularization	3c
Retinovitreal neovascularization	3c
Surface neovascularization	4c
Peripheral chorioretinal tumors	
Retinoblastoma	3a
Malignant melanoma	3b
Angiomatosis retinae	4c
Choroidal hemangioma	4c
Macular interretinal defects	
Macular serous detachment of the pigment epithelium	3c
Central serous choroidopathy	4d
Macular hemorrhage detachment of the pigment epithelium	4d
Macular hemorrhage detachment of the sensory retina	3c
Macular intraretinal abnormalities	
Branch retinal artery occlusion	3b
Central retinal artery occlusion	1a
Branch retinal vein occlusion	3c
Central retinal vein occlusion	2a
Irvine-Gass syndrome	2a
Vitreitis	1a
Miscellaneous macular diseases	
Macular hole	3c
Preretinal fibrosis	2a
Toxoplasmic retinochoroiditis	3c
Toxocara canis infestation	2c
Pigment epitheliopathy	3b
Angioid streaks	3c
Choroidal neovascularization	3c
Iris abnormalities	
Photocoreoplasty	4d
Photomydriasis	4d
Photoiridotomy	4c
Iris cysts	4c
Iridocyclitic membranes	4c

tion. The technique appears promising and should be considered if an iridotomy is required in an eye where surgical correction might be difficult.

Iris cysts

Epithelial or implantation cysts, usually secondary to trauma or surgery, can be destroyed effectively by argon laser or xenon-arc photocoagulation. These cysts can be destroyed in the phakic or aphakic states without surgical intervention.

Iridocyclitic membranes

Occasionally, a dense iridocyclitic membrane will form secondary to trauma, Still's disease, or other anterior segment problems and will require discission. Discission can be difficult if the iridocyclitic membrane is vascularized, and photocoagulation has proved to be very useful by obliterating the blood vessels in the membrane in the central area of proposed discission. When the blood vessels have been destroyed, the discission is made through the membrane without the hazard of extensive bleeding into the vitreous or anterior chamber.

Summary

In summary, the clinical responses of various ocular abnormalities to argon laser, ruby laser, and xenon-arc irradiation have been briefly presented. The effectiveness, limitations, and hazards of each method will be discussed in each particular section. A compilation of results of the treatment of ocular lesions by these three methods of photocoagulation is presented in tabular form, and the preferred treatment is suggested (Table 3).

PHOTOCOAGULATION EFFECTIVENESS CLASSIFICATIONS

The status of photocoagulation of various ocular diseases can be gradated on the basis of 1 to 4, and on the basis of a to d. The classification 1 to 4 is used to denote the therapeutic result in patients who have been treated under ideal conditions. In this classification, 1 means poor; 2, fair; 3, good; and 4, excellent. The second part of the photocoagulation effectiveness classification is concerned with the stage of investigation and the certainty with which investigation teams consider photocoagulation therapy successful for various ocular diseases. This portion of the classification is labeled by a small letter and is designated as: a, experimental; b, controversial; c, promising; and d, effective. A combination of the Arabic numeral and the small letter should give the reader an idea of the effectiveness of the therapy and the extent of the documentation of this particular stage of effectiveness (Table 4).

Part II

PHOTOCOAGULATION TECHNIQUES

SECTION ONE

Peripheral chorioretinal diseases

Chapter 6

Peripheral retinal structural abnormalities

RETINAL TEARS

Clinical symptoms. The symptoms attributable to retinal tears may be varied and include metamorphopsia, micropsia, wavy vision, burning lights, a sudden shower of spots and opacities, and lightning flashes. Many retinal tears are discovered during routine examination and are not signaled by previous disturbances.

Ophthalmoscopic appearance. Retinal breaks are divided into holes and tears. Holes are characterized by a roughly circular or oval dehiscence in the retinal layer and a small, attached, oval, shrunken operculum that may be resting near the retina or detached into the vitreous body. Retinal tears may be elongated, linear, radial, or circumferential in nature, or they may be represented by a typical U shaped horseshoe tear. The operculum of the horseshoe tear may be highly elevated into the vitreous body or resting close to the choroidal surface.

Ancillary diagnostic examinations. Indirect ophthalmoscopy with scleral depression and precorneal and contact lens biomicroscopic examinations of the fundus, as well as direct ophthalmoscopy, can be of great value in the investigation of retinal breaks. The Goldmann three-mirror lens can be used during biomicroscopy for the accurate diagnosis of peripheral retinal tears and holes.

Fluorescein angiography and visual field examinations offer little assistance in the diagnosis of this disease.

Indications for photocoagulation. Some of the factors *strongly suggesting* that a retinal tear should be treated by photocoagulation are:

1. Moderate vitreous traction on the operculum or edges of the tear
2. Preretinal or vitreous hemorrhage associated with the retinal break
3. Presence of a slight retinal detachment or subretinal fluid
4. A history of retinal detachment in the fellow eye
5. Persistent and progressively more severe symptoms relating to vitreous opacities and peripheral light flashes

In addition, certain circumstances *militate for* early photocoagulation of a retinal break. These particular indications are:

1. Presence of more than 5 diopters of myopia

2. Location of the break above the horizontal meridian
3. Absence of pigment proliferation around the tear, or other indications that the retinal break is of short duration
4. A high degree of physical activity in the patient's daily life
5. A family history of retinal detachment or other structural ocular abnormality

Photocoagulation approach. The basic photocoagulation approach is the production of an exudative choroiditis by photocoagulation around the retinal break; this choroiditis eventually heals to produce an adhesive chorioretinitic scar. In this way the sensory retina is bound firmly to the pigment epithelium and underlying choroid with a small but strong attachment. The retina and the choroid must be in close approximation in the area around the retinal tear for effective healing to take place. With peripheral breaks near the equator of the eye and with more posteriorly located retinal tears and holes, solitary, interrupted, linearly placed coagulations ranging from **500μ to 1,000μ** are produced in the area of attached retina in such a manner that they surround the retinal tear on its posterior and anterior aspects (Fig. 6-1). Coagulations should be strongly visible but not chalk white (Grade 3). Powers ranging from **400 to 600 mw** usually are required with these spot sizes at exposures of **0.2 to 0.5 sec.** If the break is under moderate traction from the vitreous body, a double or triple row of linear coagulations should be applied in a barrier fashion around the retinal tear (Fig. 6-2). The operculum of a horseshoe tear must not be coagulated directly, nor should the photocoagulation beam be directed along a path that would intercept the vitreous attachment to the tip of the operculum. The most anterior aspect of the tear is usually coagulated first, and the more easily accessible posterior portion of the tear area is coagulated later. Only topical anesthesia is required when patient cooperation is average. Preoperative and postoperative photographs of the treated area should be taken for comparison during later evaluation visits (Figs. 6-3 to 6-5).

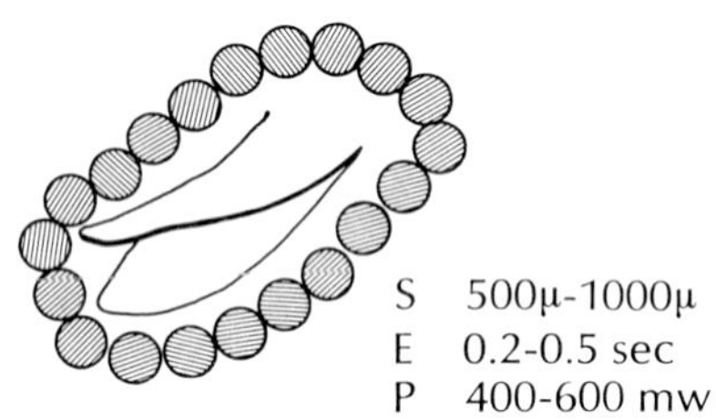

Fig. 6-1. Punctate, linear, contiguous coagulations (500μ to 1,000μ) around the border of a retinal tear in an area of attached retina.

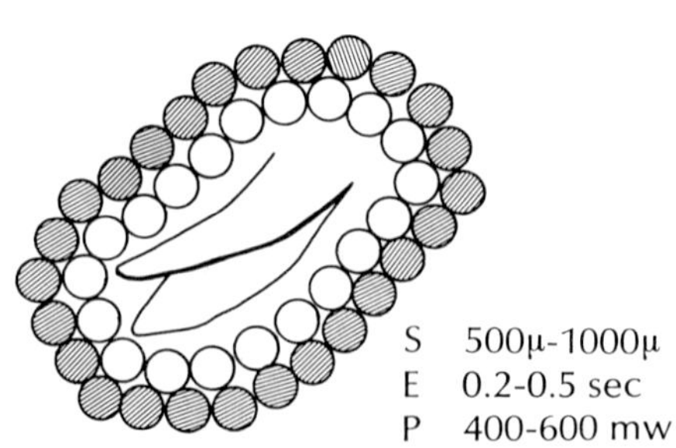

Fig. 6-2. Secondary coagulations of the same size and intensity outside the row of coagulations shown in Fig. 6-1, producing a double linear row of barrier impacts. The tip of the operculum and the vitreoretinal strands should be avoided at all times during photocoagulation.

The power intensity should be reduced in retinal areas where there is subretinal or preretinal blood. Blood or pigment flecks in the edges of the retinal tear or operculum will absorb large amounts of argon laser energy and an excessively severe coagulum will be produced. Anteriorly placed tears can be located and treated in most cases by proper utilization of the Goldmann three-mirror lens or the diagonal low-vacuum contact lens. The central portion of the Goldmann contact lens or the plano–low-vacuum contact lens can be used for more posterior retinal tears. Scleral depression with a contact lens can be

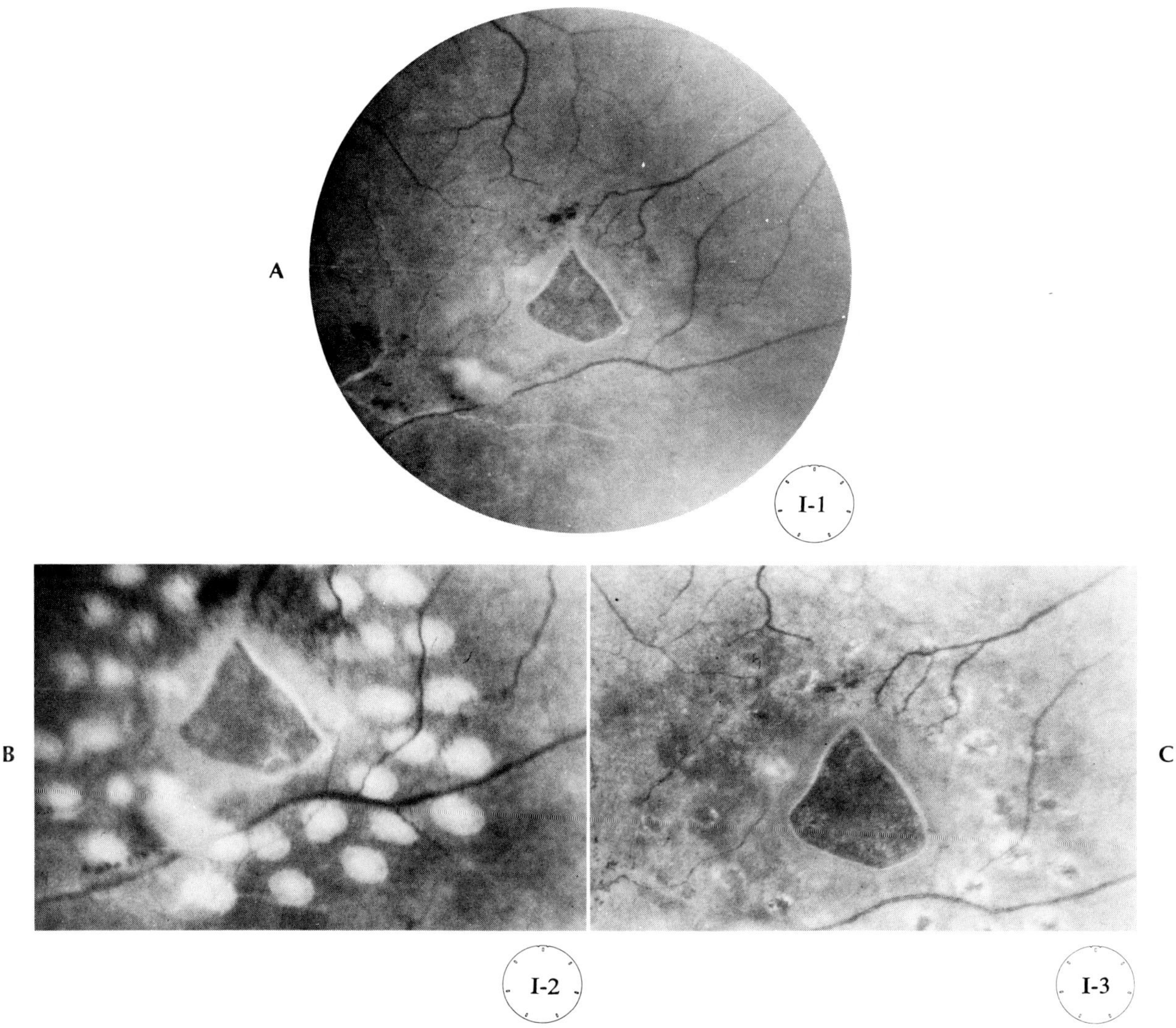

Fig. 6-3. A, A 45-year-old man who complained of having blurred vision in both eyes was found to have a branch vein occlusion in his right eye and a triangularly shaped retinal tear with a free-floating operculum in his left eye. A small area of surrounding retinal detachment and punctate intraretinal hemorrhages could be seen. **B,** Magnified view of the double linear row of punctate, interrupted coagulations placed around the retinal tear to produce a tight barrier between the retinal tear and the normal retina. **C,** The retinal tear 6 weeks after photocoagulation, showing hyperpigmentation and surrounding chorioretinal atrophy at the photocoagulation site. The retinal tear remains unaffected.

used in some cases for better positioning of the coagulation; if the retinal break is far anterior, however, transconjunctival cryocautery is usually preferred.

In the treatment of retinal breaks or any peripheral retinal disease, caution should be observed that the laser beam is not interrupted by cortical cataract opacities or corneal opacities; a high-power laser beam might be directed off anterior segment opacities, and the large amount of energy striking the retinal surface could cause devastating retinal hemorrhage or coagulum. In some cases a free-floating or highly retracted operculum will prevent adequate photocoagulation of one section of the retinal area surrounding the

A

B

C

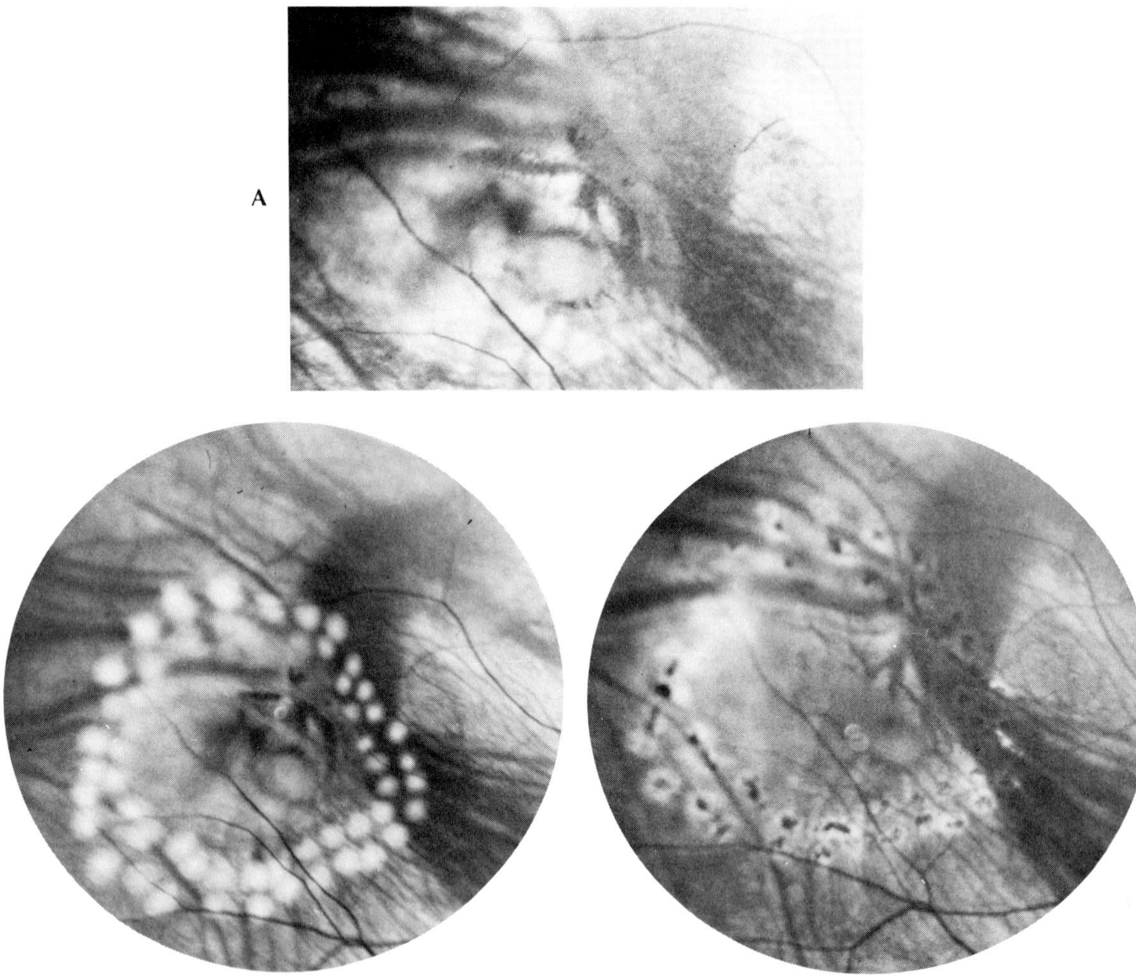

Fig. 6-4. A 60-year-old man with a 1-week history of floaters and occasional lightening flashes was found to have a retinal tear in the superonasal quadrant of his right eye. The large horseshoe tear with an operculum and a slight, surrounding retinal detachment can be seen. **B,** A double row of 500μ coagulations was placed around the retinal tear area in the zone of attached retina. **C,** The retinal tear 7 weeks after argon laser photocoagulation, showing marked hypertrophy of the pigment epithelium in the region of the coagulations. This hypertrophy effectively sealed the retinal tear from the intact retina.

break. A free-floating operculum in the vitreous can usually be momentarily moved by a sudden rotation of the eye to an extent that allows the proper coagulations to be created. A highly retracted operculum still attached to the retinal surface should not be photocoagulated, even if it shields or obscures an important retinal area to be photocoagulated. In these few instances additional cryotherapy can be considered.

Complications

Extension of the retinal tear caused by increased vitreoretinal traction. If energy has been absorbed by the vitreous body or if the tip of the operculum or the vitreous strand to

A

B

C

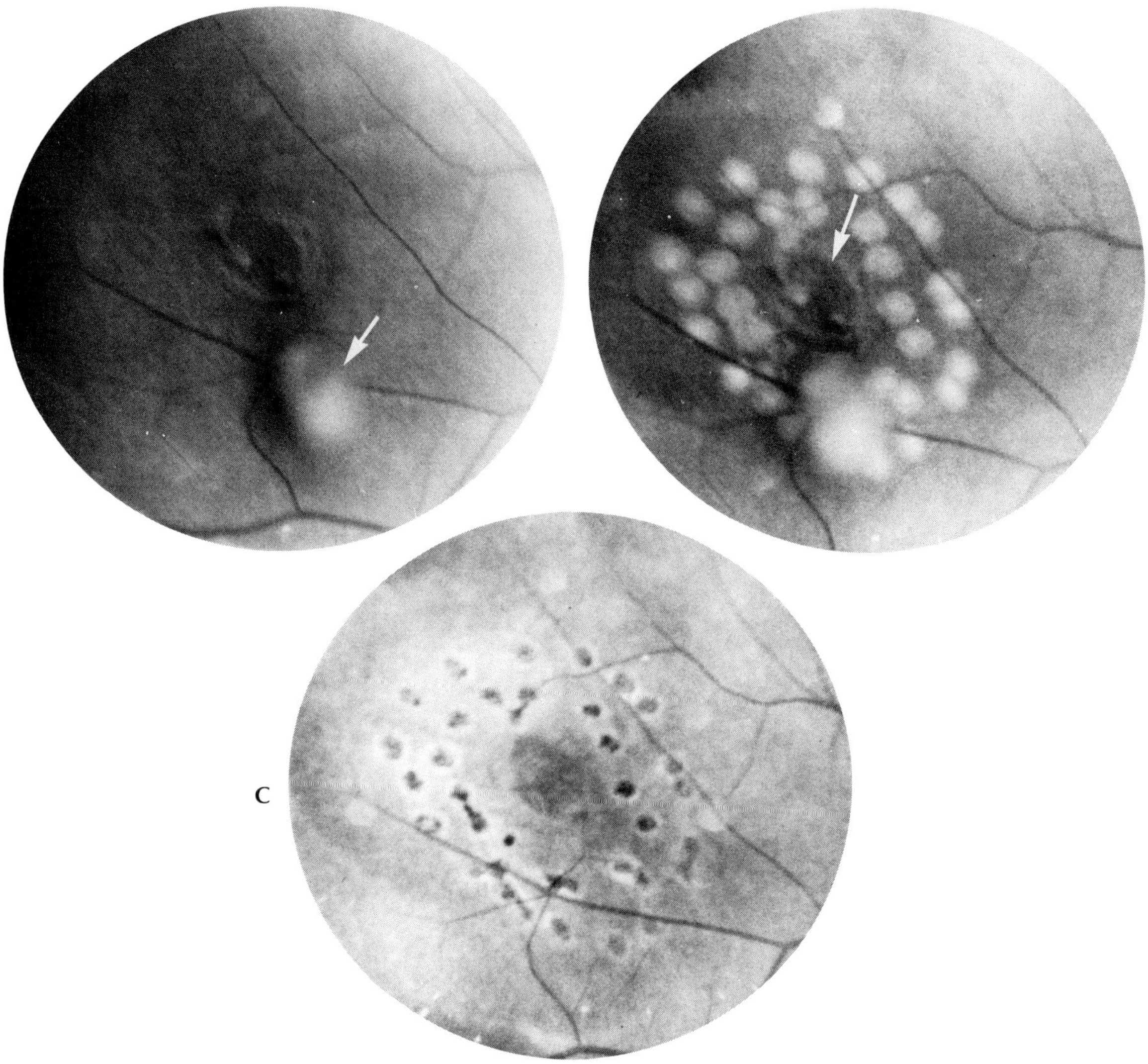

Fig. 6-5. A, A 33-year-old woman complained of having slightly blurred vision of 2 weeks' duration and was found to have a retinal tear with a completely detached operculum (arrow) in the superotemporal quadrant. There was no evidence of a surrounding retinal detachment. **(B),** A double row of 500μ interrupted Grade 3 coagulations was placed around the retinal tear (arrow). The region of the operculum and the associated vitreoretinal strands were avoided. **C,** The retinal tear area 2 months after argon laser photocoagulation, showing an effective seal around the flat retinal tear.

the operculum was inadvertently photocoagulated or absorbed some of the incident scattered light energy, the increase in vitreoretinal traction will cause an extension of the retinal tear. If an increase in traction on the retinal tear and operculum and an increase in the degree of surrounding retinal separation are noted during the initial visit 3 to 7 days after photocoagulation, a localized retinal buckling procedure to release the vitreous traction should be considered. If pigmentation has started to take place at the coagulation site, it is entirely justifiable to monitor the case closely and not intervene surgically, because the adhesive chorioretinitis may be sufficient to withstand the vitreoretinal traction.

Vitreous hemorrhage. If the vitreoretinal traction on an operculum or retinal tear area containing a retinal vessel increases following photocoagulation, this vessel can be ruptured by the shearing action of the vitreoretinal contraction. Photocoagulation of a retinal vessel in the treated area can cause necrosis of the wall of that vessel and eventually result in a severe blowout hemorrhage. If the hemorrhage is small and it can be determined that the vessel is a vein, further photocoagulation to the more distal distribution of the vein into the tear area can be done to decrease or eliminate the blood flow into the weakened and ruptured area of the vein. If the vessel is an artery, one should consider occluding the artery with the sausage-type coagulations mentioned in the section on diabetic retinovitreal neovascularization (pp. 141 and 142).

Choroidal rupture. Choroidal rupture is extremely rare; but if it occurs at the time of photocoagulation because of an excessively severe coagulum, the spot size (≅ doubled) and the intensity (≅ tripled) should be increased, and the entire zone around the area of choroidal rupture should be coagulated intensely to interrupt any choroidal flow into the ruptured zone.

Retinal detachment. Although extremely unlikely, if a retinal detachment occurs postoperatively, surgical intervention with the usual techniques for retinal surgery should be employed.

Follow-up. The patient is routinely placed on a regimen of homatropine hydrobromide 2% and dexamethasone 0.1% administered 3 times a day to the treated eye for a period of 10 days. The patient should be examined within 3 to 7 days following photocoagulation so that it can be determined whether increased vitreous traction or any other complication has occurred. The patient may then be followed at 1- to 2-week intervals until adequate pigment proliferation and chorioretinal adhesions have formed. Thereafter, treated patients should be evaluated at 3- to 6-month intervals until it has been determined that the retinal defect and vitreous condition are stable. Examinations are then repeated at yearly intervals after quiescence of the condition has been ascertained.

PERIPHERAL RETINAL DEGENERATIONS

Clinical symptoms. Symptoms similar to those outlined under the section on retinal tears (p. 73) may be experienced by the patient. Unfortunately, symptoms do not occur in the majority of cases, and the peripheral defect is discovered during routine examination.

Ophthalmoscopic appearance. Peripheral retinal degenerations can be seen as accumulations of pigment and glial proliferation involving the retina and the choroid, with atrophy or edema of the overlying retina and occasional tenting of the diseased retina at the site of a localized vitreoretinal adhesion. Lattice degeneration of the retina can be most easily recognized by the linear, circumferential accumulations of glial and pigmented tissue, particularly in the superotemporal and inferotemporal quadrants anterior to the equator. Opacified, sheathed, and occluded vessels can be seen in the area of hyperpigmentation; plaques of glial tissue, an atrophied and irregular retina, and retinal breaks can also be noted. The retinal breaks are usually in the form of small round holes located at the posterior and distal extent of the lattice degeneration plaques.

"Paving stone" degenerations of the retina are seen as atrophic retinal areas through which the sclera can be seen prominently; occurring along the equatorial and preequatorial regions, these degenerations look much like blocks of pavement stones. Retinal breaks are not as common as those occurring with pigmentary and lattice degenerations, but the defective areas must be examined carefully.

Ancillary diagnostic examinations. Indirect ophthalmoscopy and careful biomicroscopic evaluation with the Goldmann three-mirror contact lens or a similar lens are indispensable for the careful evaluation of these zones of peripheral retinal degeneration. Retinal breaks are extremely small and occasionally can be located only with the high magnification afforded by slit-lamp and contact lens evaluation.

Indications for photocoagulation. If the fellow eye has experienced a retinal tear or retinal detachment caused by a break in an area of peripheral retinal degeneration, it is more probable that the eye under consideration should be treated prophylactically when a degenerative process exists peripherally. If retinal tears or holes are present, photocoagulation should be employed as soon as this condition is recognized. The presence of surrounding retinal detachment, however slight, usually militates against the use of photocoagulation; a scleral buckling retinal surgical procedure should then be considered.

As with retinal breaks, peripheral retinal degenerations too anterior to be seen easily with the three-mirror contact lens should be treated by a retinal surgical procedure, such as scleral or transconjunctival cryocautery. The anterior areas are more accessible with direct intervention and under these conditions should be treated by these methods.

The various indications mentioned under the section on retinal tears (p. 73) regarding the structure, location, and other factors concerning the eye should be taken into consideration, and treatment should be instituted if there is concern. Quiescent lattice degeneration without retinal breaks and paving stone degenerations usually need not be treated, but they should be checked carefully at 3- to 6-month intervals. However, any change or progress in the configuration of the peripheral retinal degeneration, surgical aphakia in that eye, a history of retinal detachment in the patient's other eye, or the onset of subjective symptoms experienced by the patient should make one consider the possibility of employing prophylactic laser photocoagulation.

Photocoagulation approach. Extreme care must be taken in photocoagulating peripheral retinal degenerations because the vitreous is closely approximated and usually adherent to the region of degeneration. Photocoagulation should not be placed closer than one disc diameter (DD) or approximately $1,500\mu$, to the border of an area of lattice, pigmentary, or paving stone degeneration. In this way the production of heat at the chorioretinal interspace will have less chance of shrinking the overlying vitreous and its attachment to the area of degeneration.

An anesthetic is employed topically, and the Goldmann three-mirror lens is used to reflect the laser beam into the periphery of the retina. The anterior aspects of the retinal degeneration are photocoagulated first, because this area may be more difficult to visualize and patient cooperation may be better during the early portion of the treatment session.

Coagulation sizes of approximately **500μ to 800μ** should be used in an interrupted, solitary, linear manner; an interval approximately half the diameter of a coagulation should be allowed between each coagulation spot (Fig. 6-6). Power intensities are usually in the range of **400 to 600 mw**, depending on the coagulation size and the degree of peripheral location of the defect (Fig. 6-7). More peripheral lesions usually require slightly higher

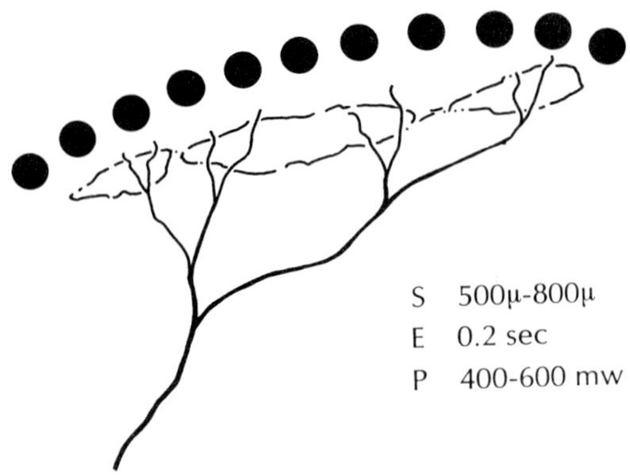

Fig. 6-6. Punctate, linear, interrupted Grade 3 coagulations of 500μ to 800μ, produced approximately 1,500μ distal to the peripheral border of the area of retinal degeneration.

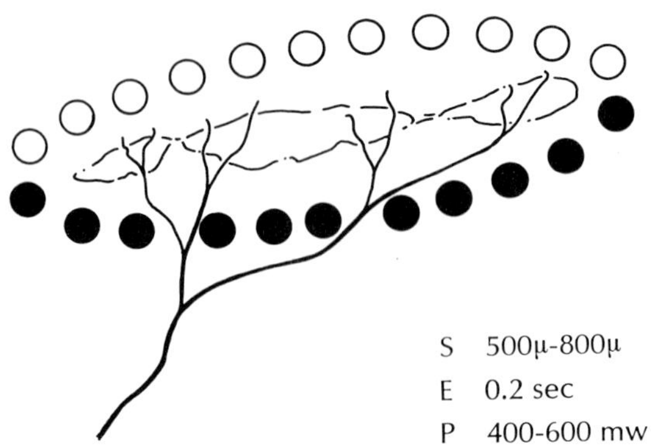

Fig. 6-7. Coagulations of the same intensity as those indicated in Fig. 6-6 are continued 1,500μ or more from the proximal border of the area of peripheral retinal degeneration. A single row of coagulations is usually effective, although a double linear row of interrupted impacts can be considered when degeneration is extensive.

powers because of optical aberrations present during the photocoagulation procedure. Coagulation exposure intervals are kept below **0.2 sec** because patients experience a slight amount of discomfort at longer exposure intervals (Figs. 6-8 and 6-9).

A double row of interrupted, linear photocoagulations can be applied around the initial barrage line, depending on the degree of vitreous traction considered to be present. If vitreous traction has caused retinal tenting in the area of lattice degeneration or in other sections of the eye, a secondary or tertiary row of coagulations should be strongly considered.

Complications. All of the complications described under the section on retinal tears (p. 77) can occur and can progress in a more rapid and devastating fashion.

Follow-up. The patient should be treated with cycloplegic and steroid drops and followed in a manner similar to that described for patients with retinal tears (p. 78). The eye should be examined with a contact lens to determine the nature of the vitreoretinal adhesion and the amount of vitreous traction present after photocoagulation as compared with the situation before photocoagulation. If the vitreoretinal traction on other retinal areas increases, transconjunctival cryocautery to these regions may be required to strengthen

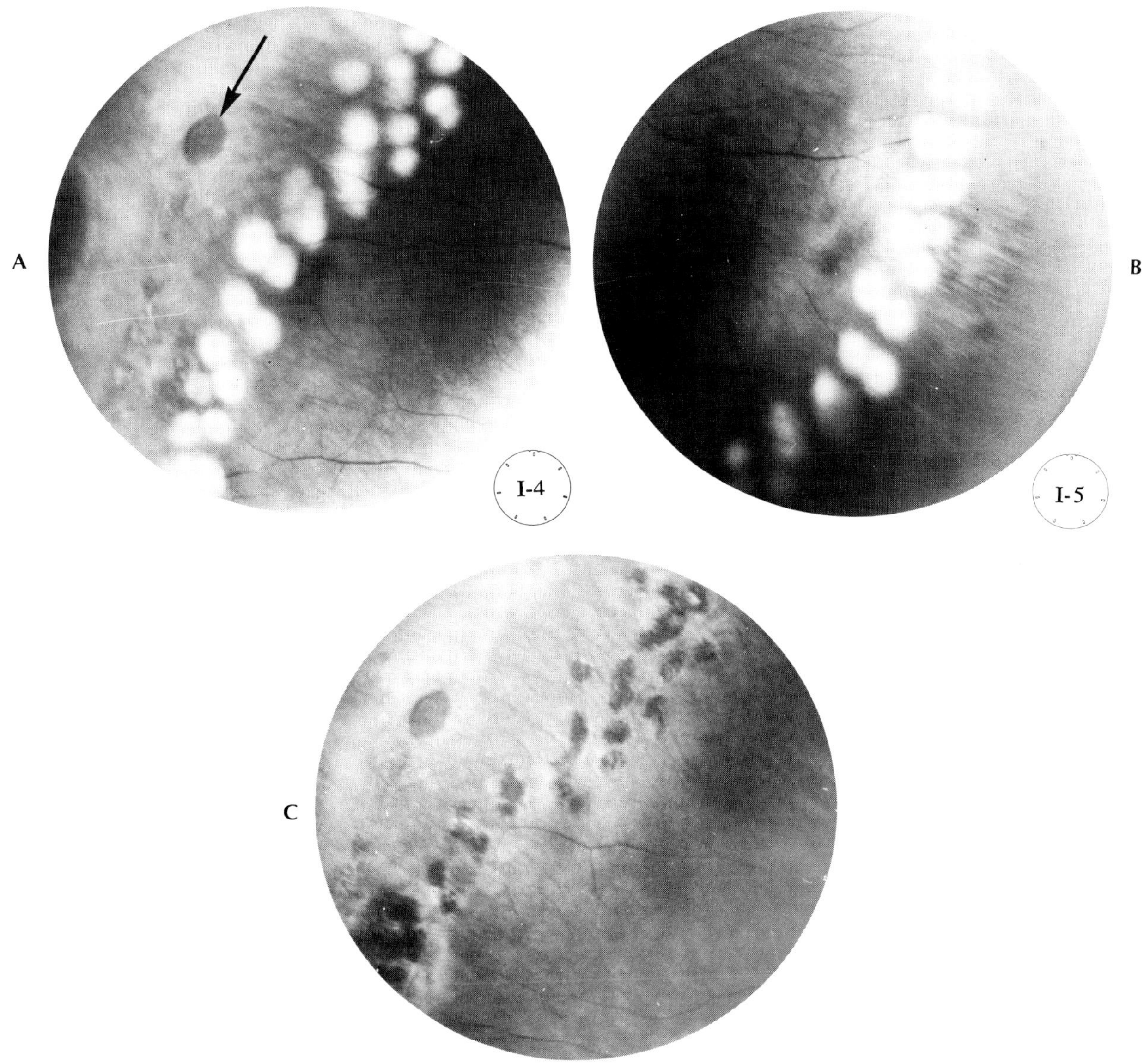

Fig. 6-8. A, Multiple areas of lattice degeneration and an open retinal hole (arrow) in the superonasal quadrant were found in a 27-year-old woman during routine examination. A double linear row of interrupted 500μ coagulations was placed around the area of retinal degeneration. **B,** A double row of interrupted coagulations was placed proximal to an area of mixed pigmentary and lattice degeneration in the inferotemporal quadrant of the same eye. **C,** The photocoagulation impact area (similar to that shown in **A**) proximal to the zone of lattice degeneration in the superonasal quadrant 2 months after treatment. Slight gliosis and pigment proliferation can be noted in the photocoagulated region.

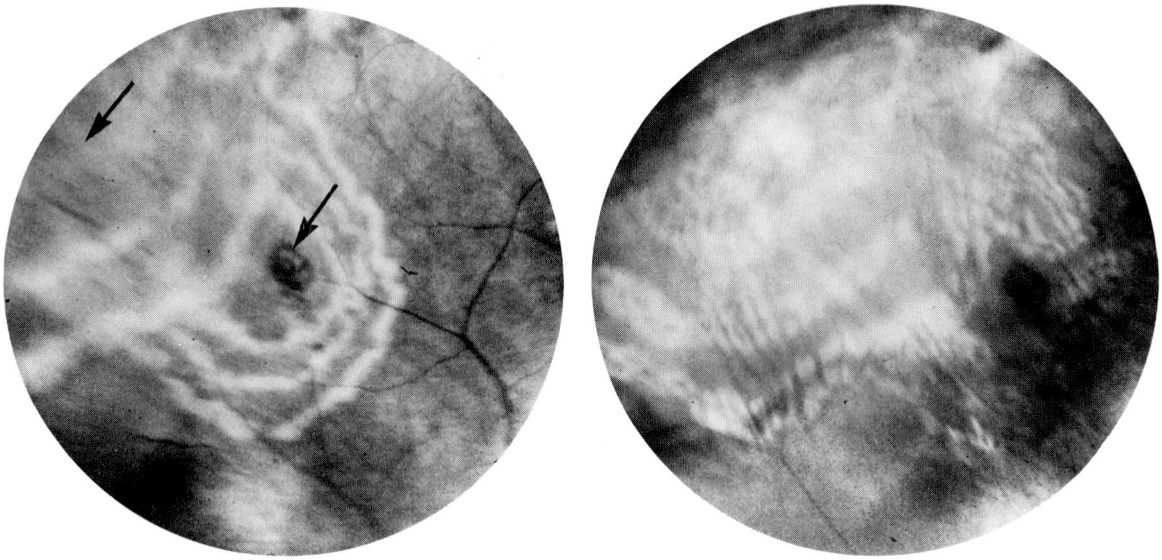

A B

Fig. 6-9. A, During routine examination a 57-year-old woman was found to have an extensive area of lattice degeneration (arrows) in the superotemporal quadrant of her right eye. A triple linear row of streaked 500μ coagulations was placed around the area of lattice and pigmentary degeneration. **B,** Healed appearance of the zone of lattice and pigmentary degeneration and barrier coagulations 9 weeks after photocoagulation. The streaks of chorioretinal adhesion produced an adequate barrier to seal off the disease process.

the chorioretinal adhesion. Localized scleral buckling procedures to the area of most marked vitreous traction may be advisable for patients with more severe disorders.

RETINAL DETACHMENTS

Clinical symptoms. Blurred vision, metamorphopsia, a veillike blurring in one field of vision, multiple lightning flashes, and a myriad of dots or spots may be observed by the patient with a retinal detachment.

Ophthalmoscopic appearance. A large bullous or shallow detachment of the retina may be seen occupying a quadrant or larger zone. Retinal breaks of the horseshoe tear, round, or oval variety can be detected in most cases of rhegmatogenous detachments. The choroid can usually be visualized behind the detached retina, although this view may be obscured. Moderate amounts of glial proliferation on the surface of the retina and microcystic changes in the periphery of the retina can be seen, and the presence of pigment proliferation and vitreous hemorrhage may be noted.

Ancillary diagnostic examinations. Thorough evaluation by indirect ophthalmoscopy and precorneal or contact lens biomicroscopy should be done. The existence of retinal tears, pigment and glial accumulations, retinal atrophy, and demarcation lines are important factors affecting the decision to treat this abnormality by photocoagulation.

Perimetry will reveal a relative scotoma in the area of the retinal detachment. This relative scotoma will differentiate the lesion from retinoschisis, with which an absolute scotoma can be demonstrated.

Fluorescein angiography will offer little assistance in the differential diagnosis unless an exudative process, such as Harada's disease, or a pooling and staining condition consistent with a malignant melanoma, metastatic carcinoma, or choroidal hemangioma is to be ruled out as the underlying cause.

Indications for photocoagulation. A small, peripheral retinal detachment can be treated by photocoagulation in which a barrier is produced around the area of retinal elevation to limit the extent and further dissection of the process. This procedure can be done as the primary one if the individual cannot undergo more definitive treatment, such as cryopexy, retinopexy, or one of the scleral buckling operations. Surgery to release the vitreous traction and seal the retinal hole or tear permanently should be considered before photocoagulation is employed.

If retinal detachment surgery cannot be performed because of systemic contraindications, photocoagulation can be employed if the retinal detachment has not extended beyond the equator posteriorly and involves less than a quadrant of the retina. A barrier around the retinal detachment to limit its spread should not be created if there is extensive vitreoretinal traction in the area of detachment or in any other region of the eye. Photocoagulation intervention for retinal detachments is usually considered only in patients with retinal elevations that are less than quadrantic, that do not extend posterior to the equatorial region, and that demonstrate only limited vitreous contraction.

Occasionally, an area of old, atrophic, and degenerated detached retina, usually with an existing demarcation line, can be reinforced by an encircling barrier of photocoagulation, even though it extends posterior to the equatorial region. In these instances the purpose of photocoagulation is to prevent a degenerated portion of the retina from detaching further, although this possibility is lessened by the long-standing nature of the retinal detachment.

Photocoagulation approach. A three-mirror Goldmann lens is most useful for the placement of barrier coagulations, particularly in the most anterior aspects of the retinal detachment. A retrobulbar injection may be needed to decrease discomfort but has not been found to be necessary in the majority of cases.

The rows of photocoagulations must approach the ora serrata closely on both lateral extents, as well as surround the entire retinal detachment posteriorly. Photocoagulations of **200μ to 500μ** at **0.05- to 0.1-sec** exposures and **250- to 450-mw** power intensities are placed in a linear, contiguous manner around the existing retinal detachment in such a way as to be located in an area of attached retina (Fig. 6-10). The coagulations should not be more intense than hazy mucoid (Grade 2), so that they affect only the chorioretinal junction and minimize the total energy transmitted through the unstable vitreous. The coagulation sizes should be smaller as they approach the posterior pole (200μ) and can be larger (500μ) more anteriorly. These coagulations can be painted linearly rather than being punctate in nature, although the latter technique appears to produce a more stable and consistent coagulum (Fig. 6-11).

A second row of coagulations can be placed outside the previous contiguous row of coagulations so that a double line of barrier coagulations will result. It may not be possible to produce this double row of coagulations in the most anterior aspects of the retinal detachment because of a lack of proper visualization. In several cases transconjunctival cryocoagulation of the most anterior portions of the retinal detachment has been required to be certain that the entire retinal detachment extending to the ora serrata is surrounded by a coagulum (Figs. 6-12 to 6-15).

Care must be taken not to coagulate the area of retinal detachment or the zones of retinal holes or tears. The vitreous should be evaluated carefully so that the photocoagulation beam is not directed, if possible, through the region of vitreous attachment to the

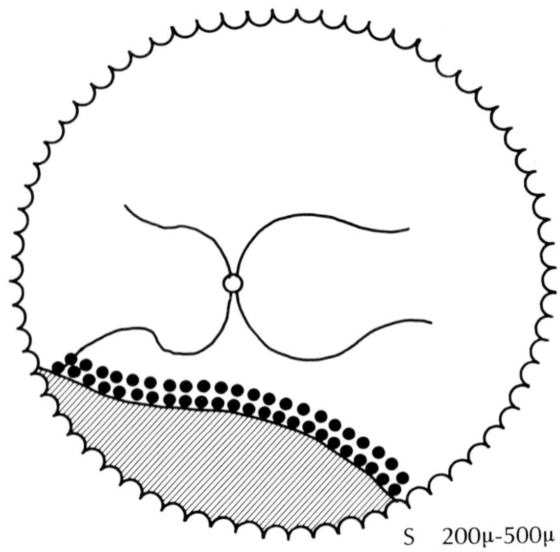

Fig. 6-10. A double linear row of punctate, interrupted 200μ to 500μ coagulations placed along the proximal border of an inferior retinal detachment and extending to the posterior ora serrata region along both lateral extents of the retinal detachment.

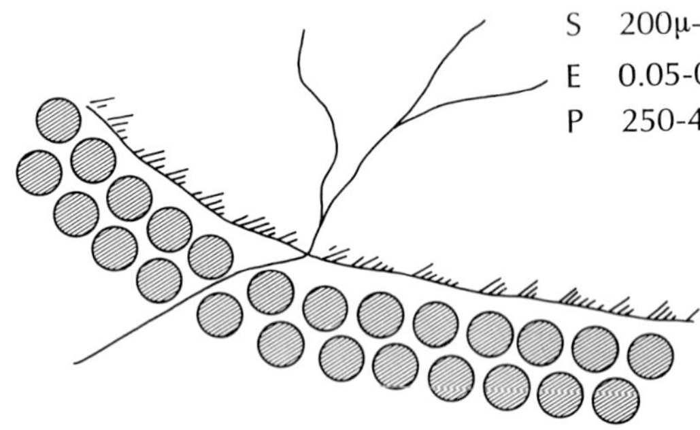

Fig. 6-11. Enlarged view of the typical positioning of interrupted, punctate coagulations in the zone of attached retina posterior to the border of a superior retinal detachment.

operculum. In this instance heat could be generated in the vitreoretinal attachment area, resulting in further contraction of the vitreous body and separation of the retina.

Complications. The retinal tear can be increased in dimensions because of an increase in vitreoretinal traction following photocoagulation. This complication usually occurs because of inadvertent heating of the vitreous strands leading to the region of the retinal tears. A great effort must be made to avoid these areas of retinal disease.

The retinal detachment itself can extend because of a small amount of heating of the vitreous or a breakdown of the areas of attachment near the retinal detachment site. This situation is not common if power densities appropriate for producing a mucoid coagulation (Grade 2) are not exceeded.

Occasional hemorrhage from the retinal vessels or the production of macular striae have been observed, although rarely. This complication can be obviated by reducing the

A B C

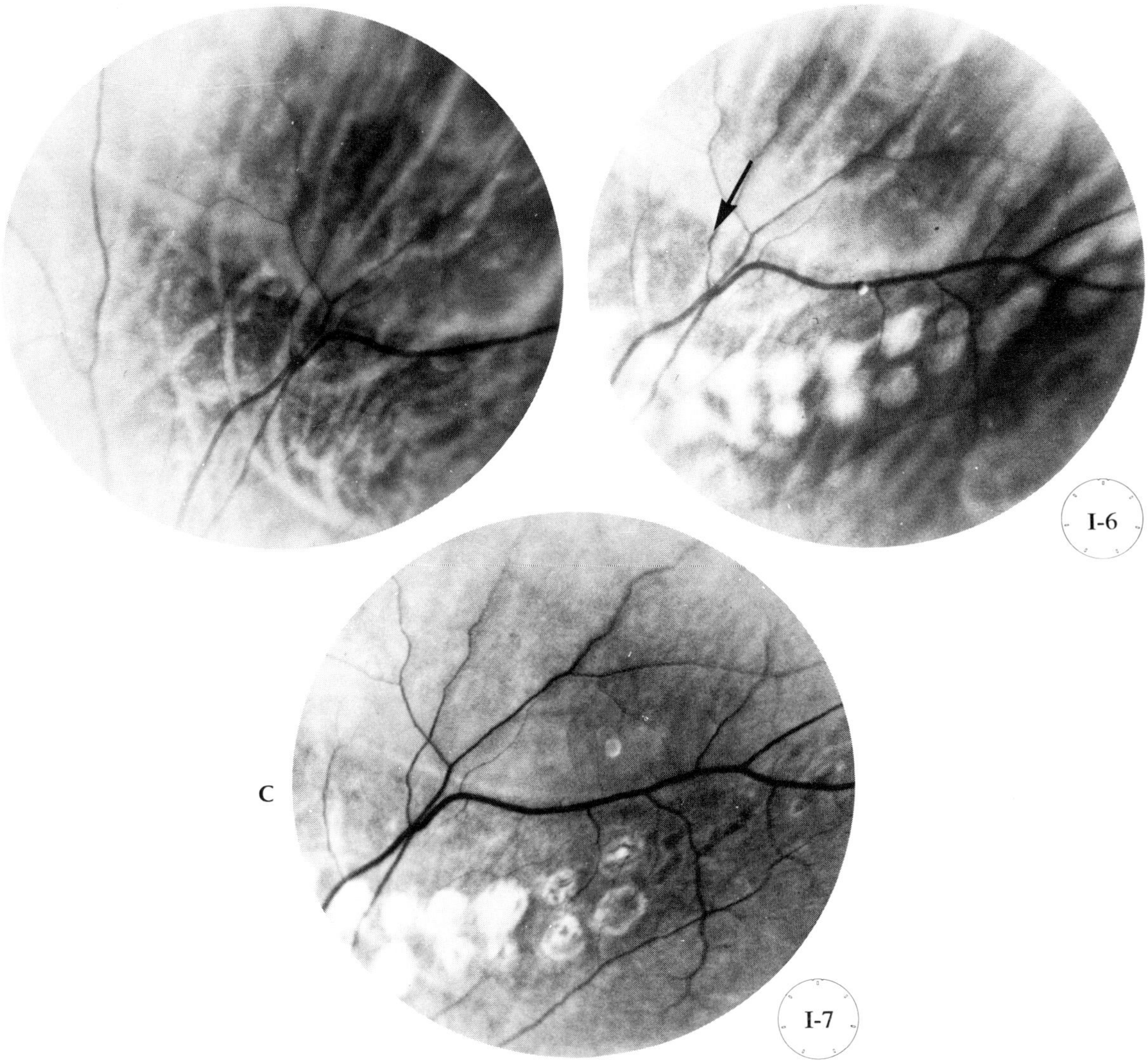

Fig. 6-12. A, An 87-year-old woman complained of photopsia and multiple vitreous floaters and was found to have an area of degenerated and atrophic detached retina in the superotemporal quadrant of her left eye. She refused retinal surgery but permitted argon laser photocoagulation. **B,** A double linear row of punctate, interrupted 500μ coagulations was placed posterior to the border of the retinal detachment (arrow) and extended to the ora serrata region. **C,** The photocoagulation barrier 2 months after treatment, showing hyperproliferation of the pigment epithelium, as well as areas of chorioretinal atrophy in the region of the laser impacts. All coagulations were produced in areas of attached retina posterior to the border of the retinal detachment.

A 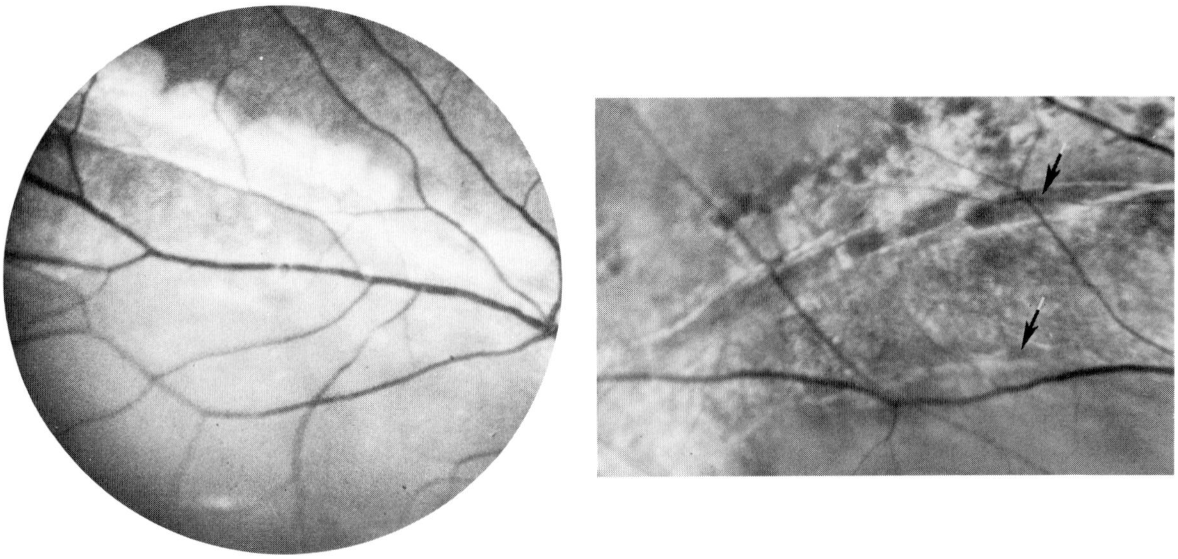 B

Fig. 6-13. A, A single linear row of punctate 500μ coagulations was placed posterior to a demarcation line, walling off an inferior retinal detachment. **B,** Magnified view (2 months after photocoagulation) of the glial and pigment proliferation produced at the photocoagulation sites posterior to the two demarcation lines (arrows), forming a reinforced barrier to the inferior retinal detachment.

A 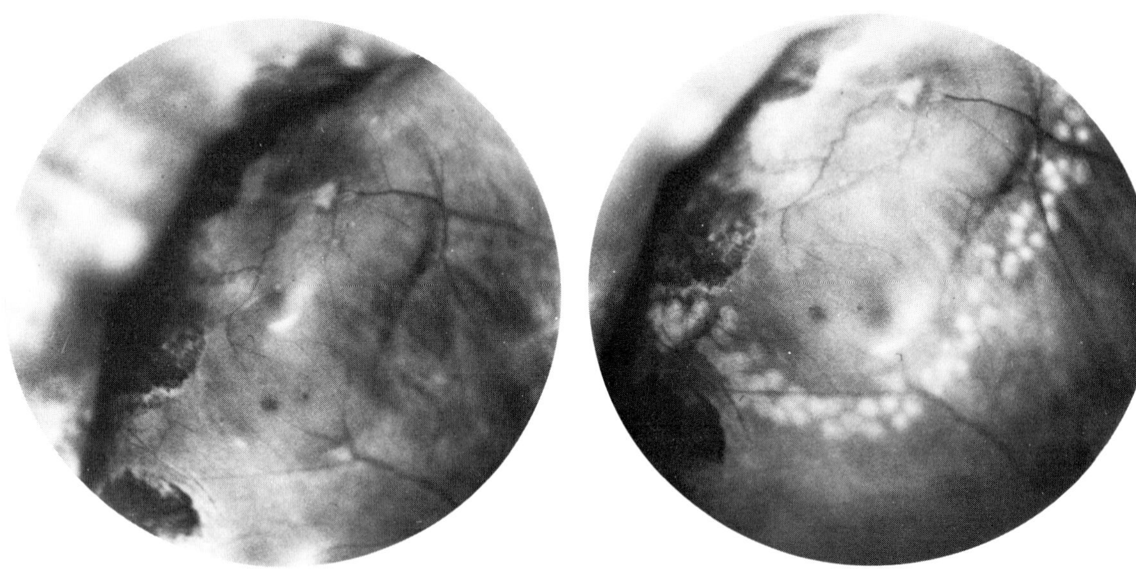 B

Fig. 6-14. A, A small retinal detachment in the periphery of a 41-year-old man who had previously undergone retinal detachment surgery. **B,** A double, and sometimes triple, linear row of punctate, interrupted 500μ coagulations was placed around the small retinal detachment bullae. The condition healed without incident and without extension of the retinal detachment.

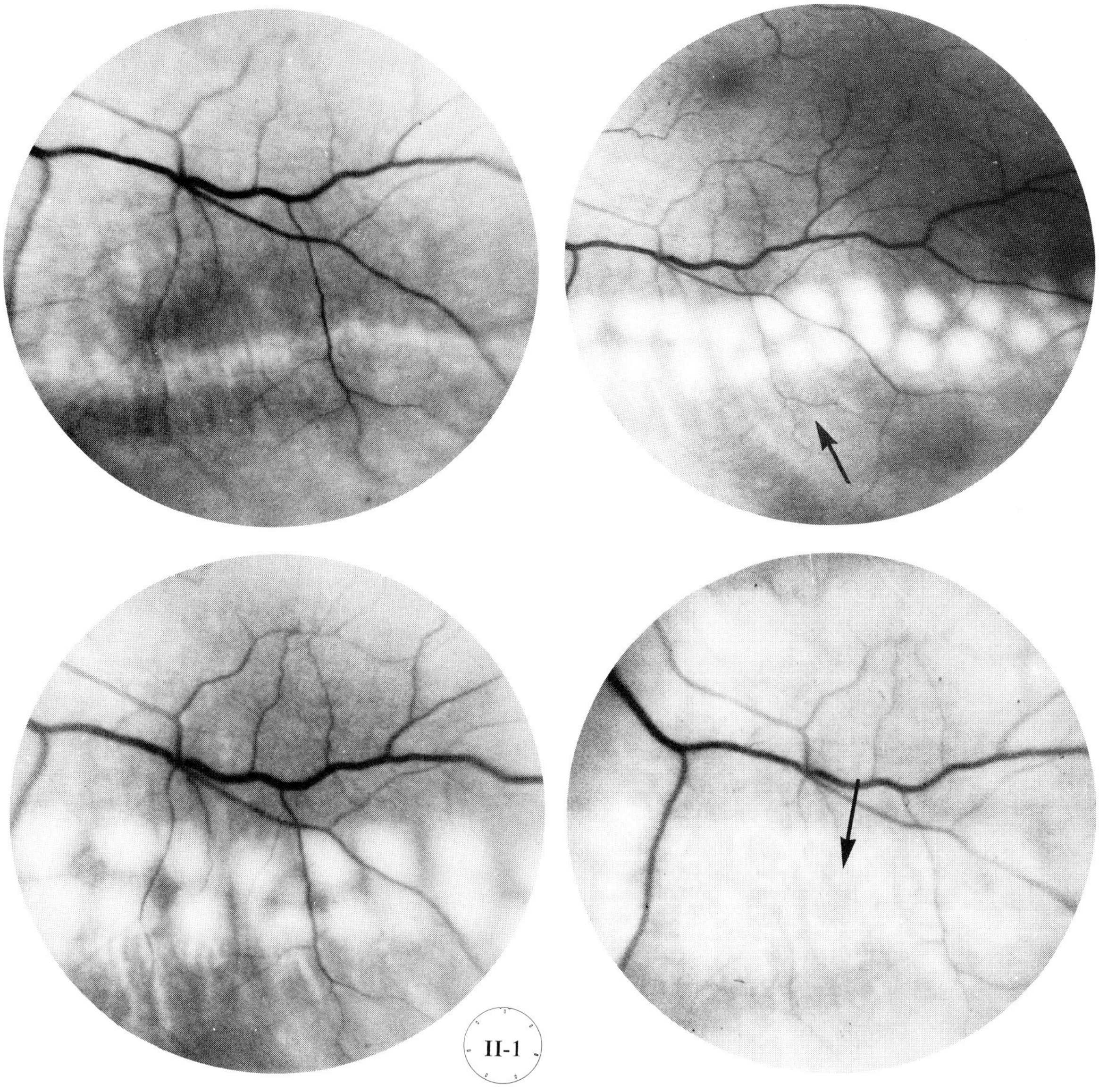

Fig. 6-15. A, During routine examination an inferior retinal detachment was found in the left eye of a 65-year-old woman who had lost the vision in her right eye from a previous retinal detachment. The retinal detachment was atrophic and gliotic. She refused surgical intervention. **B,** Wide-angle view of the 500μ coagulations in a double linear row posterior to the posterior border of the inferior retinal detachment (arrow). **C.** Magnified view of the coagulations, showing the punctate and interrupted nature of the Grade 2 to 3 coagulation intensities. **D,** Healed appearance of the argon laser photocoagulation barrier (arrow) produced between the atrophic retinal detachment and the posterior polar region.

power density in the region of the retinal vessels and particularly in any areas near the temporal vascular arcade or paramacular area.

Follow-up. At the time of photocoagulation the patient should be given cycloplegics and steroids topically to decrease possible anterior segment inflammation and discomfort.

The patient should be seen within 1 week of photocoagulation to assess the nature of the coagulations. If the retina appears to be well surrounded by adequate photocoagulations and there have been no complications or extension of the retinal tears or detachment, the cycloplegic-steroid combination is continued for a total of 2 weeks. The patient should return 2 weeks after the initial posttreatment visit for monitoring of the pigment epithelial and chorioretinal adhesive reaction. Evaluations at 4-week intervals for 2 months are recommended, and rephotocoagulation is considered if a moderate pigment and glial response is not seen at the photocoagulation sites. Care must be taken to uncover any increase in vitreoretinal traction during a period of 6 months to 1 year following photocoagulation so that more definitive retinal surgery can be considered.

RETINOSCHISIS

Clinical symptoms. The individual with retinoschisis may have no complaints. Some patients have noticed a decrease in the peripheral visual field, but this symptom is not common. Lightning flashes, floaters, and photopsia occasionally have been observed by the patient. If the retinoschisis is combined with a retinal detachment, the clinical symptoms described in the section on retinal detachments (p. 82) become apparent.

Ophthalmoscopic appearance. Senile retinoschisis is usually first seen in the lower temporal periphery of the retina and may, over a period of months or years, slowly dissect posteriorly. During this time the other quadrants of the retina become involved at their anterior aspects. The microcystic changes commonly seen in the peripheral retina become confluent, and the retinoschisis may appear as a large area of thin, bullously displaced retina with the inner retinal layer containing the retinal blood vessels and the outer retinal layer consisting of the receptor elements and outer nuclear cells. Multiple accumulations of saltlike spots and projections extend into the retinoschisis cavity and can be seen by careful observation with any of the diagnostic instruments. The visualization of the inner and outer retinal layers should be accomplished for absolute verification of retinoschisis.

Ancillary diagnostic examinations. Careful evaluation by indirect ophthalmoscopy, contact lens biomicroscopy, and perimetry should be done. Perimetry will show an absolute field defect in the region of the retinoschisis, caused by interruption of the nerve fibers and impulses from the receptor layer to the inner retina. Fluorescein angiography is not particularly useful for this condition.

A trial photocoagulation in the area with the suspected disorder will show a coagulum in the outer retinal layers produced by the heat generated in the juxtaposed pigment epithelium. Such a coagulum would not be produced if the entire sensory retina were detached and elevated away from the pigment epithelial surface. This test usually serves to differentiate a retinal detachment from retinoschisis.

Indications for photocoagulation. If very peripheral retinoschisis can be shown to be progressing and extending toward the posterior pole by visual field or ophthalmoscopic examination, photocoagulation can be considered in an attempt to stabilize the disease.

If the retinoschisis is first observed within 2 DD of the macular region, photocoagulation to prevent further posterior spread of the diseased area should be considered immediately.

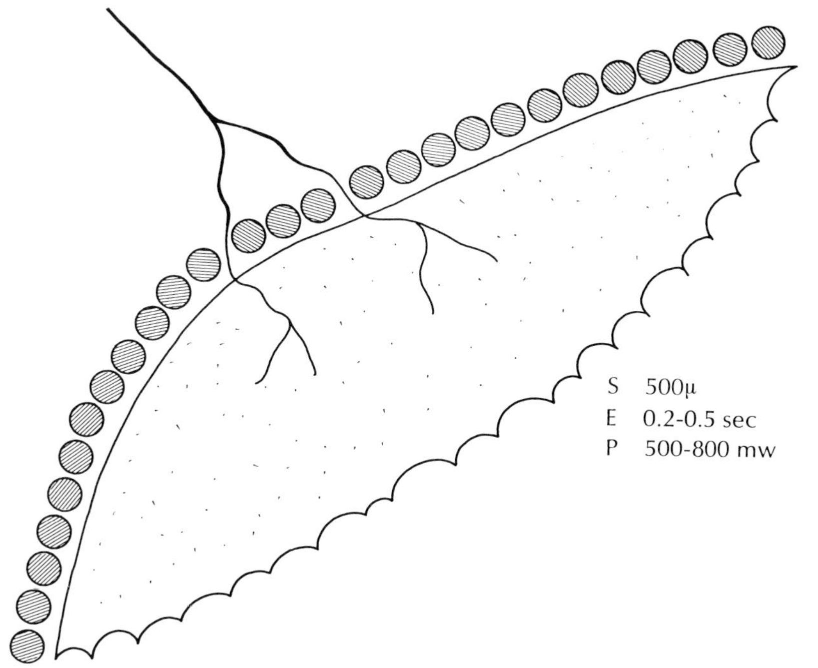

Fig. 6-16. *Barrier* photocoagulation technique with 500μ punctate, interrupted, linear coagulations in normal retina approximately 1 DD posterior to the edge of an inferotemporal retinoschisis area. The barrier extends as far anterior as possible along the lateral extent of the retinoschisis bleb.

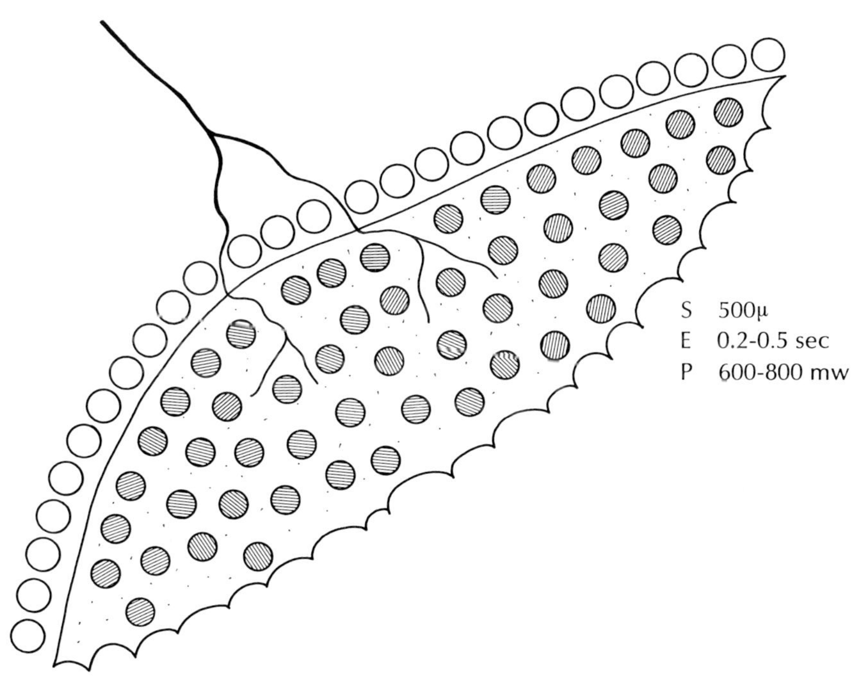

Fig. 6-17. *Barrage* photocoagulation technique (employing the barrier approach initially) barraging the retinoschisis bleb with solitary 500μ Grade 3 coagulations. This combined technique tends to collapse the retinoschisis cavity.

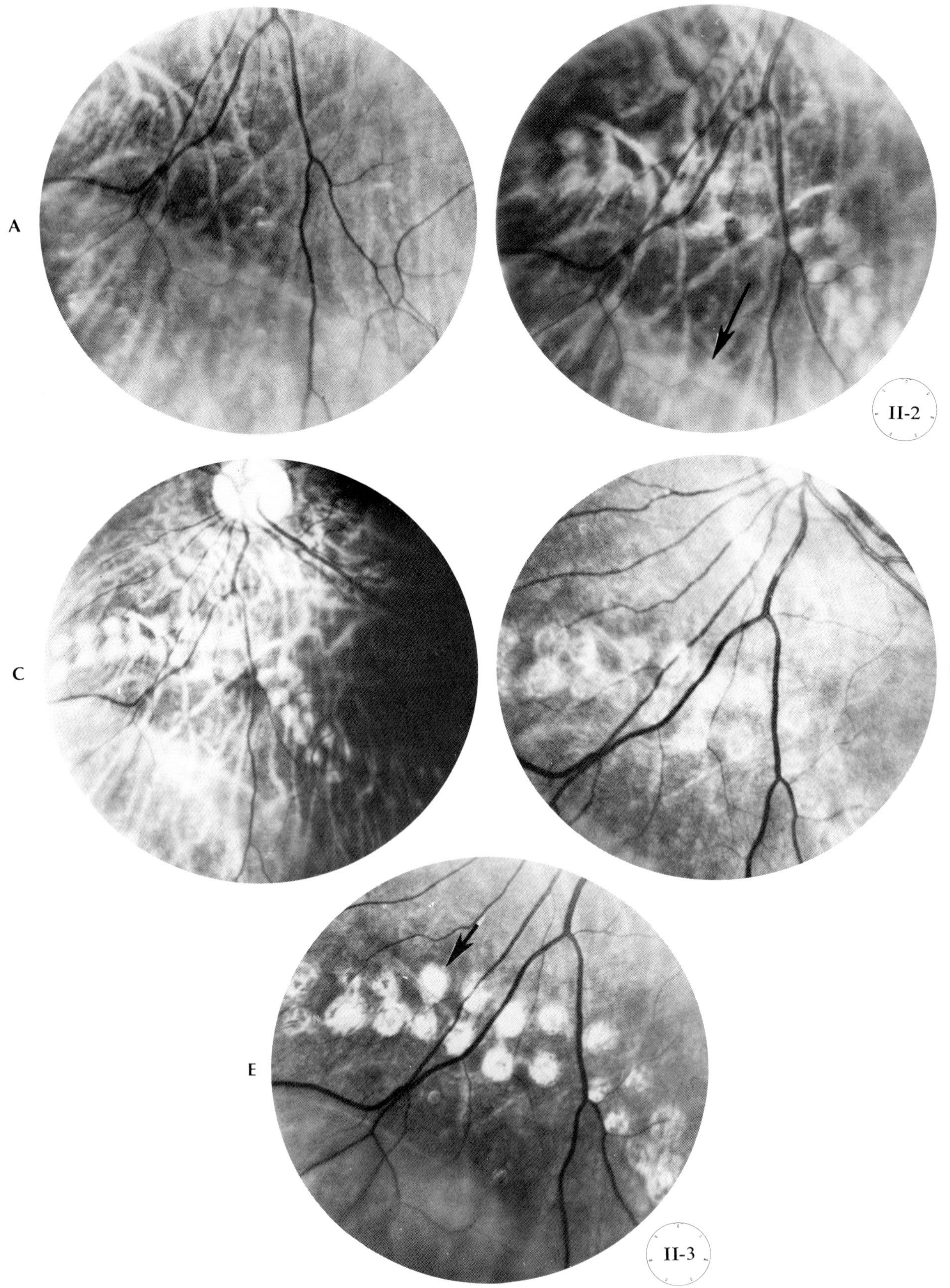

Fig. 6-18. For legend see opposite page.

If considerable traction exists on the area with retinoschisis or if the bulla is markedly elevated, a scleral buckling procedure in addition to photocoagulation therapy is advisable.

If the retinoschisis has not been shown to be progressive and has not changed, the condition should be evaluated carefully by photography and perimetry at 3-month intervals without photocoagulation intervention.

Photocoagulation approach. A three-mirror Goldmann contact lens, Jungner contact lens, or diagonal low-vacuum contact lens is used with the patient under topical anesthesia only.

A *barrier* posterior to the retinoschisis junction with the normal retina can be produced to limit its posterior dissection in a manner similar to that described in the section on retinal detachments (p. 83). However, the photocoagulations should be larger, encompassing a minimum diameter of **500μ** and retaining a sufficient power density to produce a mucoid to moderately white coagulum (Grade 3). This procedure usually entails exposures of **0.2 to 0.5 sec** and power ranges in the vicinity of **500 to 800 mw.** The barrier coagulations must be placed at least 1 DD posterior to the retinoschisis cavity margin into normal retina to delimit and contain the disease process properly (Fig. 6-16).

A

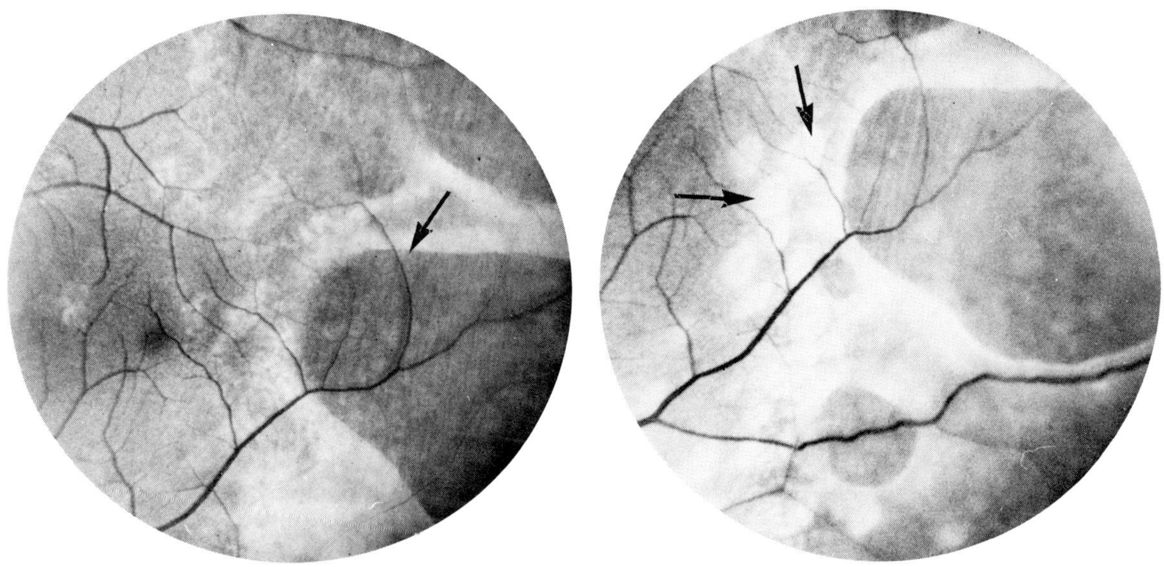

B

Fig. 6-19. A, A 19-year-old man with juvenile retinoschisis and marked retinal cystic areas (arrow) surrounded by regions of glial proliferation. **B,** Barrier-type, 500μ coagulations were placed around the extent of the posterior retinoschisis bullae (arrows).

Fig. 6-18. A, A 32-year-old woman was found to have asymptomatic retinoschisis in the inferior portion of the retinas of both eyes. **B,** A double linear row of interrupted, 500μ punctate barrier coagulations was produced approximately 1 DD from the posterior edge of the retinoschisis bulla (arrow). The coagulations were extended to the preequatorial region. **C,** Wide-angle view showing the extent of inferior retinoschisis into the posterior polar region. **D,** Appearance of the photocoagulated area 6 weeks after treatment; early pigment proliferation has occurred in the center of the impact area. **E,** Photocoagulation sites (arrow) 10 weeks after treatment; chorioretinal atrophy and hypertrophy of the pigment layer are more pronounced.

If the retinoschisis cavity is more extensive and if a moderate amount of vitreous traction exists, the retinoschisis bleb can be photocoagulated directly with a *barrage* pattern (Fig. 6-17). Coagulations of **500μ** can be produced with sufficient intensity to cause the outer retinal layer to be denatured to an off-white appearance (Grade 3). This barrage technique is used in conjunction with the barrier technique described previously; the barrier photocoagulations are created before the barrage method is utilized. Adequate barrage coagulations creating an off-white dense coagulum usually require **0.2- to 0.5-sec** exposures at power intensities of **600 to 800 mw** (Figs. 6-18 and 6-19).

If the vitreous traction on the area of retinoschisis is extensive, the area can be buckled with a solitary explant or an encircling silicone band. Cryocautery can be employed at the time of surgery, and supplemental photocoagulation can be used during the postoperative period if the coagulation produced by the cryosurgery is not adequate. In these cases **500μ to 1,000μ** coagulations are used along the scleral buckling at exposure of **0.2 to 0.5 sec** with sufficient intensities (usually **600 to 1,000 mw**) to produce a distinct off-white coagulum (Grade 3).

Complications. Complications are similar to those outlined under the section on retinal detachment (p. 84). In addition, retinal tears can be produced by extensive and excessive photocoagulation, and these tears can lead to the development of a retinal detachment. The patient should be closely watched during the postoperative period for the development of a retinal detachment, and appropriate surgical measures should be taken if one occurs.

In some individuals photocoagulation can cause an excessive exudative response resulting in elevation of the retina or an increase in the size of the retinoschisis cavity. Steroids given systemically may be indicated if the exudative response is excessive or prolonged.

Follow-up. The patient should be followed in the manner outlined under the section on retinal detachment (p. 88) to determine whether an increase in vitreous traction or exudation has occurred. If the retinoschisis cavity has not collapsed during a 1- to 2-month period following the barrier or the barrier-barrage technical approach, further photocoagulation can be considered. The amount of pigment epithelial hypertrophy and glial proliferation following photocoagulation should also be monitored to ensure that an adequate scarring response has been produced and that the retinoschisis process has been stabilized.

Chapter 7

Peripheral retinal vascular abnormalities

EALES' DISEASE

Clinical symptoms. Blurred vision may occur gradually or suddenly, depending on the degree of hemorrhage into the preretinal space or vitreous cavity from the abnormal vasculature. Metamorphopsia, floaters, reduction in peripheral vision, and photopsia may be observed by the patient during various stages of the disease.

Ophthalmoscopic appearance. The earliest stages of Eales' disease are manifested by dilated arteriovenous vessels and shunt capillaries, which make their appearance in the periphery and move posteriorly, leaving behind a vessel-free periphery. The most peripheral portions of these capillaries become occluded by an embolic, thrombotic, or endarteritic process, which leads to hypoxia; the hypoxia, in turn stimulates the proliferation of new vessels. There may be beading of the involved vessels, as well as saccular aneurysms and venous swelling. Feeder vessels, similar to those found in von Hippel's angiomatosis, can be observed entering an area of dilated and arcuate vessels that are commonly associated with the aneurysms in Eales' disease. Multiple hemorrhages, as well as evidence of periphlebitis, sheathing of vessels, and new vessel formation, can be seen in the retina, choroid, and vitreous cavity.

Ancillary diagnostic examinations. Fluorescein angiography is extremely useful for the documentation of telangiectatic, saccular, and arcuate vessels, particularly in the posterior retinal region. Fluorescein leakage from the areas of active vascular change may be considerable. Feeder vessels into the area of dilated and saccular vessels can usually be located accurately for photocoagulation purposes. Stereo fluorescein angiography can be valuable for the evaluation of the depth and extent of the vascular process. Wide-angle fluorescein angiography can also be employed as a screening procedure to detect changes in larger areas of the fundus during the fluorescein transit. Attention can then be directed to those zones of new leakage or new regrowth of neovascular tissue.

Stereo color photography is of considerable assistance in following the course of the disease. Serial wide-angle photography (45°), especially stereoscopic photography, can document any subtle changes in the retinal vasculature and help indicate areas for possible treatment by photocoagulation.

Indications for photocoagulation. When the diagnosis of Eales' disease is suggested, either by the character of the vessels or by the occurrence of retinal and vitreous hemorrhages, photocoagulation should be considered. If new vessel formation exists or if arteriolovenous shunting complexes can be isolated, photocoagulation should be directed toward these abnormal areas.

If the neovascularization has widely proliferated throughout the posterior pole or has extended to a great degree into the vitreous body, photocoagulation probably would not be beneficial and may be contraindicated. Therefore, most photocoagulation attempts should be limited to those cases of Eales' disease that are early or only moderately advanced.

Photocoagulation approach. With the patient under topical anesthesia, the central portion of the Goldmann three-mirror contact lens, the Goldmann posterior fundus contact lens, the Jungner contact lens, or the plano–low-vacuum contact lens can be used for adequate photocoagulation in most circumstances.

All aneurysms and newly formed vessels should be treated at the time of photocoagulation. These abnormal vessels are usually located at the periphery of the sheet or cluster of vessels near the avascular or infarcted zone. Circumferential, sometimes telangiectatic vessels are commonly located at the border of the avascular retinal area, separating the patent vasculature from the midperiphery. Many of these vessels will be seen much more clearly at the time of photocoagulation because of the brightness of the visualization beam and the contrast created by the background coagulation. As with the feeding vessels in cases of von Hippel's angiomatosis, one should avoid treating markedly dilated, arcuate vessels associated with the aneurysms in Eales' disease, since the effect tends to be transitory and may be dangerous because of necrosis and rupture of these high-flow channels. Following treatment of the aneurysms and neovascularization, the caliber of these feeder vessels gradually returns to a more normal state. The treatment should be limited to one quadrant of the retina at a time, and an interval of 2 weeks should be allowed between quadrant treatments.

The aiming beam spot size diameter should be approximately twice the size of the involved vessel, and the coagulum produced should be slightly whiter (Grade 3) than mucoid. An average coagulation requires the use of **300μ** spot sizes with power levels between **200 to 350 mw** at **0.2 to 0.5 sec** (Fig. 7-1).

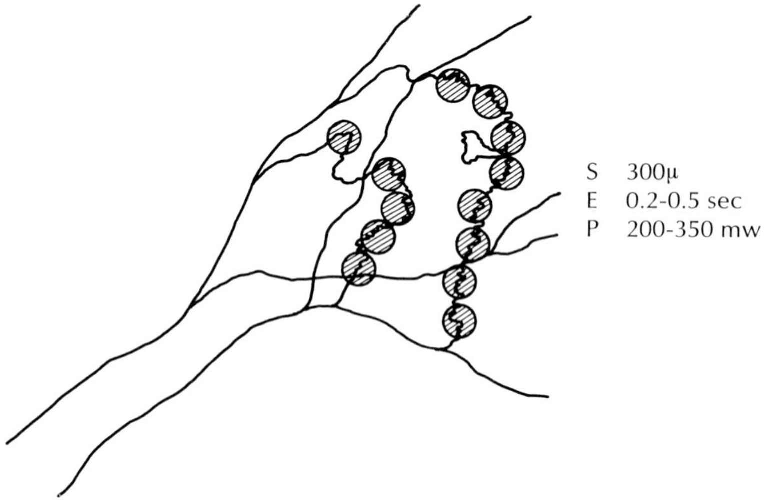

Fig. 7-1. Application of random, interrupted, or contiguous 300μ punctate coagulations in the area of the telangiectatic or saccular abnormal vessels.

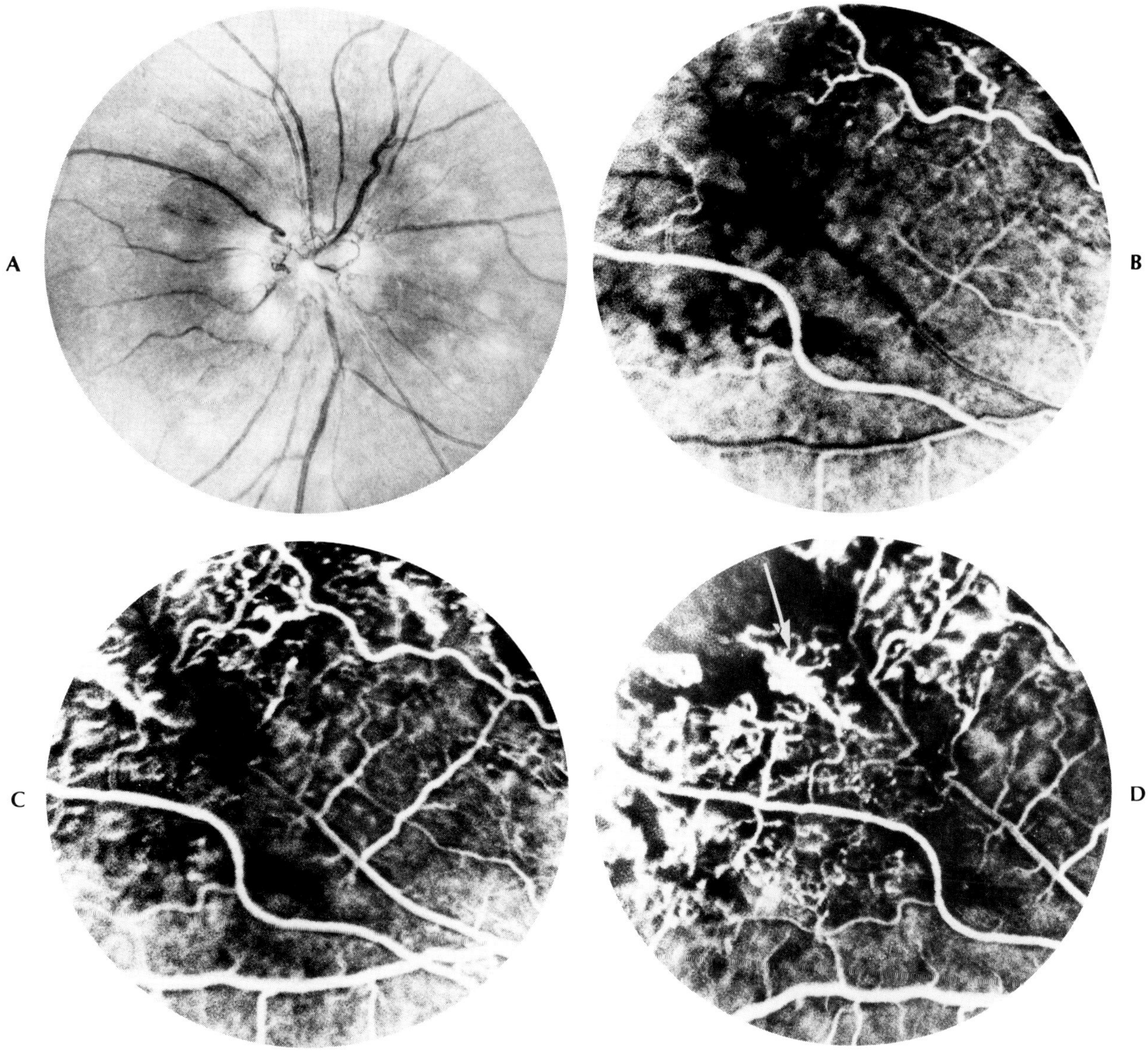

Fig. 7-2. A, Slightly dilated and tortuous retinal vein and a small patch of neovascularization over the disc of a 48-year-old woman with a 1-year history of perivasculitis and mild papilledema. Her condition progressed until obliteration of vessels in the midperiphery and neovascularization of the border of the nonperfusion zone were noted. Neovascularization later developed on the optic disc. **B,** Fluorogram of the zone of neovascularization during the very early laminar flow stage of transit. **C,** Arteriolovenous stage of the fluorescein angiographic transit, showing the peripheral area of nonperfusion and increased staining of the vessels at the junction of the vascularized and obliterated blood vessels. **D,** Fluorogram 3 sec later, showing early dye leakage from the neovascularization (arrow).

Continued.

E F G H

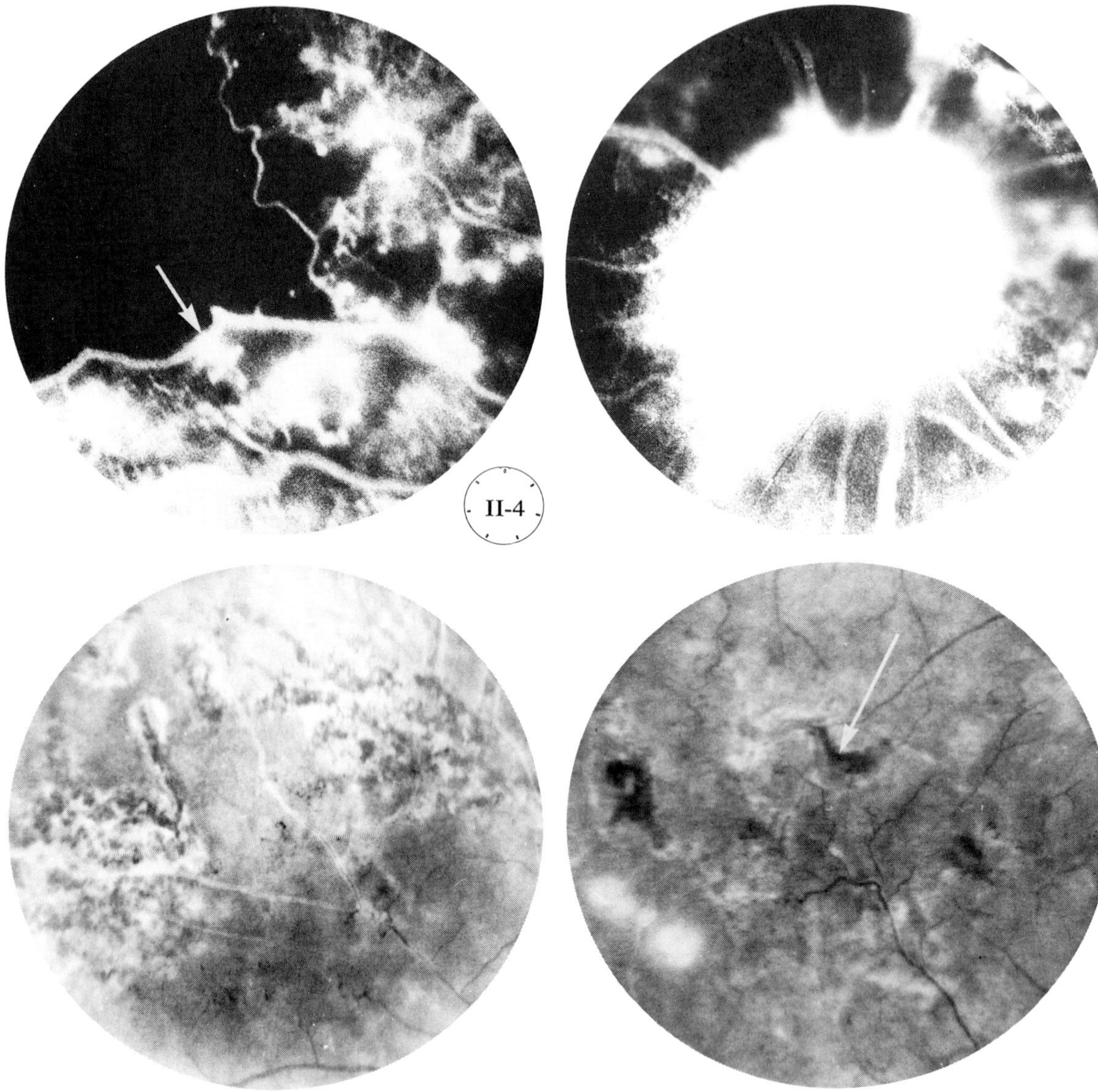

Fig. 7-2, cont'd. E, Fluorogram demonstrating heavy leakage of fluorescein in the retina from the neovascularization approximately 23 sec later. Note the sharp border of the area of perfused and nonperfused retina (arrow). **F,** Venular phase of the fluorescein angiographic transit, showing profuse leakage of dye from disc neovascularization. **G,** Areas of argon laser photocoagulation 2 months after treatment, showing areas of pigmentation at the site of obliterated neovascularization at the border of perfused and nonperfused retina. **H,** Hyperpigmentation and gliosis in the areas of treatment 2 months after argon laser photocoagulation (arrow). (Courtesy Arnall Patz, M.D.)

Coagulations can be interrupted and contiguous, or they can be placed in a continuous or streaked fashion directly on the vascular lesions. A "soft" coagulation should be produced; the coagulation energy is applied gently, with slightly longer exposure times and lower energy (Fig. 7-2).

All abnormal vessels in the quadrant, including those near the peripapillary area, should be treated. After 2 weeks, further photocoagulation can be directed toward another quadrant to destroy completely the neovascular elements in that area.

Complications. The most serious complication is massive vitreous or preretinal hemorrhage from the treated vessel area. The production of soft or gentle coagulations by the use of longer exposures will usually prevent this type of complication.

A late complication of loss of vision due to traction and exudate formation in the macula can occur. Again, the soft coagulations, particularly in the region of the paramacular zone or the temporal vascular arcades, should be minimal and not intense.

Follow-up. One must examine the fundus in patients with Eales' disease as meticulously as one does in patients with other telangiectatic and exudative retinal abnormalities, since the tendency for rapid development of further vascular changes, with attendant new vessel formation and hemorrhage, is marked in Eales' disease. The patient should be seen approximately 1 week following photocoagulation and then observed at intervals of 2 to 3 months following successful obliteration of the abnormal vessels throughout the fundus.

If a large vitreous hemorrhage does occur and the blood in the vitreous body does not clear over a 6-month period, vitrectomy should be considered. Photocoagulation can then be attempted following vitrectomy, to stabilize the vascular process.

LEBER'S MILIARY ANEURYSMS

Clinical symptoms. The patient may experience a sudden decrease in vision as a result of a vitreous hemorrhage, or the presence of macular and perimacular exudation may cause a slow decrease in vision, onset of metamorphopsia, micropsia, or scotomas.

Ophthalmoscopic appearance. The abnormality is generally localized to one area of the fundus and consists of numerous sacculations and fusiform swellings of the terminal arteriolar tree and perhaps of the capillaries. Often, associated hard, white, intraretinal exudates surround the clustered aneurysms. These aneurysmal changes occupy areas in the retina that are generally posterior to the equator. Often, exudates are deposited above the macular region in a circinate fashion. The lesions are usually found in younger persons and most frequently are unilateral and slowly progressive; they seem to occur more often in men.

Increased brilliance of the light reflex, whitening, and thickening of a short segment of a major, secondary, or tertiary artery is first noted. A few microaneurysms may be seen nearby in association with small retinal hemorrhages. Fatty yellow exudates usually begin to form in a ring centered on the arteriole lesion and several disc diameters from it. As the arteriole segment continues to enlarge and whiten, deep edema thickens the retina within the ring and aneurysms hyalinize, becoming first a lighter red, then a yellowish white. As the exudative ring thickens, the bulbous segment of the artery becomes 2 to 3 times its normal width, resembling a whitish, aneurysmal dilation that can be likened to an electric light bulb.

Ancillary diagnostic examinations. Stereo color photography will show the progression of any of the lesions and any changes in the surrounding retinal edema or exudate formation.

Fluorescein angiography will demarcate the areas affected by the process and indicate the zones of most extensive leakage and active proliferation of the small vessels. The saccular and fusiform dilations of the affected vessels are readily apparent, especially during the arteriolovenular phase of the fluorescein transit.

Indications for photocoagulation. The existence of moderately advanced telangiectatic vessels of Leber's variety is sufficient indication for treatment by photocoagulation. Since many of these herniated and saccular vessels will rupture, it is important that they be obliterated when found.

All areas afflicted by the aneurysms should be treated directly with the possible exception of the perifoveal zone. Those aneurysms can be approached by more indirect methods, but the overall use of photocoagulation is still indicated.

Photocoagulation approach. A plano–low-vacuum or Goldmann contact lens is usually used after a topical anesthetic has been given. The eyes of an unreliable patient or eyes with foveal vascular lesions should be stabilized by the use of a retrobulbar anesthetic.

The individual arteriolar aneurysm is gently photocoagulated with a spot size larger than the largest diameter of the fusiform swollen portion. Off-white coagulations of the adjacent retina (Grade 3) and some slight constriction of the aneurysm itself should occur (Grade III). A painting or brushing movement of the photocoagulation beam can be used to cover uniformly spaced, isolated, or clustered aneurysms. Spot sizes vary from **200μ to 600μ**, and power settings range from **200 to 700 mw,** depending on the area of the coagulation beam. Exposure intervals range from **0.2 to 1.0 sec,** depending on whether punctate exposures or the painting technique is utilized (Fig. 7-3). In most cases the aneurysms will gradually disappear in several weeks, becoming shrunken and engulfed, with adjacent retinal pigmentation and gliosis (Fig. 7-4).

Aneurysms located in the perifoveal zone cannot usually be considered for direct treatment; in this precarious location it is advisable to coagulate the paramacular feeder vessel to the perifoveal macroaneurysm, rather than the aneurysm itself. The feeder vessel to the foveal aneurysm is coagulated in the paramacular area by intense off-white impacts (Grade III) along the vessel in an attempt to occlude this vessel permanently.

Retreatment should be directed to the areas of persistent aneurysm formation and possibly to any areas adjacent to vessels showing a beaded or irregular appearance. If the argon laser photocoagulation appears to be ineffective for the larger and more saccular aneurysms, xenon-arc photocoagulation should be considered. The polychromaticity of the output beam, particularly in the infrared area, makes the xenon-arc source more destructive and more penetrating.

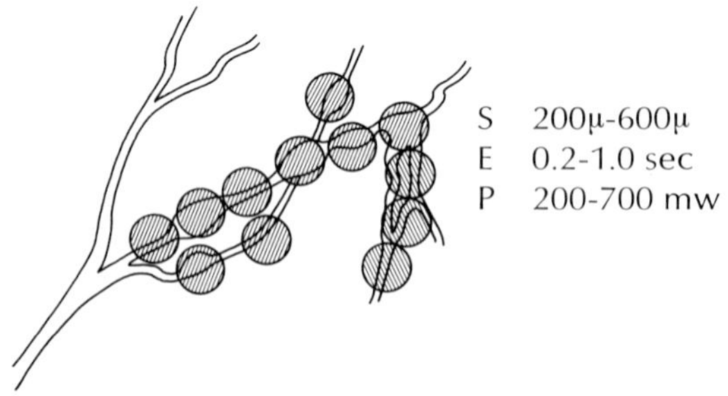

Fig. 7-3. Placement of random, interrupted 200μ to 600μ coagulations along the telangiectatic and fusiform herniations of the abnormal vessels. The coagulations should be 50% larger than the vessel to be treated; exposures longer than 0.2 sec are needed for a Grade III vascular coagulation.

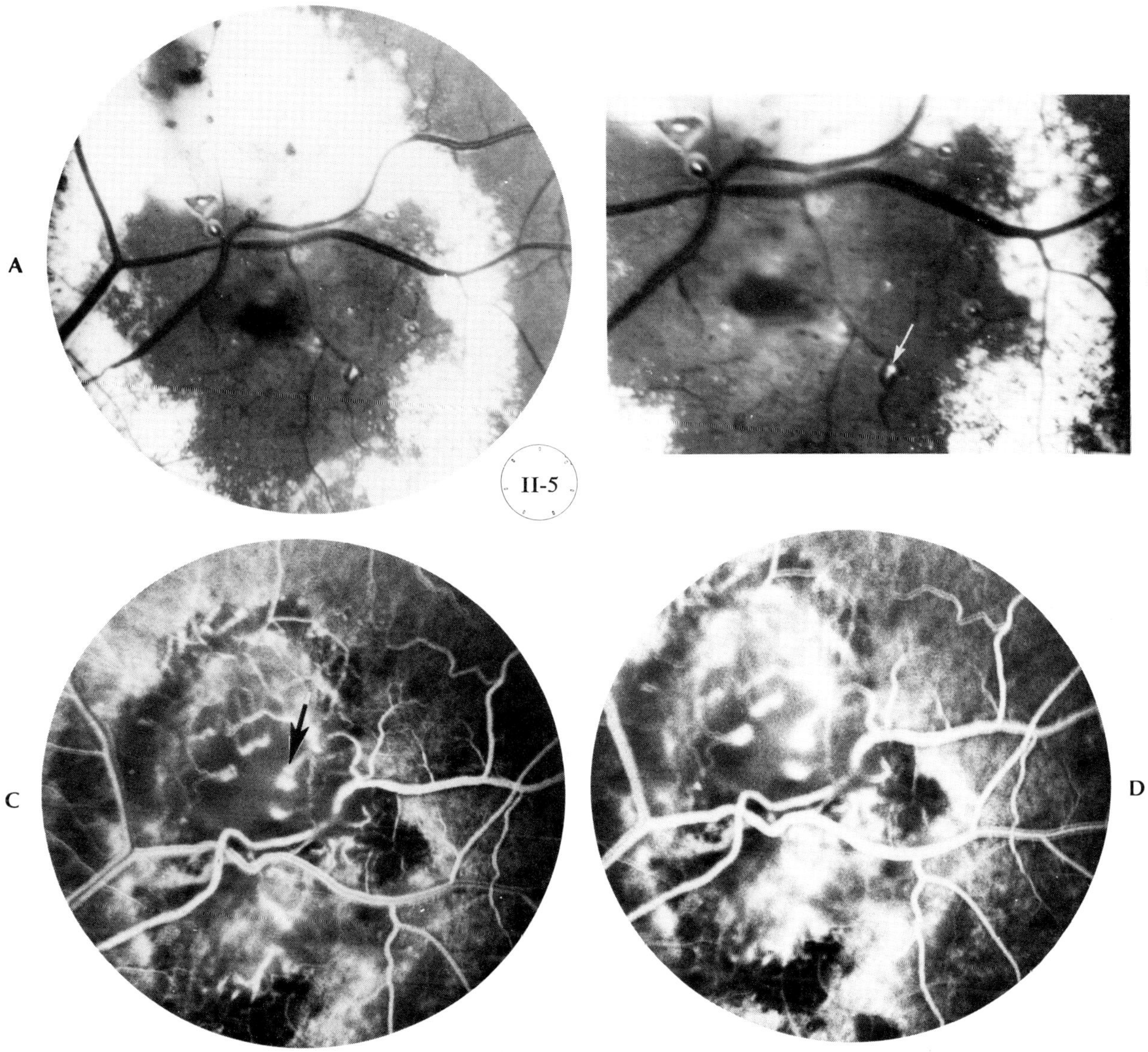

Fig. 7-4. A, A 32-year-old man complained of the gradual onset of blurred vision in his left eye and was found to have classical Leber's miliary aneurysms, marked retinal edema, and exudate formation. **B,** Enlarged view of the fusiform light bulb–like swellings (arrow) of the vessels in the affected area and the marked amount of retinal edema and exudates surrounding the edematous zone. **C,** Fluorogram during the arteriolovenular phase, showing marked filling of the fusiform, herniated areas of the vasculature and leakage into the retinal space (arrow). **D,** Fluorogram during the early venular phase, showing more extensive leakage from the abnormal retinal vasculature into the surrounding retinal tissue.

Continued.

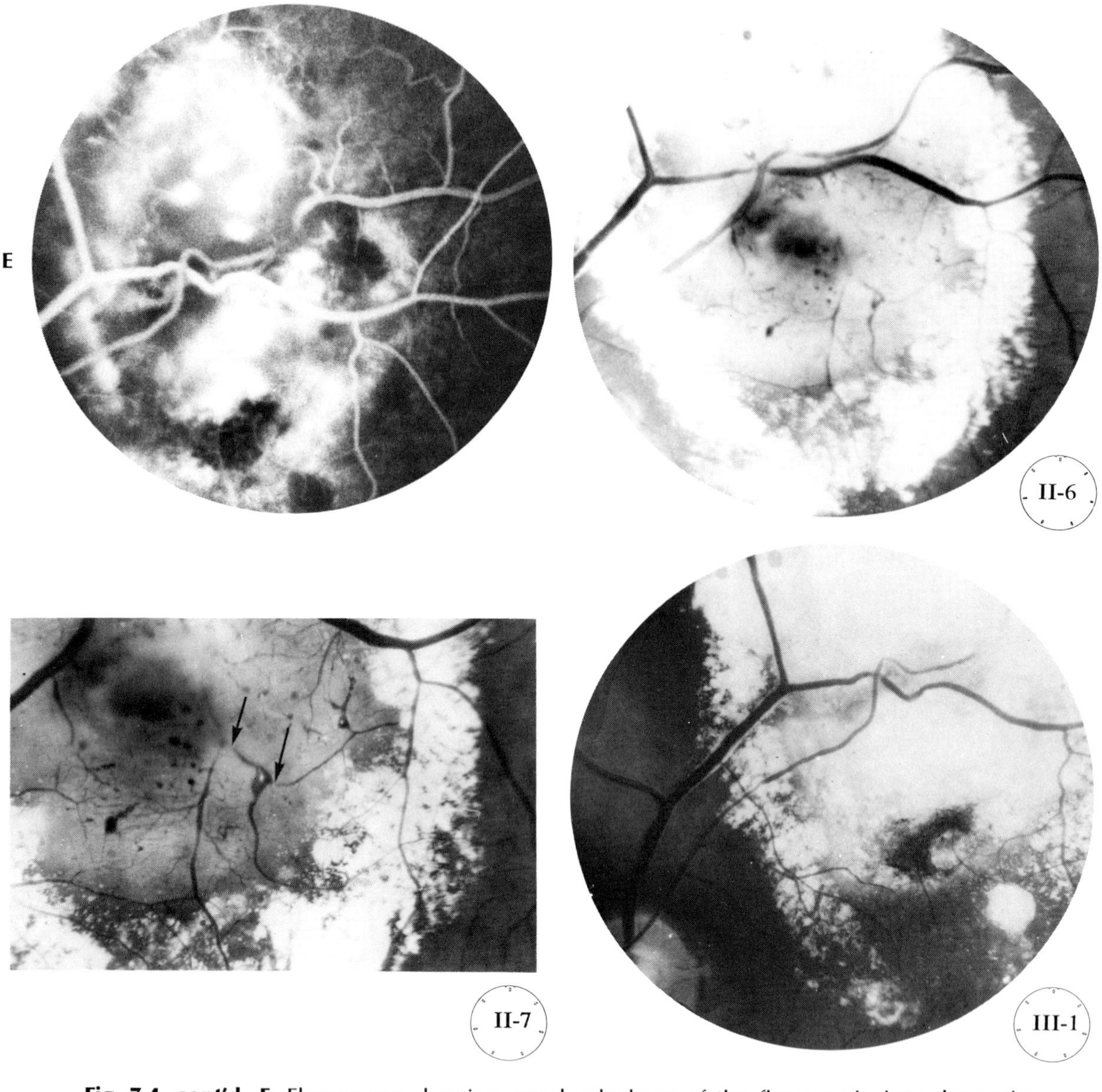

Fig. 7-4, cont'd. E, Fluorogram showing smudgy leakage of the fluorescein into the entire portion of the retina affected by the abnormal vasculature. **F,** Complete overlapping or contiguous Grade 3 coagulations in the region of the fusiform or saccular swellings of the retina vasculature. The areas of exudates and retinal edema are not treated. **G,** Magnified view of the abnormal vessels immediately after photocoagulation. Marked constriction, spasm, and obliteration of these vessels can be seen at this time (arrows). **H,** Healed area of treatment 9 weeks after argon laser photocoagulation, showing complete disappearance of the abnormal herniated segments of the retinal vasculature, absence of retinal edema, and partial absorption of the surrounding exudates. The visual acuity improved from 20/100 to 20/40 several months after treatment.

Complications. The most serious complication can be the rupture of an aneurysm, resulting in a large preretinal, intraretinal, or intravitreal hemorrhage. One is advised to use large coagulations at weaker powers with longer exposure intervals so that the target tissue is photocoagulated more gently. The complication of hemorrhage should be rare under these circumstances.

The location of a macroaneurysm near the nerve fiber layer should be carefully evaluated, since coagulations at this point will damage and perhaps interrupt the nerve fiber layer communication over the area of coagulation. Therefore, macroaneurysms in the papillomacular bundle should be evaluated carefully; photocoagulation should not be considered unless a gross enlargement of the aneurysm has been noted.

Retinal striae can be produced if one area of the paramacular region or the temporal arcade region is photocoagulated heavily or extensively. Photocoagulations need not be severe for obliteration of these vascular lesions, and one is advised to use a lower energy dose and repeat photocoagulation rather than attempt obliteration on the initial treatment by using an excessive amount of input energy.

Follow-up. Follow-up consists of thorough examination by indirect ophthalmoscopy and contact biomicroscopy at 2-week intervals. Fluorescein angiography to verify the obliteration of the vascular channels can be done at the 1-month stage or at a later stage. If a vascular channel remains visible following retinal pigmentation and gliosis in the photocoagulated zone, additional photocoagulation can be considered.

The patient should be followed at 3-month intervals for approximately 2 to 3 years following photocoagulation and successful obliteration of the arteriolar and capillary fusiform aneurysms. The examination must be thorough and consist of meticulous investigation of all components of the retinal vascular tree. Any abnormality consistent with the diagnosis of a regrowth of Leber's miliary aneurysms should be treated as soon as it is recognized, unless it is located in the perifoveal region.

COATS' DISEASE

Clinical symptoms. Sudden loss of vision because of hemorrhage into the vitreous and gradual loss of vision because of progressive macular edema have been reported. A veillike deterioration of a section of the visual field, lightning flashes, marked distortion, and variation in image size have been noted.

Ophthalmoscopic appearance. The clinical picture of massive intraretinal and subretinal exudation, retinal detachment, and associated vascular ectasias and aneurysms has been described as the ophthalmoscopic entity of Coats' disease. Greenish bullous retinal detachments resulting from the angiomatous malformation in the retina in young children have been described, in conjunction with an inordinate amount of intraretinal and subretinal exudation. The macula can be affected by massive retinal edema and exudate formation, leading to marked visual deterioration.

Ancillary diagnostic examinations. Ultrasonography can usually determine the nature of a retinal detachment and the presence of an underlying angiomatous lesion or otherwise solid tumor. The Coats' disease-like process can be more clearly defined if an underlying tumor mass can be ruled out.

Fluorescein angiography can show the presence of leakage patterns into the retinal or subretinal space, or any accumulation or pooling of the dye caused by vascular malformations. Massive outpouring of the dye from neovascular areas on the retinal surface and under the retinal detachment can be observed. The lipid deposits of cholesterol give a pseudofluorescence and should be differentiated from the telangiectatic areas. Angiographic studies are also used for localizing areas of vascular effusion for coagulation purposes. This information can be correlated with the ophthalmoscopic impression noted by indirect ophthalmoscopy and contact lens biomicroscopy.

Visual field examinations can determine the progress of the lesion during the early evaluation stage. Documentation of an increase in the size or density of the scotoma can be an indication for photocoagulation intervention.

^{32}P radioisotope examination can be considered if an underlying solid tumor mass, such as a malignant melanoma, is suspected. A marked uptake of this isotope can help determine that the process is neoplastic rather than exudative.

Indications for photocoagulation. If an angiomatous mass can be visualized or if telangiectatic vessels can be located in an area of massive retinal or subretinal exudation, photocoagulation should be strongly considered. Interruption of the vascular channels usually leads to improvement.

Gliosis of the retina to such an extent that the underlying telangiectatic or vascular channels cannot be visualized is usually a contraindication to photocoagulation, because the beam will be highly scattered instead of affecting the target tissue.

If the situation depicted in the preceding paragraph is encountered but the lesion has been limited to a small portion of the globe, double linear rows of delimiting coagulations can be used to contain the process.

Following cryocautery or previous photocoagulation of the angiomatous lesion, it is possible to find areas of vascular ectasia that become more noticeable following reduction of the subretinal exudation and flattening of the overlying retina. These areas should be considered for photocoagulation with the argon laser or the xenon-arc photocoagulation devices.

Photocoagulation approach. With argon laser photocoagulation a Goldmann three-mirror lens or similar contact lens is used with a topical anesthetic and occasionally a retrobulbar anesthetic. Xenon-arc photocoagulation requires no contact lens, but topical and retrobulbar anesthetics are necessary.

Xenon-arc photocoagulation should be considered in all cases as the treatment of first choice, particularly if the retina is gliotic or a moderate degree of retinal edema or other exudation exists. Argon laser photocoagulation can be used very effectively if the vessels have not developed a gliotic shield or a large amount of surrounding retinal edema.

The area of abnormal vasculature (telangiectatic or vascular ectasia, or other mac-

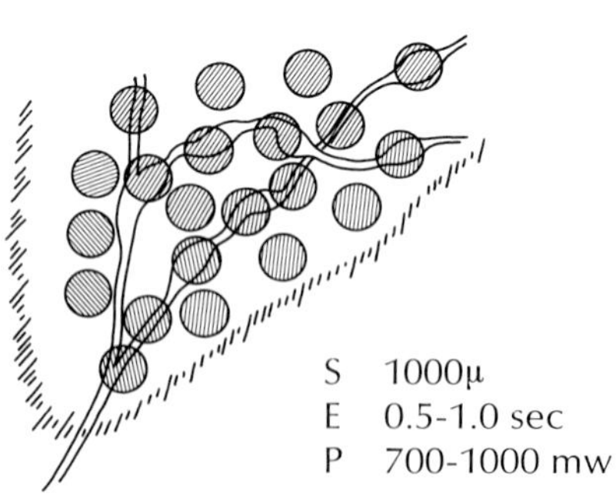

Fig. 7-5. Placement of punctate, barrage-type, 1,000μ coagulations in the region of the telangiectatic abnormal vessels to obtain a Grade 3 chorioretinal and vascular coagulation. Coagulations are confined to the abnormal telangiectatic vessels in the middle or far periphery of the eye.

A B C D

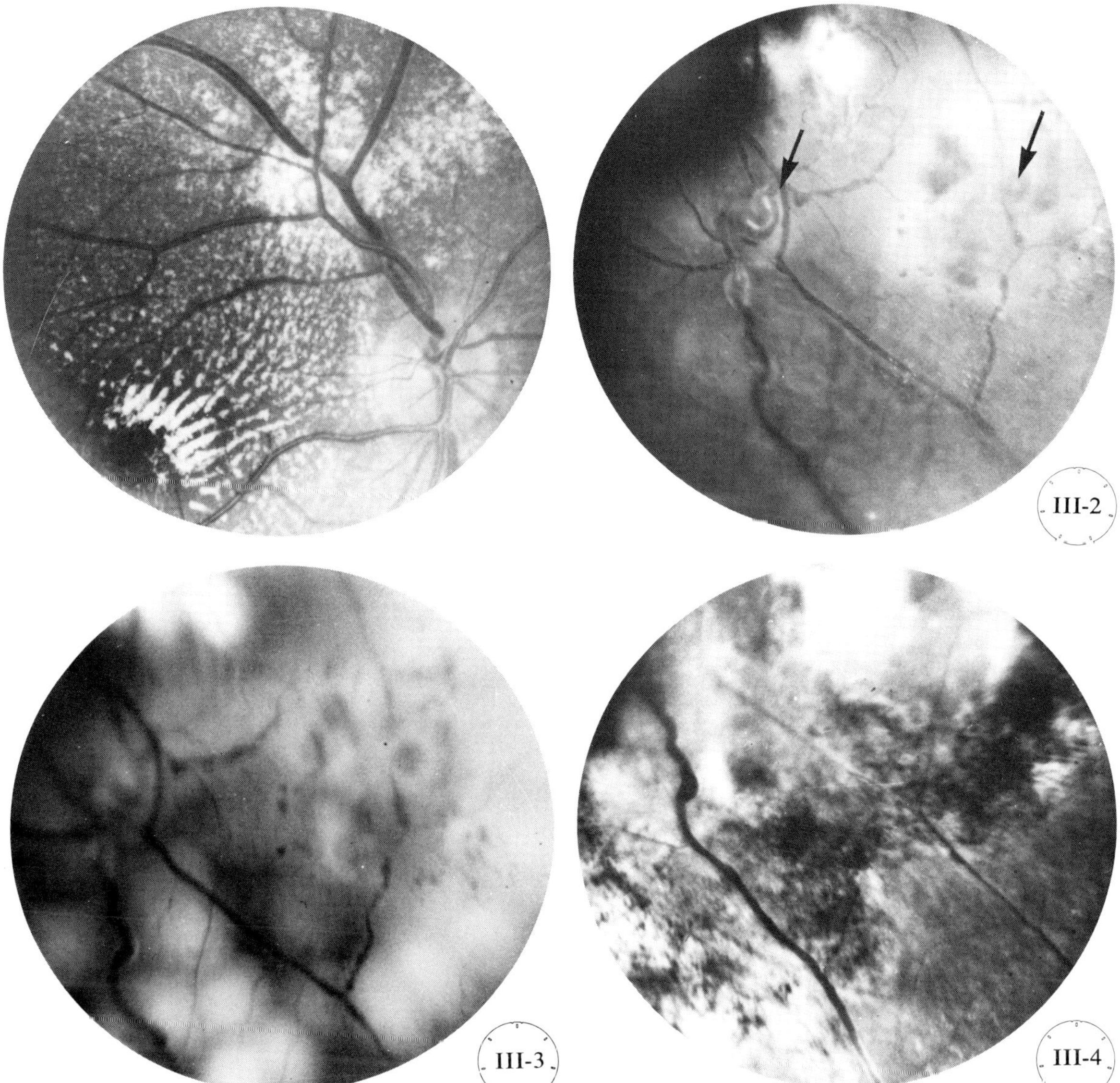

Fig. 7-6. A, Optic disc and macular and superotemporal regions of a 9-year-old boy who was found to have a peripheral area of telangiectatic and macroaneurysmal vascular changes that contributed to his early symptom of blurred vision. Note the hard exudates along the superotemporal vascular arcade and in the macular region, creating a macular star figure. **B,** Midperipheral area, showing the large fusiform and telangiectatic vessels (arrows) forming the peripheral shunting network and marked retinal and subretinal edema. **C,** Abnormal vasculature immediately following photocoagulation with 1,000μ Grade 3 coagulations of an intensity sufficient to obliterate the vessels and create a dirty-white retinal coagulation. **D,** Healed area 2 months after treatment, showing complete obliteration of the telangiectatic vessels and reduction of the retinal edema and exudate formation.

Continued.

E

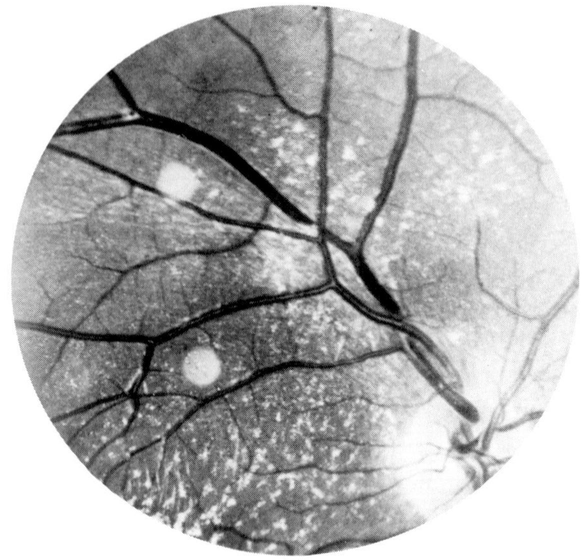

Fig. 7-6, cont'd. E, Macular area, optic nerve, and superotemporal area 10 weeks after obliteration of the peripheral shunting vascular malformation. Note the obvious decrease in hard exudates throughout this entire area.

A

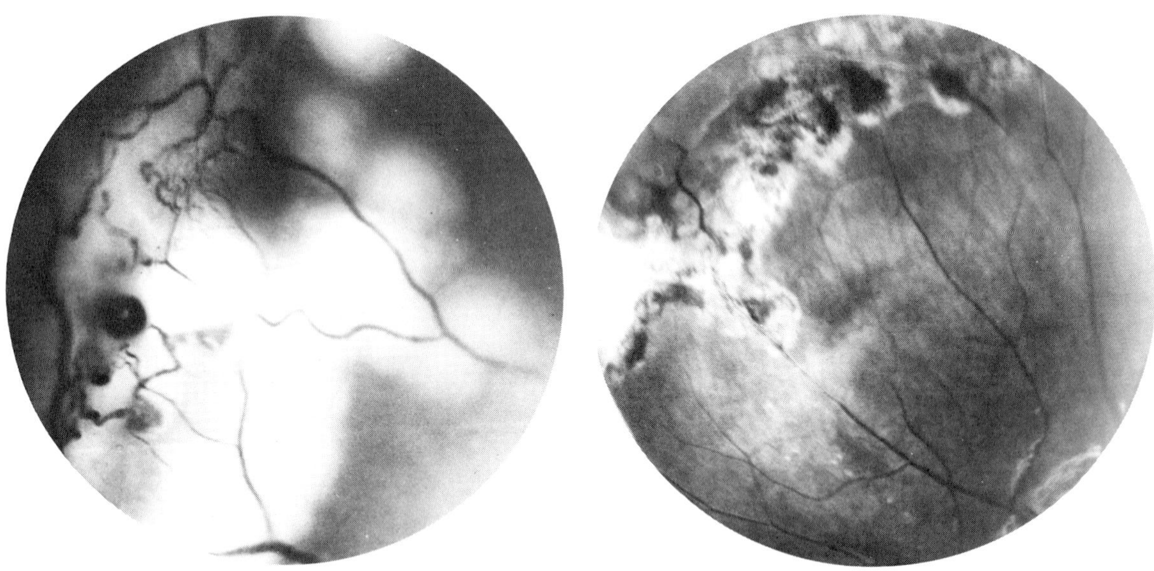

B

Fig. 7-7. A, Superotemporal area of telangiectatic vessels and neovascularization following photocoagulation in a 9-year-old boy whose complaint of a sudden loss of vision was caused by a small vitreous hemorrhage. Treatment was with 6° (1,800μ) xenon-arc coagulations at a Red II intensity for 0.5 sec. **B,** Healed area 2 months after xenon-arc photocoagulation, showing complete destruction of the abnormal vasculature, secondary gliosis, and pigment proliferation. Vision improved from $20/80^{-2}$ to $20/20^{-1}$ following absorption of the blood and obliteration of the vascular abnormality.

roaneurysmal change) should be treated with large coagulations sufficient to cover the vascular abnormality with a moderately white coagulum (Grade 3). A 6° spot is used with a xenon-arc instrument at a power setting of **Red II,** or a **1,000μ** spot is used with the argon laser at a power setting of **700 to 1,000 mw** (Fig. 7-5). Usually, exposures of **0.5 to 1.0 sec** are used with either machine to create the proper coagulation appearance (Figs. 7-6 and 7-7). All of the lesion is coagulated during the initial treatment session, and the fundus is searched carefully for any small, early changes suggestive of incipient Coats' disease.

Complications. Hemorrhage at the time of coagulation or during the period immediately following photocoagulation is the most common, and perhaps the most devastating, complication. A light but even coagulation of the vascular malformation and the surrounding retinal tissue is most important. Overcoagulation of the abnormal vessels will cause necrosis of the vascular wall and a high probability of hemorrhage during the week after photocoagulation. The patient must be cautioned against any type of strenuous activity or initiation of Valsalva's maneuver.

Macular gliosis and striae have occurred because of excessive photocoagulation to the temporal arcade and more peripheral regions. In many cases, the extensive photocoagulation was justified to destroy the vascular malformation and unfortunately resulted in a great deal of traction laterally along the plane of the retina into the macular zone. Usually, multiple photocoagulation treatments with an adequate intervening period for complete healing, scarring, and atrophy of the vascular lesion is recommended as the proper method of treatment.

Failure of photocoagulation because of scatter of the impinging photocoagulation beam by the protective glial tissue also occurs. In these cases one should consider cryocautery to the vascular malformation in repeated doses during several sessions for destruction of the vascular tissue.

Macular pucker or traction on the macular region sometimes occurs because of the large amount of energy that is necessary to destroy these vascular lesions. Theoretically, the vitreous shrinks, pulling on the foveal and macular region and causing the macular pucker. If macular pucker or a semicontracted state of the vitreous is suspected as a potential risk before treatment, argon laser photocoagulation should be employed as the method of choice because of the smaller amount of total energy necessary for effective therapy of these vascular lesions.

Follow-up. The patient should be carefully followed and evaluated at monthly intervals. Further photocoagulation will be necessary if any telangiectatic vessels or areas of exudation are located. After the lesions have been obliterated, the patient should be seen at 6-month intervals for a period of at least 3 to 4 years.

PROLIFERATIVE SICKLE RETINOPATHY

Clinical symptoms. The sudden onset of blurred vision is the most common complaint of individuals with sickle retinopathy. Floaters, scotomas, metamorphopsia, and photopsia can be observed.

Ophthalmoscopic appearance. Sickling disorders, particularly sickle cell hemoglobin C disease (SC disease) and sickle cell thalassemia (S thal), are complicated by patches of retinal neovascularization. So-called sea fans and fronds can be seen in the midperiphery in association with dusky red or salmon-colored angiomatous vascular channels. These large telangiectatic and irregular vessels emerge into the vitreous and usually have one or more feeder vessels that supply the distal angiomatous tuft. Supportive glial tissue is frequently seen in the area of the vascular malformation, and occasional hemorrhages into the retina and the preretinal space are noted. Neovascular changes on the surface of the retina, including the formation of shunt vessels and aberrant channels, can be observed in various portions of the midperipheral fundus. Black sunburst patterns, obstructed arterioles, and vitreous membranes can be seen throughout the equatorial and postequatorial regions.

Ancillary diagnostic examinations. Fluorescein angiography may show obvious perfused neovascular sea fans, areas of ischemia peripheral to the neovascular tissue, large areas of fluorescein leakage into the vitreous, and areas of tortuous vessels leading to the angiomatous sea fans. The fluorescein leakage and areas of nonperfusion can be extensive and must be evaluated carefully.

Perimetry with the Goldmann hemispherical projection perimeter or other perimetric devices can show areas of scotoma formation or arcuate field defects.

Indirect ophthalmoscopic and contact lens biomicroscopic examinations are most important for documenting, with drawings, the exact location and extent of the proliferative sickle retinopathy.

Stereoscopic and regular Kodachrome fundus photography with the ordinary 30° or wide-angle 45° camera is most important for documenting the progress of the disease and for postphotocoagulation evaluation.

Indications for photocoagulation. The observation of areas of proliferative sickle retinopathy, particularly with large angiomatous channels, is an indication for immediate photocoagulation of the lesion. Since most cases of sickle-related retinitis proliferans are progressive, these disease areas should be photocoagulated as soon as they are recognized.

Areas of ischemia or tortuous vessels in the midperiphery of patients with sickling disorders should be considered for photocoagulation, particularly if the lesions have been shown to be progressive during recent evaluations.

Photocoagulation approach. Usually, only the topical use of an anesthetic is necessary for adequate photocoagulation. A Goldmann three-mirror lens or Jungner contact lens is used to approach the sickle retinopathy in the midperipheral portions of the eye. The plano–low-vacuum contact lens can be used for photocoagulation of the more posterior diseased retinal portions. Occasionally, a retrobulbar injection of lidocaine will be required during the procedure to alleviate pain felt during photocoagulation.

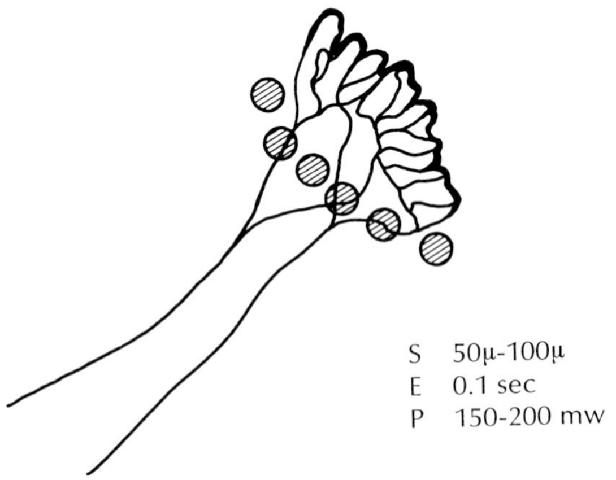

Fig. 7-8. Placement of 50μ to 100μ coagulations along the feeder vessels to the distal sea fan. Coagulation and obliteration of these afferent and efferent vessels should be clearly perceptible.

Photocoagulation should be directed primarily toward permanent occlusion of the feeding arteriolar vessels and secondarily toward obliteration of the entire neovascular lesion. Vascular channels will show interruption of their blood columns when the instrument is set at a spot size of **50μ to 100μ**, with an exposure of **0.1 sec** and a power level of **150 to 200 mw** (Fig. 7-8). The feeder vessels can be interrupted without difficulty if they remain in the retinal plane close to the pigment epithelium. However, if the feeder vessels are elevated into the vitreous, the power density level must be increased for adequate photocoagulation and occlusion of these particular channels.

The neovascular sea fan lesions are photocoagulated directly following occlusion of the feeder vessels to the sea fan. Typical settings required to interrupt blood flow in the larger vessels are a power level of **300 to 350 mw**, an exposure interval of **0.5 sec**, and a beam diameter of **100μ** (Fig. 7-9). A larger beam diameter should be employed for larger angiomatous lesions or for more diffuse or extensive patches of neovascularization. In these cases the power level required for adequate neovascular obliteration may reach **600 to 700 mw**.

All visible areas of proliferative sickle retinopathy should be photocoagulated to obliteration. Either xenon-arc or argon laser photocoagulation is adequate for the destruction of these areas, although argon laser photocoagulation appears to be the more effective treatment for elevated neovascular fans (Fig. 7-10).

Complications. The most common complication is hemorrhage into the preretinal space and vitreous body, this problem can be caused by rupture of the large angiomatous lesions or the high-flow feeder vessel channels and can be minimized if the power density is increased slowly, until the proper photocoagulation level is reached.

Macular striae, glial proliferation from the site of vascular occlusion, delayed hemorrhages into the vitreous, and macular edema have been observed following photocoagulation. These complications can be decreased by the use of minimal amounts of argon laser or xenon-arc photocoagulation energy during the therapeutic session.

Follow-up. The patient is given steroids and cycloplegics topically for a period of approximately 10 days to 2 weeks following photocoagulation.

The patient should be seen several weeks following photocoagulation, and fluorescein

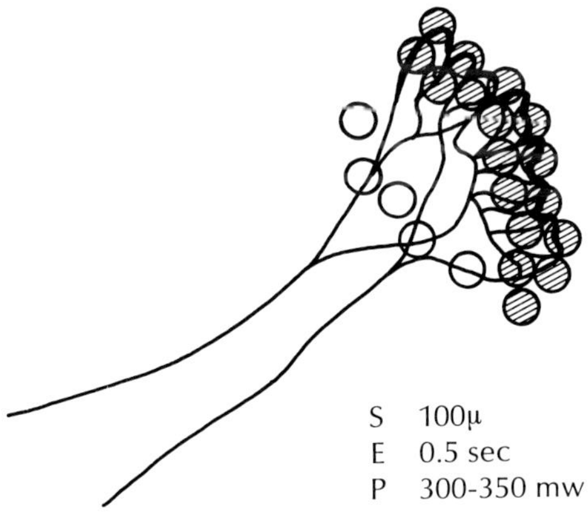

Fig. 7-9. Interrupted, barrage-type, punctate 100μ coagulations to the distal portion of the sea fan that may be elevated into the vitreous. Caution should be exercised and low powers used initially. The entire neovascular area should be treated during the photocoagulation session.

A

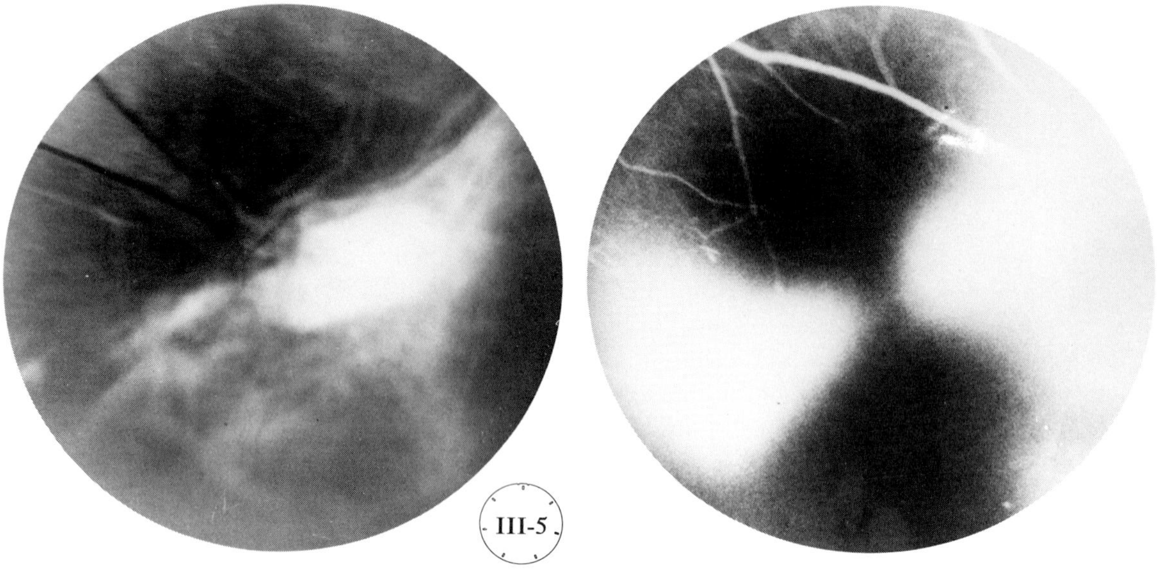

B

C

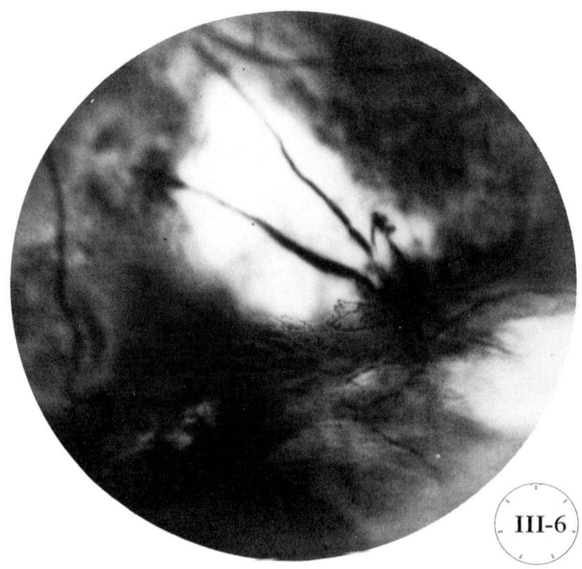

Fig. 7-10. A, An area of proliferation in a patient with SC disease with multiple episodes of bleeding and secondary glial proliferation. **B,** Fluorescein angiogram demonstrating the area of neovascularization and leakage into the vitreous from the distal portions of the sea fan tufts. **C,** Contiguous and overlapping argon laser photocoagulations to the feeder vessels just proximal to a large sea fan. **D,** Fluorogram demonstrating absence of filling of the photocoagulated feeder vessel (arrow) during the late venular phase. **E,** Treated area, showing pigment proliferation, gliosis, and complete destruction of the afferent and efferent vessels from the distal sea fan. **F,** Fluorogram showing absence of filling of the neovascular area and some late staining of the glial and pigmented tissue in the area of previous photocoagulation. **G,** A typical salmon patch of angiomatous tissue (arrow) in proliferative sickle retinopathy immediately after photocoagulation with 600μ coagulations at a 0.5-sec exposure and a 600-mw power intensity. Deep penetration of the photocoagulation energy into the area surrounding the salmon patch is important. **H,** Healed area 2 months after photocoagulation, showing complete obliteration of the neovascularization and angiomatous vessels. **I,** A typical sea fan 2 months after argon laser photocoagulation, showing obliteration of the feeder and collector vessels and of the vascular channels at the root of the sea fan. (Courtesy Morton Goldberg, M.D.)

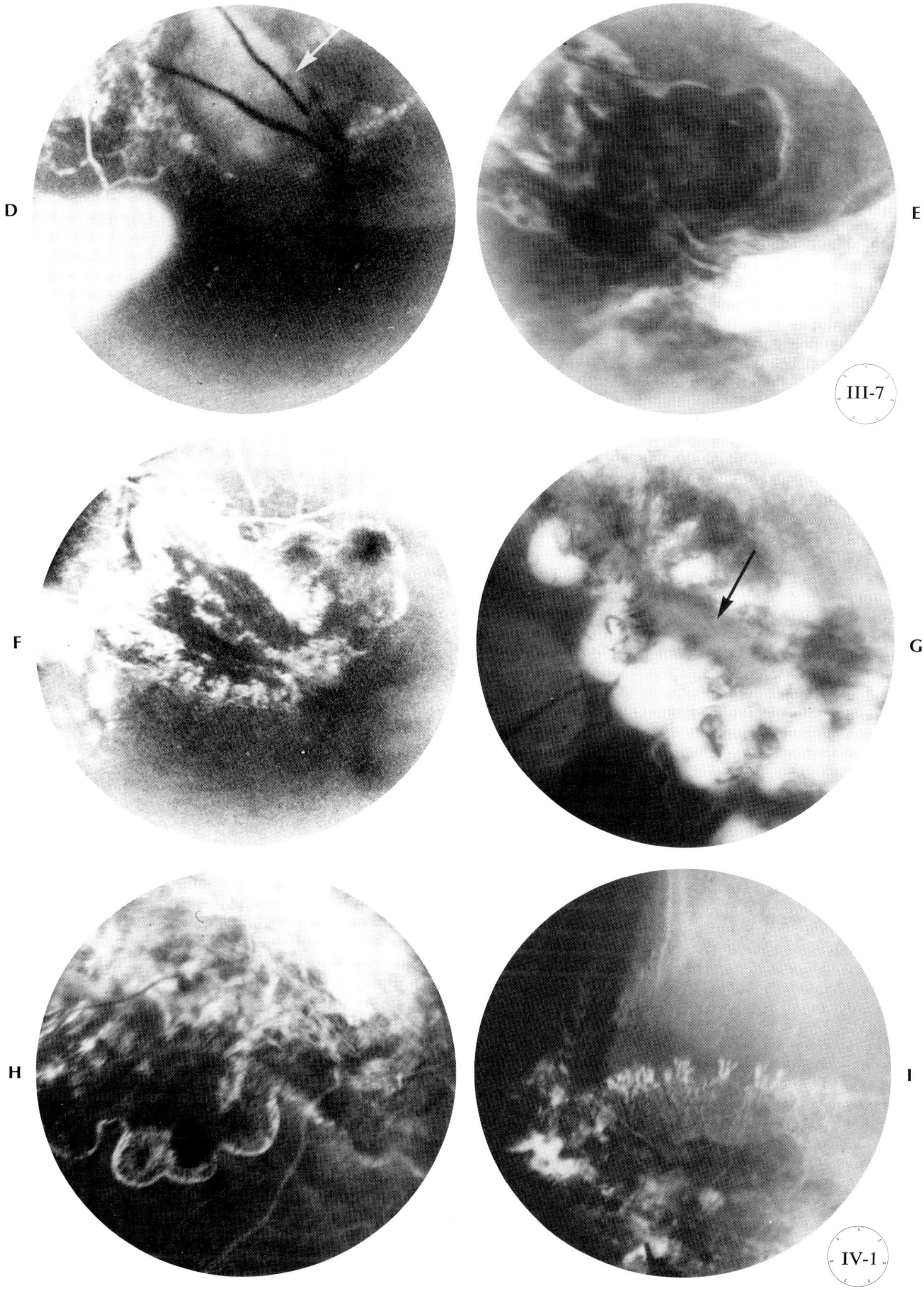

Fig. 7-10, cont'd. For legend see opposite page.

angiography should be performed at that time to evaluate whether the neovascular tissue continues to carry blood. Simple ophthalmoscopy has often been misleading, and perfused neovascular channels have been camouflaged by a mantle of healed scar tissue following photocoagulation. Fluorescein angiography can help detect these areas of neovascular perfusion, and photocoagulation should be attempted as soon as they are recognized.

Wide-angle fundus photography is performed on each visit, and the patient is examined carefully by indirect ophthalmoscopy and contact lens biomicroscopy.

After it has been determined that the condition has been arrested, the patient should be evaluated by fluorescein angiography at 6-month intervals. The fundus should be scanned meticulously for any regrowth of the neovascularization or proliferation of glial or pigmented tissue.

RETROLENTAL FIBROPLASIA

Clinical symptoms. Clinical symptoms are few because of the age of the babies. Older children may notice blurred vision or loss of a portion of the visual field secondary to glial proliferation, vitreous traction, or retinal detachment.

Ophthalmoscopic appearance. A bilateral retinal disease of premature infants, retrolental fibroplasia is characterized by wildly disorganized growth of the fetal retinal tissue. In 1954 the cause was found to be an excessive amount of oxygen given to premature infants during the first few weeks of life; an excess of oxygen causes an abnormal response of the underdeveloped capillary network of the fetal retina. Initially, there is edema of the peripheral retina, followed by vascular dilation and tortuosity, and peripheral retinal detachment. Fibrous tissue replacement of the retina and total retinal detachment can occur later. Retrolental fibrosia usually has its onset in the first few days of life and progresses rapidly over a period of weeks.

The retina is seen as a white retrolental membrane in the pupillary aperture. A few surface vessels on the membrane are evident. The anterior chambers are shallow, and the pupillary light reflexes may be absent. In severe cases the contracting retrolental tissue can draw the ciliary body anteriorly, and the normal ciliary processes can be seen with the ophthalmoscope along the circumference of the periphery of the dilated pupil.

Indications for photocoagulation. Although photocoagulation is an extremely experi-

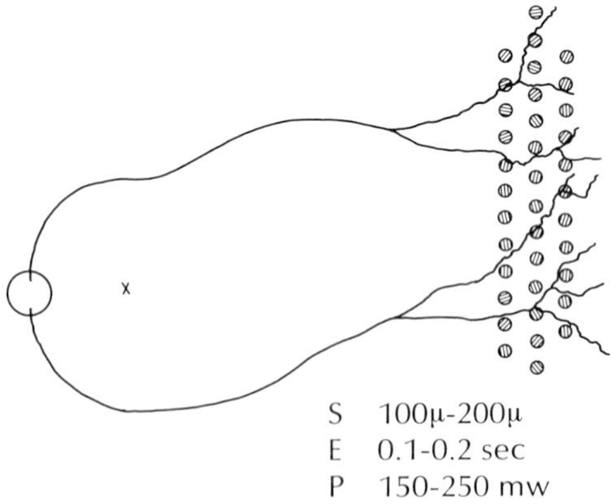

Fig. 7-11. Placement of punctate, interrupted, linear argon laser coagulations in the temporal periphery of the affected eye in the region of proliferating retinopathy. The neovascular channels can be considered for photocoagulation if progression of the disease has been documented.

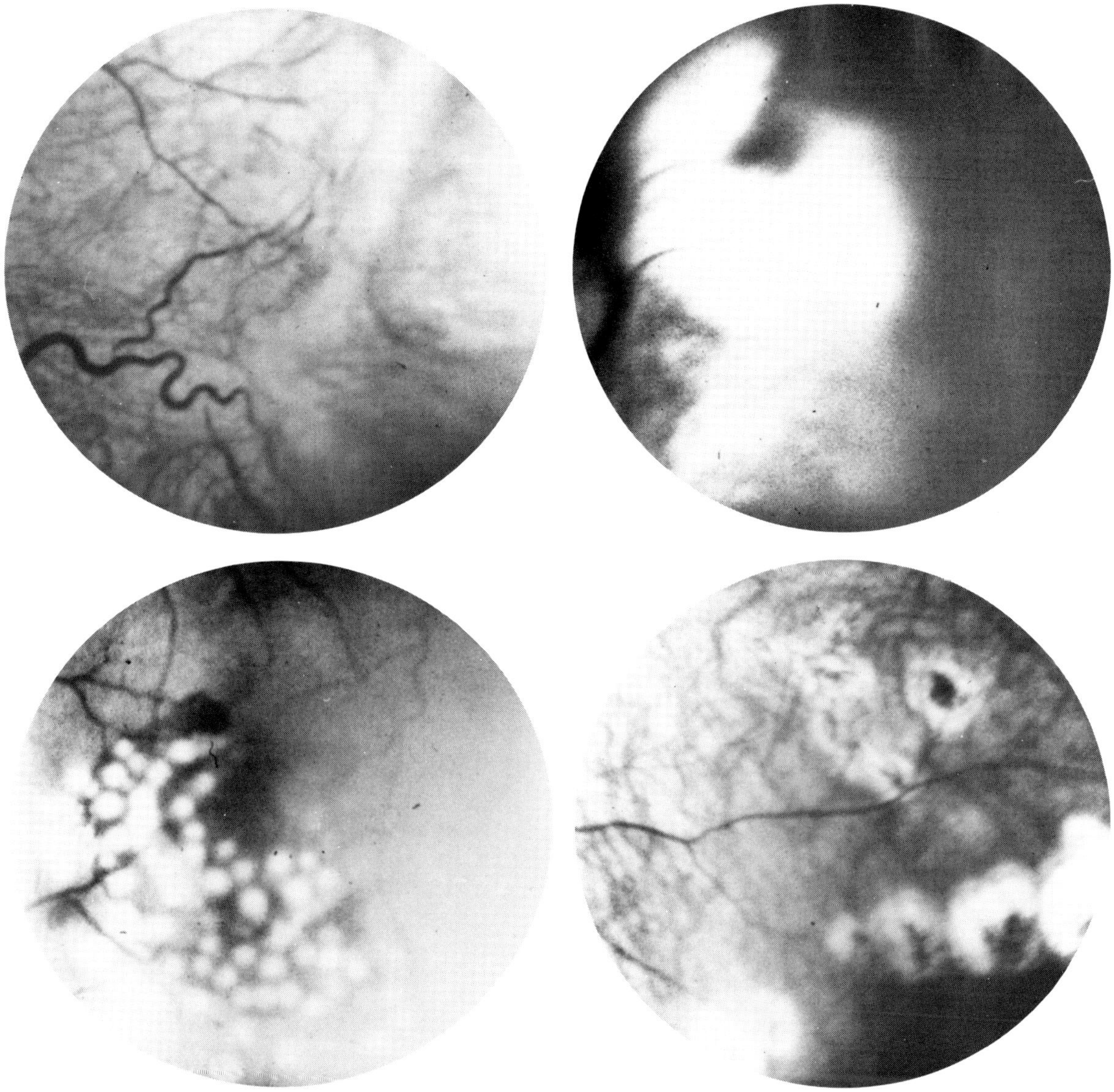

Fig. 7-12. A, Bilateral retrolental fibroplasia with neovascularization just temporal to the equator was noted in a 3½-month-old girl with a history of premature birth. (Birth weight was 2 lb, 9 oz; gestational age was 7½ months.) Follow-up examination 2 weeks later showed further increase of proliferative activity. **B,** At 4½ months of age a large vitreal hemorrhage was noted. The vitreal hemorrhage involved the temporal periphery and extended posteriorly near the region of the optic disc. **C,** Under anesthesia, the child was tilted nasally to allow the blood to migrate posteriorly. Argon laser photocoagulation was then applied to the area of neovascularization near the equator. Multiple 100μ and 200μ coagulations were used. **D,** Pigmented scars at the site of the argon laser photocoagulation, 4 months later. The vitreous has cleared completely, and the remainder of the fundus appears normal. The condition of the fellow eye, which was then treated, had progressed to "dragged" vessels, a heterotopia of the macular area, and a temporal traction detachment of the retina. (Courtesy Arnall Patz, M.D.)

mental procedure for retrolental fibroplasia, it has been apparent that photocoagulation of the proliferating vessels, particularly in the temporal aspect of the eye, can be beneficial (Fig. 7-11). If the proliferation of neovascular tissue can be observed on the surface of the retina, the area should be photographed or accurately drawn for later evaluation.

The eye should then be examined 1 to 2 weeks after the photograph or drawing has been made; if progression of the disease with an increase in the fibrovascular tissue in the area of concern can be documented, photocoagulation of this region can be considered. The disease process should be determined to be progressive before photocoagulation intervention since 85% to 90% of eyes with observable fibrovascular tissue will enter a stage of regression.

If the disease is clearly progressing with an increase of neovascularization and fibrous tissue elements, photocoagulation should be considered for one eye only; the fellow eye is thereby given the opportunity to regress spontaneously (Fig. 7-12). The experimental nature of the photocoagulation procedure also militates for the treatment of one eye only.

Photocoagulation approach. The areas of neovascularization and fibrovascular proliferation, as well as the retinovitreal fronds extending into the vitreous body, should be photocoagulated by a technique similar to that employed for proliferative sickle retinopathy (p. 106). The power intensities and energy dosages are also similar and should be sufficient to create a Grade 3 chorioretinal coagulation. All areas of suspected fibrovascular proliferation should be treated during the photocoagulation session.

Complications and follow-up. The complications encountered and the postoperative management of the patient are similar to those of proliferative sickle retinopathy (p. 107). These babies should be evaluated carefully for further progression of the disease at any future time.

DIABETIC RETINOPATHY

CLASSIFICATION

A classification of diabetic retinopathy that embodies both the ophthalmoscopic appearance and the dynamic factors affecting the ultimate prognosis for each particular eye with diabetic retinopathy is presented. This classification is useful for determining which patient might benefit from photocoagulation treatment.

Nonproliferative diabetic retinopathy

Diabetic retinopathy can be divided basically into two categories: the nonproliferative phase and the proliferative phase. The nonproliferative phase consists of a continuum involving venous dilation, microaneurysm formation, the appearance of small intraretinal hemorrhages, the formation of patches of edema, and the later formation of exudates, particularly in the macular and paramacular regions. These changes may progress to involve most of the posterior polar region, resulting in markedly decreased visual acuity.

The nonproliferative portion of the classification is designed so that the appearance of one of these abnormalities signals a particular stage in the evolution of the retinopathy process. It is assumed, for purposes of simplification and with clinical justification in the majority of cases, that one disease category or stage leads to the next and has arisen from a previous stage. The first probable change in diabetic retinopathy that can be visualized is a slight dilation of the veins; this stage is followed, in most cases, by scattered microaneurysm formation. Microaneurysms eventually lead to intraretinal hemorrhages that may or may not occur from the microaneurysm sites. As the retinopathy progresses, breakdown of the vessel wall permits serum transport into the surrounding retinal tissue,

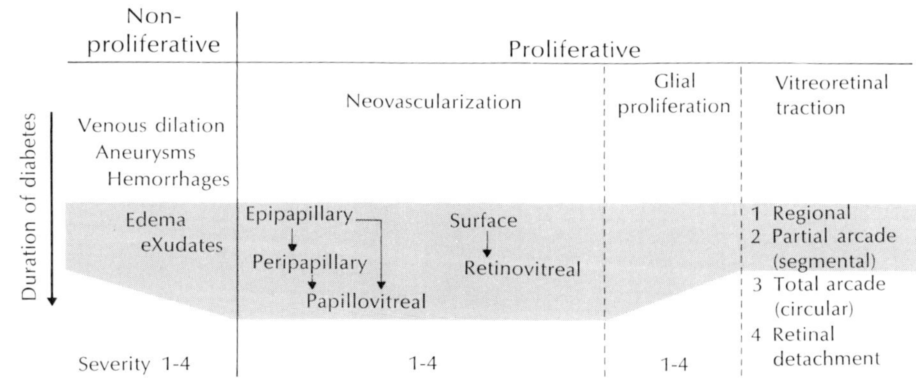

Fig. 7-13. Classification for nonproliferative and proliferative diabetic retinopathy involving gradation of the type of neovascularization, glial proliferation, and vitreoretinal traction for the latter category. Shaded zones indicate the type and severity of those retinal abnormalities that can be considered for photocoagulation treatment.

and edema is produced. When the retinal tissue is affected directly by the edematous process, cellular death and serum transport derangement through the retina can be anticipated, and exudates may begin to accumulate in various parts of the posterior pole. Therefore, with few exceptions the progression, although gradual, from venous dilation to exudate formation in the nonproliferative phase of diabetic retinopathy can be classified by the observation and documentation of each stage of the pathologic process (Fig. 7-13).

The stages of nonproliferative diabetic retinopathy can be remembered most easily by the acronym VAHEX (V, venous dilation; A, microaneurysm formation; H, hemorrhagic activity; E, retinal edema; X, exudate formation). These five stages are then classified according to a 1 to 4 severity rating. As each earlier stage of proliferative diabetic retinopathy increases in severity, the next more pathologic component appears, and the classification then shifts into that category. Therefore, classifications 3 and 4 usually involve only the production of the end phase exudates. Exudate formation can be quite extensive; there can be intraretinal hemmorrhages and edema throughout the posterior regions of the fundus. However, there may be no sign of neovascularization or glial tissue proliferation.

Proliferative diabetic retinopathy

Proliferative diabetic retinopathy is a large classification that includes the production or proliferation of new tissue, supportive or neovascular in nature, in the chorioretinal area secondary to injury by the diabetic process. The amount and type of neovascular and glial tissue proliferation, as well as the relationship between the vitreous and the retinal structures, must be evaluated. If these three components of the proliferative stage of diabetic retinopathy (vitreoretinal neovascularization, glial proliferation, and vitreoretinal traction) can be accurately classified, the condition of the eye can be determined more precisely on a pathophysiologic basis. This classification provides a more accurate assessment of the desirability for photocoagulation therapy and offers a more exact prognosis for the particular eye.

Neovascularization

Neovascularization must first be categorized as one of the five types seen in diabetic retinopathy: epipapillary, peripapillary, papillovitreal, retinovitreal, or preretinal (surface). Each neovascular type is described more completely in the section dealing with that entity.

Epipapillary neovascularization can progress to the more advanced and more extensive papillovitreal type of neovascularization, or it can extend to the peripapillary form with growth along the shallowly detached posterior hyaloid. Surface neovascularization can become extremely extensive in some areas, and proliferation can extend into the vitreous, thereby converting preretinal or surface neovascularization to the retinovitreal neovascular type. One type of neovascularization may lead to a more advanced type (Fig. 7-13). The two primary types of neovascularization—epipapillary and preretinal (surface)—can proliferate and evolve to the more advanced forms of neovascular tissue. Therefore, classification of the neovascularization as papillovitreal indicates that the epipapillary stage was surpassed, and the designation retinovitreal indicates that the neovascularization was surface in nature at one time. All of these five types of neovascularization are graded in severity from 1 to 4 so that the patient can be ophthalmoscopically followed more accurately.

Glial proliferation

Glial tissue may proliferate alone or in combination with neovascular elements. Glial proliferation may occur on the optic disc and along the vascular arcades, particularly the temporal vascular arcade, and may not be involved with neovascularization. The proliferation may grow along the posterior hyaloid from the region of the optic disc and vascular arcades without evidence of neovascularization. Not uncommonly, glial tissue will proliferate from the optic disc over the macular region in a canopy fashion along the surface of a shallowly detached posterior hyaloid. In many cases this canopy effect causes a loss of vision, while the underlying retina remains relatively normal.

Glial tissue may also be intertwined with epipapillary or papillovitreal neovascularization. As the neovascular frond matures, the glial tissue component increases and the percentage of neovascularization decreases. Older intravitreal fronds can be heavily gliotic and have little neovascularization in or on the surface of the glial tissue. In all cases the severity of the glial proliferation should be categorized in grades 1 to 4, which need only reflect the relative quantity of glial tissue seen by ophthalmoscopic examination.

Glial proliferation on the retinal surface is graded from 1 to 4 as follows:

- GRADE 1 Patchy gliosis in the posterior retina or along the midportion of the vascular arcades, not involving the optic disc
- GRADE 2 Gliosis involving the optic disc area only
- GRADE 3 Gliosis of the arcade region and the optic disc
- GRADE 4 A circular band of gliosis involving the optic disc, vascular arcades, and temporal interarcade retinal area

Vitreoretinal traction

The condition of the vitreous body must be analyzed if one is to make an accurate evaluation of diabetic retinopathy. Knowing the state of the vitreous and the relationship of the posterior hyaloid to the retina is most significant for determining the type of photocoagulation treatment that should be employed as well as the ultimate prognosis for the particular eye.

If a portion of the posterior retinal area has become organized with glial proliferation or neovascularization and is undergoing traction toward the central vitreous, the vitreoretinal traction is designated as Grade 1. This category denotes traction of the vitreous on the retinal structures in sectional or regional areas but not along any well-organized path or zone.

Grade 2 indicates that the vitreoretinal adhesion has extended along one of the major vascular arcades, usually the temporal arcade, and that traction is exerted on the retina in that particular area. The traction is not generalized but is concentrated in one geographic or segmental zone of the posterior fundus.

Grade 3 indicates that more than one of the segmental sections of the posterior retina, usually the vascular arcades, are involved with more severe vitreous contraction. In these cases usually the inferior and superior temporal vascular arcades are under considerable traction by vitreoretinal adhesions, and the traction may form a circular ringlike area of retinal tenting.

Grade 4 indicates that the contraction of the vitreous has been sufficiently severe to pull the sensory retina from its attachment to the pigment epithelium, thereby causing a traction retinal detachment. These traction detachments are usually small at first but can proceed to total detachment of the retina.

General considerations

This classification of diabetic retinopathy attempts to categorize the various phases of diabetic retinopathy as an evolving process starting with early venous dilation and ending with gross glial proliferation, neovascularization, marked vitreoretinal traction, and total retinal detachment. The classification is purely ophthalmoscopic and does not involve the use of fluorescein angiography or any of the electrophysiologic studies. Fluorescein angiography has been found to add to the diagnostic and therapeutic information gathered before photocoagulation but does not change the overall classification or prognosis significantly; electrophysiologic tests are nonspecific and require elaborate equipment that is not readily available to all ophthalmologists.

The total designation and classification of an eye with diabetic retinopathy is accomplished by determining whether the condition can be categorized as nonproliferative or proliferative. If it is nonproliferative, one simply selects the stage of involvement and a severity gradation of from 1 to 4; for example, one might classify the condition as X2.

If the proliferative phase is observed during examination of the diabetic eye, the nonproliferative classification is made and the three proliferative components are judged individually. The predominant form of neovascularization is determined first, and the appropriate representative letter (E, epipapillary; P, peripapillary; V, papillovitreal; R, retinovitreal; and S, surface neovascularization) and severity (number) are noted. The remaining categories of glial proliferation (G) and retinovitreal traction (T) are then judged for severity (for example, G1 and T1) and noted, separated by hyphens. The entire classification would then read: X2-E2-G1-T1. In essence, these four categories serve to allow the examining ophthalmologist (or any other ophthalmologist) to have a distinct impression of the pathophysiologic nature of that particular eye with diabetic retinopathy.

In general, photocoagulation, especially with the argon laser, can be considered if the nonproliferative diabetic retinopathy process has progressed to the level of edema or exudates with a concurrent visual acuity decrease or involvement of the foveal region. An eye with Grade 3 or 4, and usually Grade 2, vitreoretinal traction should not be treated with photocoagulation. Similarly, eyes with Grades 3 and 4 glial proliferation should not be considered for photocoagulation. In these cases the small amount of heat generated by the photocoagulation energy passing through the ocular media could be sufficient to cause further shrinkage of the vitreous body and subsequent retinal detachment.

THERAPY

Focal photocoagulation

Nonproliferative diabetic retinopathy

Clinical symptoms. There may be no symptoms observed by the patient when the nonproliferative diabetic retinopathy is moderately advanced. Usually, far-advanced nonproliferative diabetic retinopathy is accompanied by progressive blurring of central vision, metamorphopsia, washing-out or dimming of vision, and decreased color sensitivity. Scotomas caused by intraretinal or preretinal hemorrhages can be observed by some patients.

Ophthalmoscopic appearance. Nonproliferative diabetic retinopathy encompasses a continuum of hemodynamic events, commencing with the dilation and irregularity and beading of the retinal veins. Capillaries herniate and form microaneurysms or macroaneurysms, and many vessels will rupture into the retina or the preretinal space. Much of the retinal vasculature will leak serum into the retinal space, forming patches of edema throughout the macular, paramacular, and posterior polar regions. Eventually, multiple exudates will form in the regions of edematous and hemorrhagic activity. As the entire condition worsens, multiple intraretinal shunting complexes can be observed, and vision frequently decreases. The visual acuity and visual field sensitivity can continue to deteriorate markedly as the nonproliferative phase of diabetic retinopathy progresses.

Ancillary diagnostic examinations. Fluorescein angiography is most helpful for determining the extent of the microangiopathy; it illustrates the areas of infarction, intraretinal and preretinal vascular leakage, microaneurysm formation, and regions of retinal edema and fluid retention. The integrity of the perifoveal capillary network, as well as some indication of the vascular decompensation of the macular and paramacular region, can also be demonstrated by fluorescein angiography.

Stereoscopic color fundus photography, as well as regular fundus photography, are helpful in documenting the progression of the nonproliferative phases of the diabetic retinopathy process.

Visual field examinations will show multiple scotomas. However, these scotomas change location commonly, and knowing their location provides little advantage in determining the severity of the retinopathy.

Indications for photocoagulation. If the integrity of the foveal and macular regions is threatened by marked retinal vessel leakage or hemorrhage, photocoagulation of these small diseased areas should be considered if they are outside the perifoveal capillary network and at least 0.5 DD from the umbo.

Larger areas of macular and paramacular leakage into the retina or zones of total infarction can be considered for photocoagulation if they are at least 0.5 DD from the umbo and do not occupy macular areas greater than 1.5 DD in extent.

Large microaneurysms or macroaneurysms located in the macular region at least 0.5 DD from the umbo can be considered for photocoagulation because of the possibility of rupture and hemorrhage into the vitreous cavity. These areas can also be considered for photocoagulation because they usually leak profusely.

Photocoagulation approach. Topical use of an anesthetic and a plano contact lens are required for photocoagulation of nonproliferative diabetic retinopathy vascular defects in the paramacular region. Macular and perifoveal defects should be treated after a retrobulbar anesthetic has been administered to produce extraocular muscle akinesia and ocular anesthesia.

If they occupy a region more than 750μ (0.5 DD) from the umbo, discrete vascular abnormalities, such as macroaneurysms and large intraretinal shunting complexes, can be treated directly with **100μ to 200μ** coagulations at **200- to 300-mw** power intensities and **0.1- to 0.2-sec** exposures (Fig. 7-14). At the time of photocoagulation the retina surrounding the vascular malformation should be coagulated to some extent and the abnormal vessel constricted (Grade III) (Figs. 7-15 and 7-16).

Areas of diffuse intraretinal leakage can be coagulated directly with similar powers and exposures if the area of proposed photocoagulation is at least 750μ from the umbo and occupies an area no greater than 20% of the total macular region. It has been shown that photocoagulation to areas of diffuse leakage or infarction should be applied carefully at

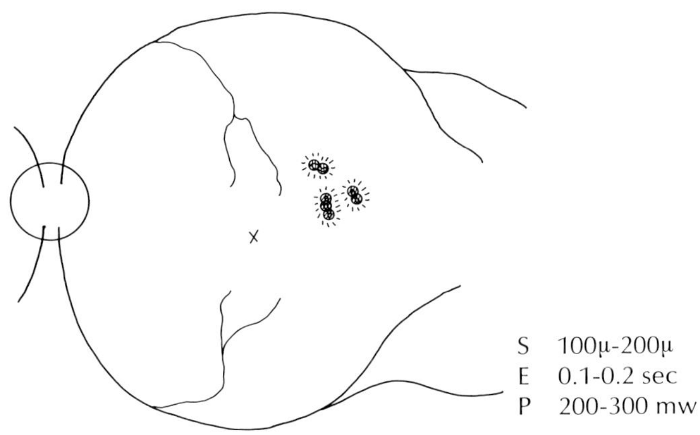

Fig. 7-14. Placement of contiguous or overlapping, punctate 100μ to 200μ coagulations in areas of advanced retinal vascular leakage. Coagulations should be at least ½ DD from the central fovea (umbo).

A

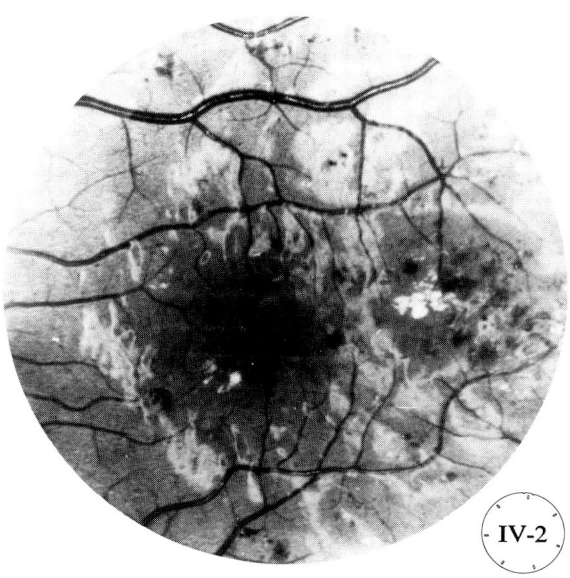

B

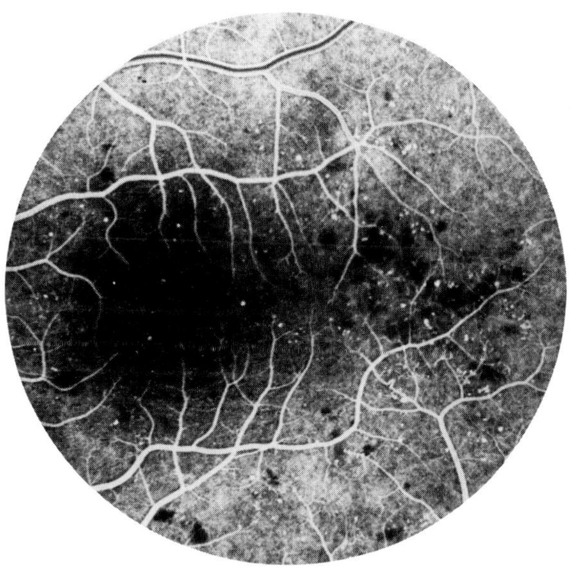

Fig. 7-15. A, Left macular and paramacular region of a 27-year-old man with diabetes of 17 years' duration, showing moderately advanced retinal edema, hemorrhagic activity, and exudate formation. **B,** Fluorogram showing multiple microaneurysm formations and early leakage temporal to the macular region during the early arteriolovenular transit phase. *Continued.*

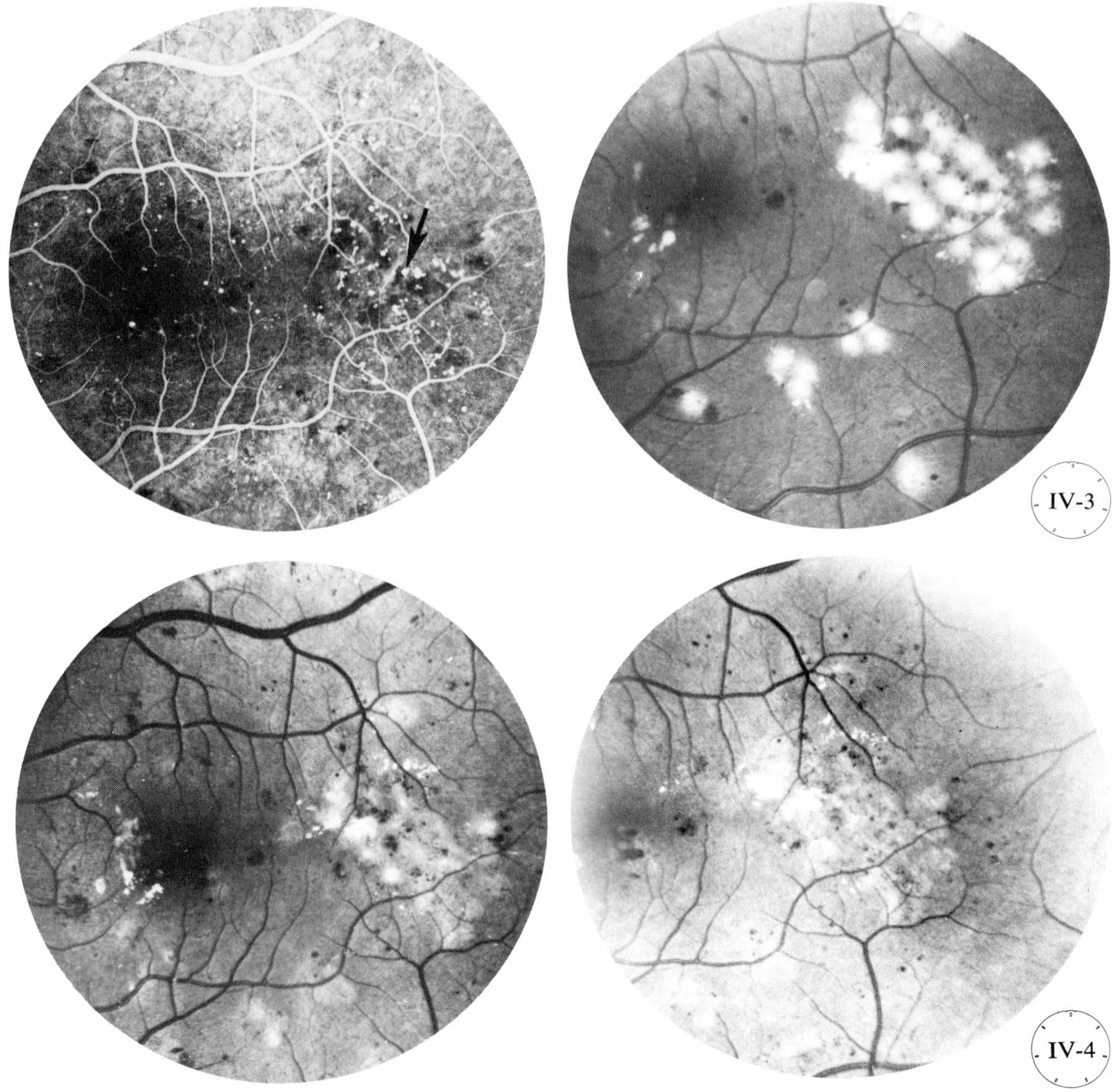

Fig. 7-15, cont'd. C, Fluorogram showing more pronounced microaneurysm and macroaneurysm formations (arrow) and moderately extensive leakage temporal to the macular region during the early venular transit phase. **D,** Treated area immediately after 200μ punctate coagulations were applied to the regions of most extensive retinal vascular leakage temporal to the macular zone. Hemorrhages and nonleaking microaneurysms were not treated. **E,** Treated area 6 weeks after photocoagulation, showing decreased edema and microaneurysm formation. **F,** Treated area 3 months after argon laser photocoagulation, showing a decrease in the edema, hemorrhagic activity, and exudate formation. The visual acuity remained at 20/20 during the treatment interval.

extended intervals, so that the macular region can acclimate to the photocoagulation therapy. If the area of photocoagulation is restricted to below 20% of the macular region, the macula appears to compensate for the photocoagulation therapy without difficulty. Photocoagulation of larger areas occasionally produces increased macular decompensation resulting in the formation of foveal microcystic edema.

At least 2 months should elapse before additional photocoagulation is considered for any retinal vascular abnormalities in the macular area. Another fluorescein angiogram

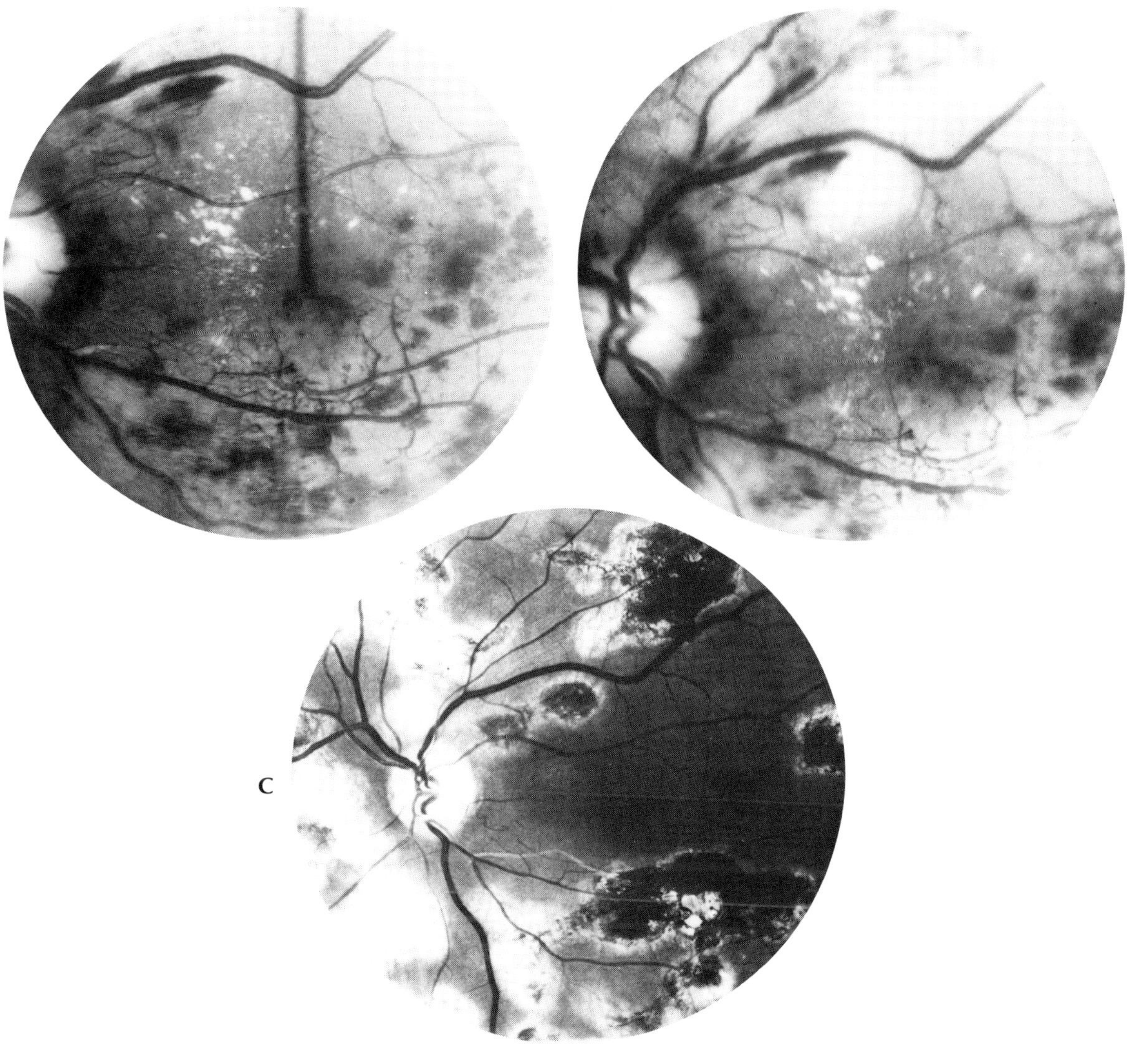

A B C

Fig. 7-16. A, A 51-year-old man with diabetes of 21 years' duration had a vision of 20/100, severe hemorrhagic activity, intraretinal shunting complexes, and marked macular edema (fixation pointer marks central fovea). **B,** Xenon-arc photocoagulation to the region of marked intraretinal shunting and edema along the vascular arcades was performed with 6° coagulations at a Red II intensity and 0.2-sec exposure interval for a Grade 3 coagulation. **C,** Healed eye 10 weeks after photocoagulation, showing complete destruction of the abnormal intraretinal shunting complexes. The macular region showed very little retinal edema and no hemorrhagic activity, although the vision improved only slightly, to $20/70^{-1}$.

taken at this time will show any areas of increased leakage or intraretinal microvascular abnormalities. These areas can then be considered for treatment; the various considerations and parameters listed in the previous paragraphs should again be followed.

Complications. The most common complication of the treatment of nonproliferative diabetic retinopathy is the formation of macular striae and observable scotomas. If treatment is employed away from the fovea and with moderate photocoagulation intensities, these complications can be minimized.

Hemorrhages at the treatment site have been observed rarely and have not been of great consequence.

Follow-up. As noted previously, approximately 2 months after photocoagulation, fluorescein angiography should be performed to document the vascular status of the macular region. Additional photocoagulation can be considered at this time if the vascular compensation has decreased. The patient should be followed by regular or stereoscopic color fundus photography at each visit.

Proliferative diabetic retinopathy

The growth and physical characteristics, the response to argon laser photocoagulation, the potential hazards encountered, and the photocoagulation technique required in diabetic retinopathy indicate that five different types of retinovitreal neovascularization exist, at least from a photocoagulation viewpoint. These five types of neovascularization are epipapillary, peripapillary, papillovitreal, retinovitreal, and preretinal.

Epipapillary neovascularization

Ophthalmoscopic appearance. Epipapillary neovascularization can be defined as new blood vessel formation extending from the central optic disc area a short distance into the vitreous (Fig. 7-17). These vessels take the form of wispy or fibrillar channels of blood that may be interspersed with more closely associated tufts or berrylike clumps of vascular tissue. This neovascularization usually carries a small volume of blood and is usually not supported by extensive glial proliferation during its early stages. At this time the new vessels are confined principally to the optic nerve area; there is little tendency for them to proliferate along the vascular arcades.

Epipapillary neovascularization usually begins with minute budding from one of the smaller vessels on the optic nerve; this budding later develops into a network of delicate

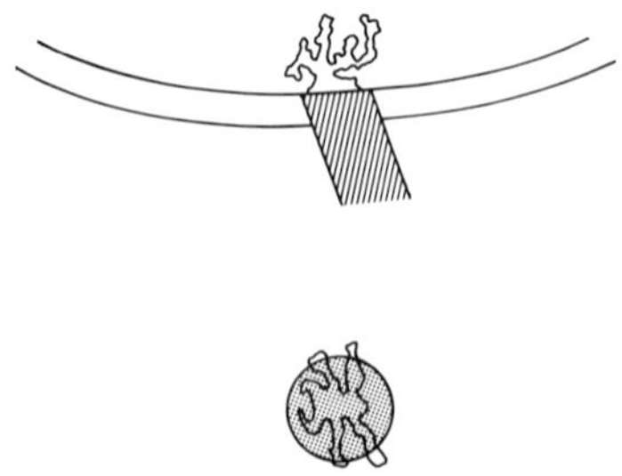

Fig. 7-17. Epipapillary neovascularization, characterized by wispy, threadlike neovascular growths from the optic nerve into the vitreous, presumably along the highly detached posterior hyaloid.

vessels that can be seen only with the magnification afforded by the direct ophthalmoscope or by biomicroscopy with the precorneal or corneal lens. More mature and later phases of epipapillary neovascularization suggest that the neovascularization is adherent to the posterior hyaloid for support. Occasionally, proliferation can extend along the vascular arcades. Neovascularization of this type tends to grow rather slowly unless it is aggravated by hypertensive episodes or other systemic problems. Ultimately, it can extend far into the vitreous, accompanied by marked glial proliferation around the vessels, and convert to the more widespread papillovitreal type of neovascularization.

Photocoagulation approach. The treatment of epipapillary neovascularization can be difficult because of the small amount of intravascular hemoglobin present with which to absorb the argon laser beam. Smaller amounts of energy are converted to heat, and relatively high input energies must be used to create satisfactory coagulations. In addition, the epipapillary neovascularization is commonly intertwined with the major vessels and may be difficult to isolate for adequate treatment.

Coagulation of epipapillary neovascularization must be sufficient to cause total obliteration during the early treatment sessions. Neovascular injury, rather than obliteration, may produce marked fibrovascular proliferation in the treatment area. It may be advisable to postpone therapy until the epipapillary frond has developed beyond the wispy neovascular stage, so that larger amounts of hemoglobin can be obtained in the treated vessels.

The diameter of the attenuated coagulation spot should be slightly larger than the largest vessel that will be treated in the neovascular area (**50μ to 75μ**).

Exposures between **0.05 to 0.1 sec** are selected, and a test photocoagulation is made to a retinal area outside the vascular arcades.

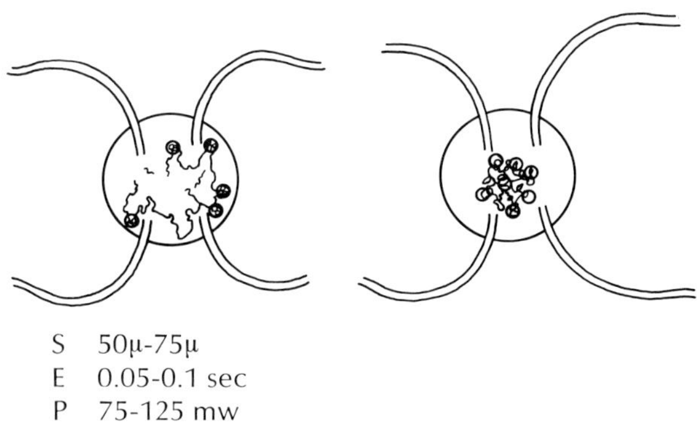

Fig. 7-18. Photocoagulation parameters used with punctate, interrupted coagulations in the areas of epipapillary neovascularization.

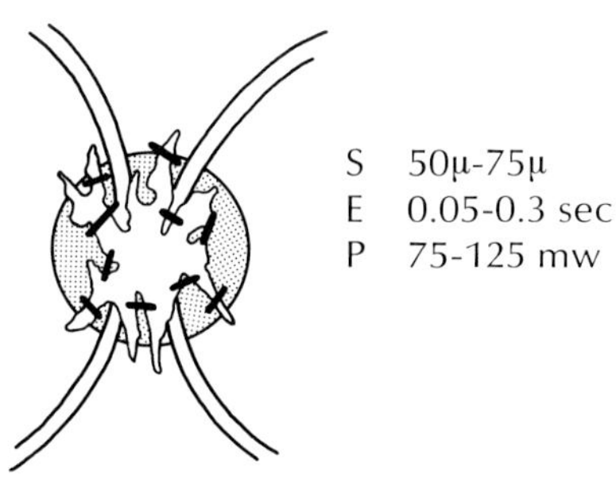

Fig. 7-19. Photocoagulation parameters used with the streaked, interrupted photocoagulation technique for epipapillary neovascularization.

The power level can then be adjusted in **25-mw** steps, starting with an initial power of approximately **50 mw,** until a mucoid white coagulation (Grade 2) is observed in this noncritical area. This power level is recorded.

The attenuated beam is directed onto the epipapillary neovascularization; the feeder vessel, if it can be found by ophthalmoscopy or by fluorescein angiography, is then treated with multiple impacts. The power input is raised in 25-mw steps until spasm of the feeder vessel can be observed through the biomicroscope (Fig. 7-18).

Photocoagulation of the remainder of the epipapillary neovascularization is conducted with slightly reduced powers at the same exposures and spot size. Photocoagulation is

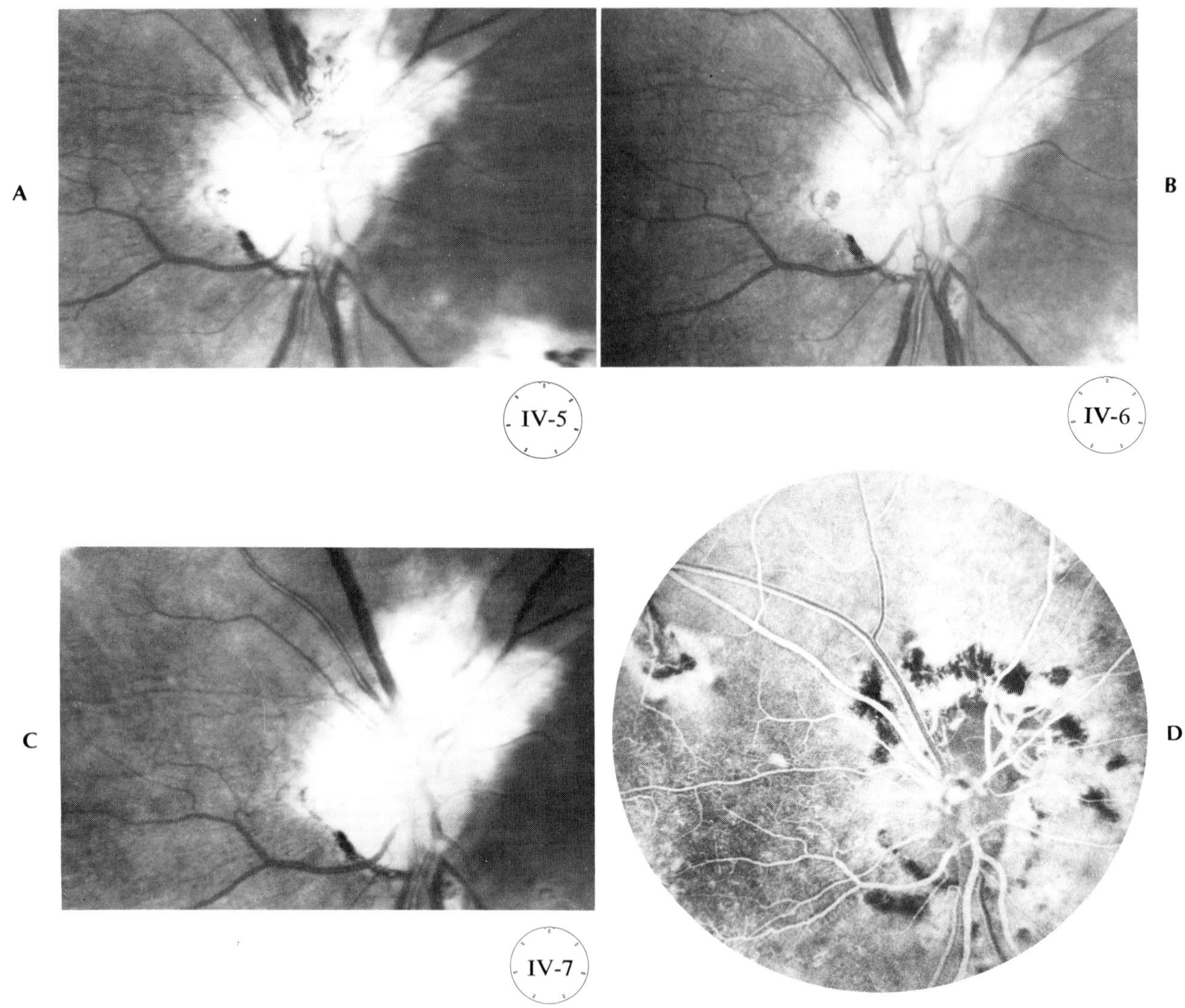

Fig. 7-20. A, Optic nerve region of a 25-year-old man with diabetes of 17 years' duration, showing moderately advanced epipapillary neovascularization. **B,** Epipapillary neovascularization immediately following argon laser photocoagulation with 75μ, streaked coagulations across the neovascular tissue. **C,** Healed optic nerve region 2 months after argon laser photocoagulation to the epipapillary neovascularization, showing complete obliteration of the neovascular tissue. **D,** Fluorogram showing the absence of perfusion of the neovascular area 2 months after argon laser photocoagulation to the epipapillary neovascularization.

restricted, when possible, to the inner rim of the optic nerve; the larger retinal vessels and the peripapillary area are avoided. Occasionally, short painting strokes can be employed across the neovascular vessels to create vascular spasm and coagulation (Fig. 7-19).

More extensive coagulation should be radial and not involve the maculopapillar bundle. Hemorrhages, segmented vessels, or areas of pigment proliferation on the optic nerve should be avoided; these areas can absorb higher amounts of energy, and the result may be possible damage to the nerve fiber layer.

The endpoint for photocoagulation of the more distal epipapillary neovascularization is the segmentation, blanching, and slightly grayish coagulation of the tissue. It is most important not to caramelize the neovascular tissue with extremely high energies (Figs. 7-20 and 7-21).

A

B

C

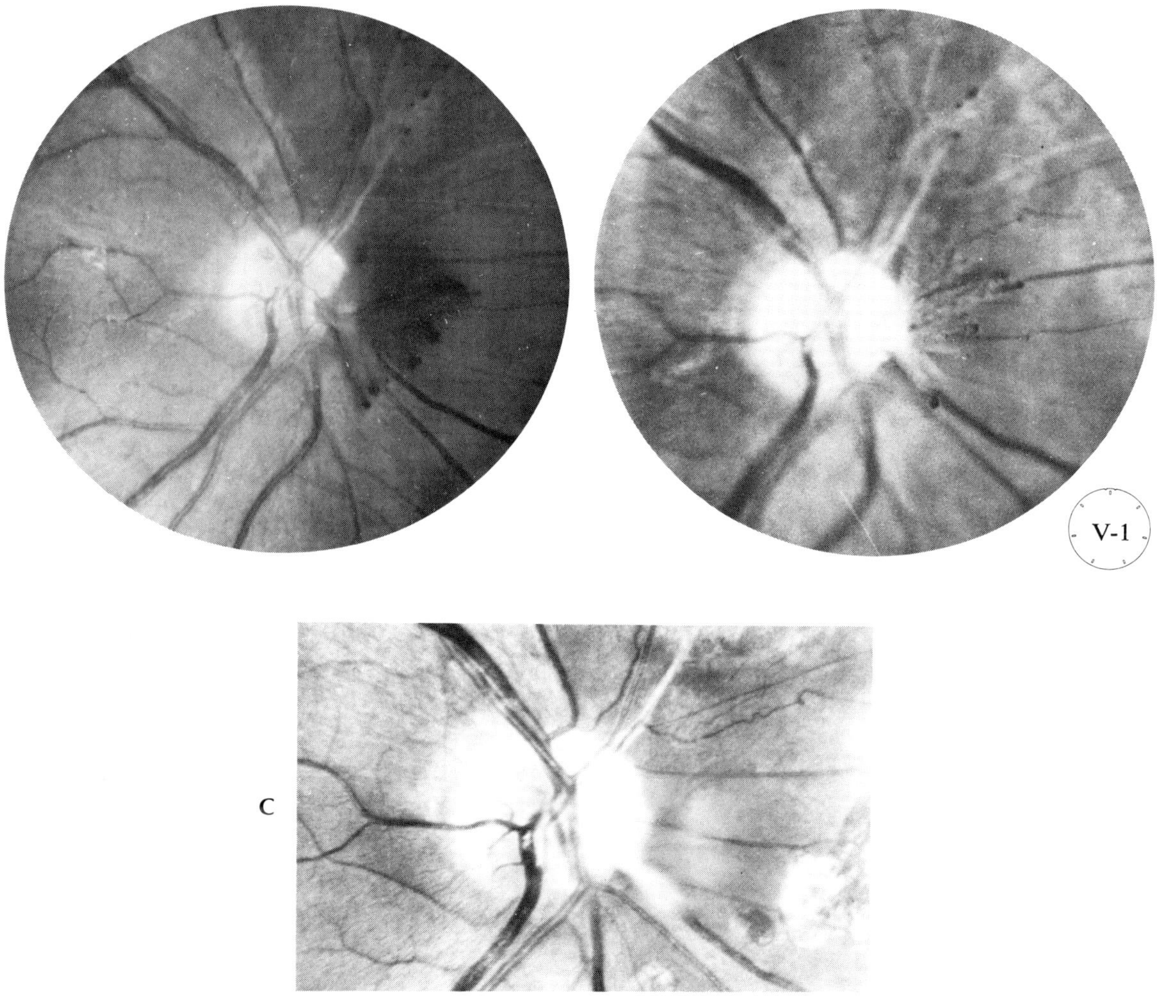

Fig. 7-21. A, An advanced epipapillary frond extending nasally from the optic disc in a 28-year-old man who had noticed blurred vision caused by repeated vitreous hemorrhages. **B,** Epipapillary frond immediately after argon laser photocoagulation, showing segmentation and obliteration of the neovascular tissue. **C,** Epipapillary neovascular area 2 months after argon laser photocoagulation, showing complete avascularity and only a suggestion of the glial stalk remaining nasally.

The epipapillary area should be evaluated in approximately 1 to 3 days, since recanalization of the treated vessels can occur. Retreatment should be instituted immediately if patent channels are observed ophthalmoscopically or by fluorescein angiography. Segmentation and slightly grayish coagulation of the tissue are then considered adequate treatment at this stage.

The eye should be examined again in approximately 2 weeks for possible recanalization or new growth of vessels. Similar examinations are conducted at 2-month intervals for 6 months, and treatment should be given if either condition exists. Fluorescein angiography should also be done at 6-month intervals to evaluate whether there is any suggestion of neovascular growth.

Peripapillary neovascularization

Ophthalmoscopic appearance. Peripapillary neovascularization can be described as neovascularization extending centrifugally from the optic nerve in a slightly elevated fashion over the surrounding retina, vascular arcades, and occasionally the macular region (Fig. 7-22). The neovascularization extends from the rim of the optic nerve to the peripapillary region and forms delicate arcades and webs of vessels with multiple arteriolar feeder and venular drainage channels. The peripapillary distribution of vessels is much like the mesenteric vessel distribution, and the progress of the neovascularization is by small endothelial tuft formation in a radial and circumferential manner. Neovascularization can originate in any quadrant of the optic disc; in early neovascularization, however, the spread of the disease appears to be toward the temporal vascular arcades. Extensive peripapillary neovascularization can extend 3 to 4 DD over the retinal surface; resembling a shallow saucer, its end curls gently toward the vitreous. The border of peripapillary neovascularization is scalloped like the arborization on a leaf; radiating channels extend from the optic disc to peripheral circumferential channels. Bleeding into the vitreous usually occurs from the distal vascular tufts along the arching channels, but decompensation may occur suddenly and massively from the more well developed central neovascular patches. The feeder vessels originate from the optic nerve region, although collateral circulation may be established later from the major vascular arcades. Little glial tissue appears between the vascular elements at first, but eventually glial proliferation becomes extensive and is closely interdigitated between the vascular elements.

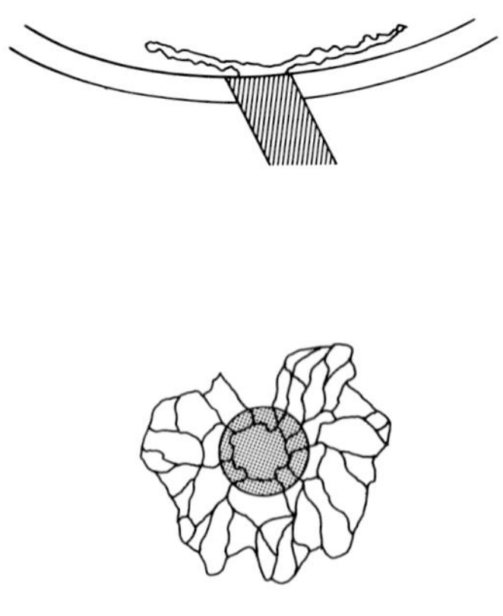

Fig. 7-22. Saucerlike configuration of the peripapillary neovascularization as it grows from the optic nerve along the posterior aspect of the shallowly detached posterior hyaloid membrane.

Photocoagulation approach. The architecture of the peripapillary fan of neovascularization should be determined carefully; approximation should be made of the width, distribution, and height of each vessel above the surface of the retina. The feeder vessel or vessels to the frond should be determined by fluorescein angiography and careful ophthalmoscopic surveillance. The amount and distribution of glial tissue in the fan, as well as areas of hyperpigmentation or hemoglobin concentration, should also be noted.

Since the destruction of large peripapillary fans by direct coagulation of all areas of neovascularization would involve destruction of a large portion of the underlying retina in a critical area, it is advisable to proceed in the following manner.

The feeder vessels are treated as they emerge from the inner rim of the optic nerve on their course into the peripapillary space. Treatment is instituted on the optic nerve with a coagulation size (**50μ to 75μ**) and power setting (usually **100 to 175 mw**) sufficient to cause spasm of the feeder vessels, thereby trapping the blood in the loops of the peripapillary fronds.

Continuous streak coagulations with spot sizes ranging from **50μ to 100μ** are then produced from the inner rim of the optic nerve peripherally in a radial fashion through the area of neovascularization to an extent of 1,000μ to 1,500μ (Fig. 7-23). The coagulations should be made, as much as possible, in the natural nerve fiber layer pattern so as to induce as little damage to this layer as possible. The radial coagulations are made between the large vascular arcades or other large background vessels with an intensity sufficient to cause interruption and segmentation of the neovascular frond (usually **150 to 200 mw**).

Smaller peripapillary neovascular arborizations can be obliterated more easily by simply interrupting the stalk vessels on the optic nerve and proceeding more peripherally with several oblique or radial coagulations designed to segment and obliterate the smaller tufts.

Larger spot sizes in the range of **100μ to 200μ** can be used to paint over the larger distal portions of the peripapillary frond in areas of definite endothelial budding. Effective obliteration of these peripheral areas has been obtained with the production of less dense, mucoid-appearing coagulations (Grade 2) (usually **150 to 225 mw**) rather than the more severe, dense, white coagulum (Grade 4) used for the radial coagulations (Figs. 7-24 to 7-27).

It is advisable to reevaluate the coagulated zone within 3 to 7 days to determine whether blood flow exists in the treated area and whether further coagulation should be performed. If it is found (either ophthalmoscopically or by fluorescein angiography) that

Text continued on p. 130.

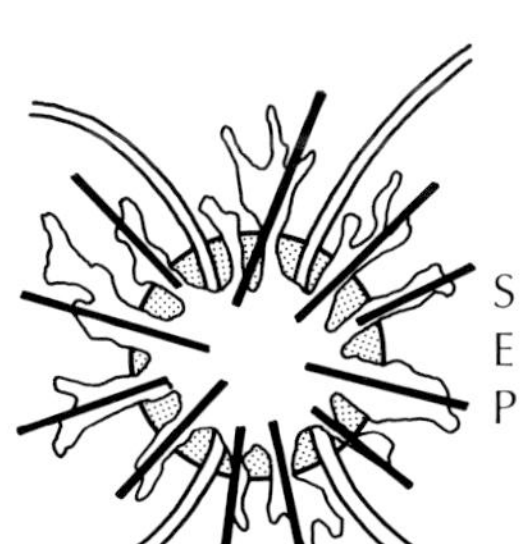

Fig. 7-23. Photocoagulation parameters and the radial photocoagulation technique utilized for peripapillary neovascularization.

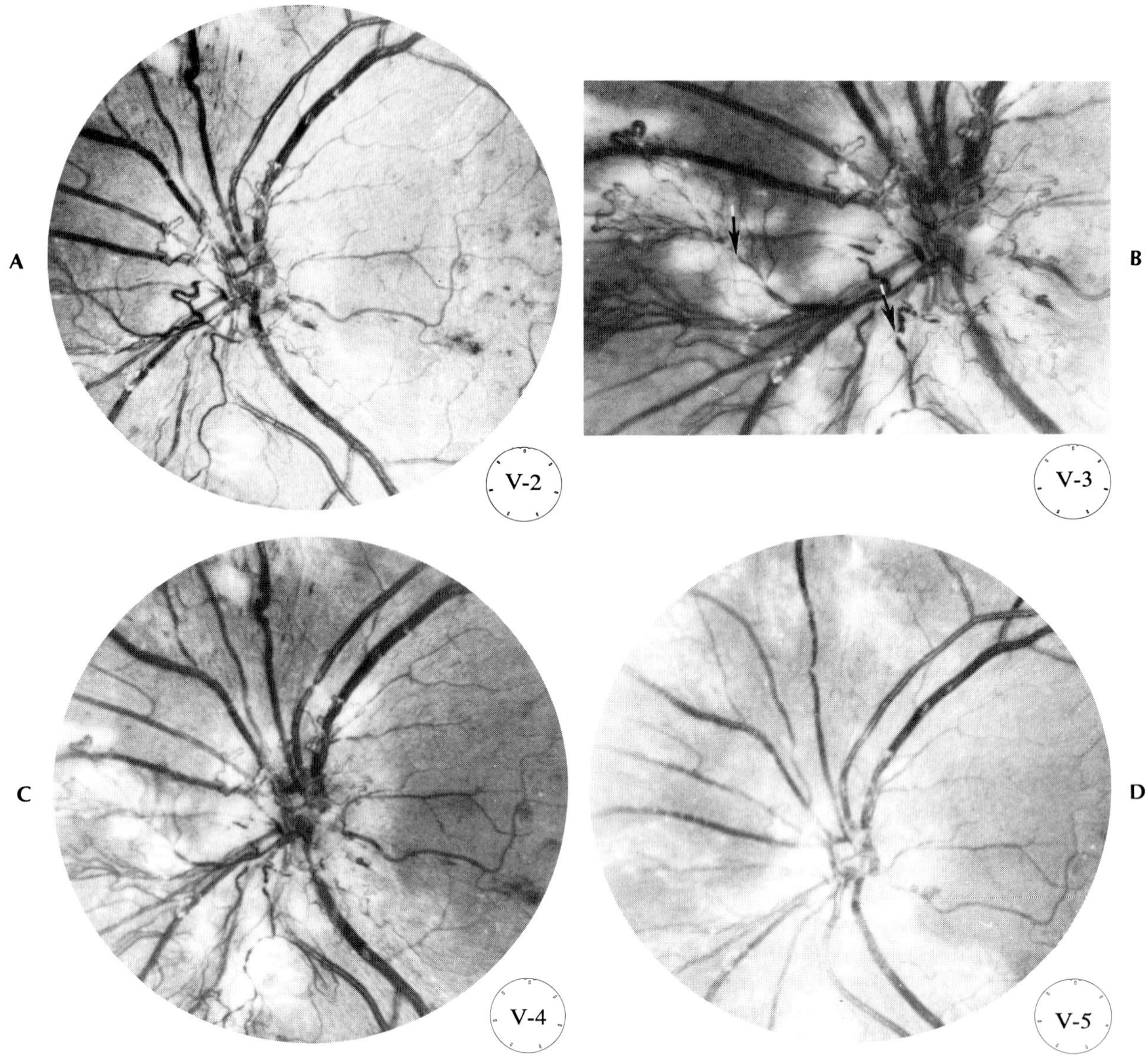

Fig. 7-24. A, Advanced peripapillary neovascularization in a 17-year-old high school girl. **B,** Radial coagulations were placed to produce segmentation and sequestering of the blood (arrows) in the distal aspects of the peripapillary neovascularization. **C,** Wide-angle view of the advanced peripapillary neovascularization immediately after argon laser photocoagulation, showing segmentation and obliteration of the vascular channels. **D,** Optic nerve region 7 weeks after argon laser photocoagulation to the peripapillary neovascularization, showing complete obliteration of the neovascular tissue.

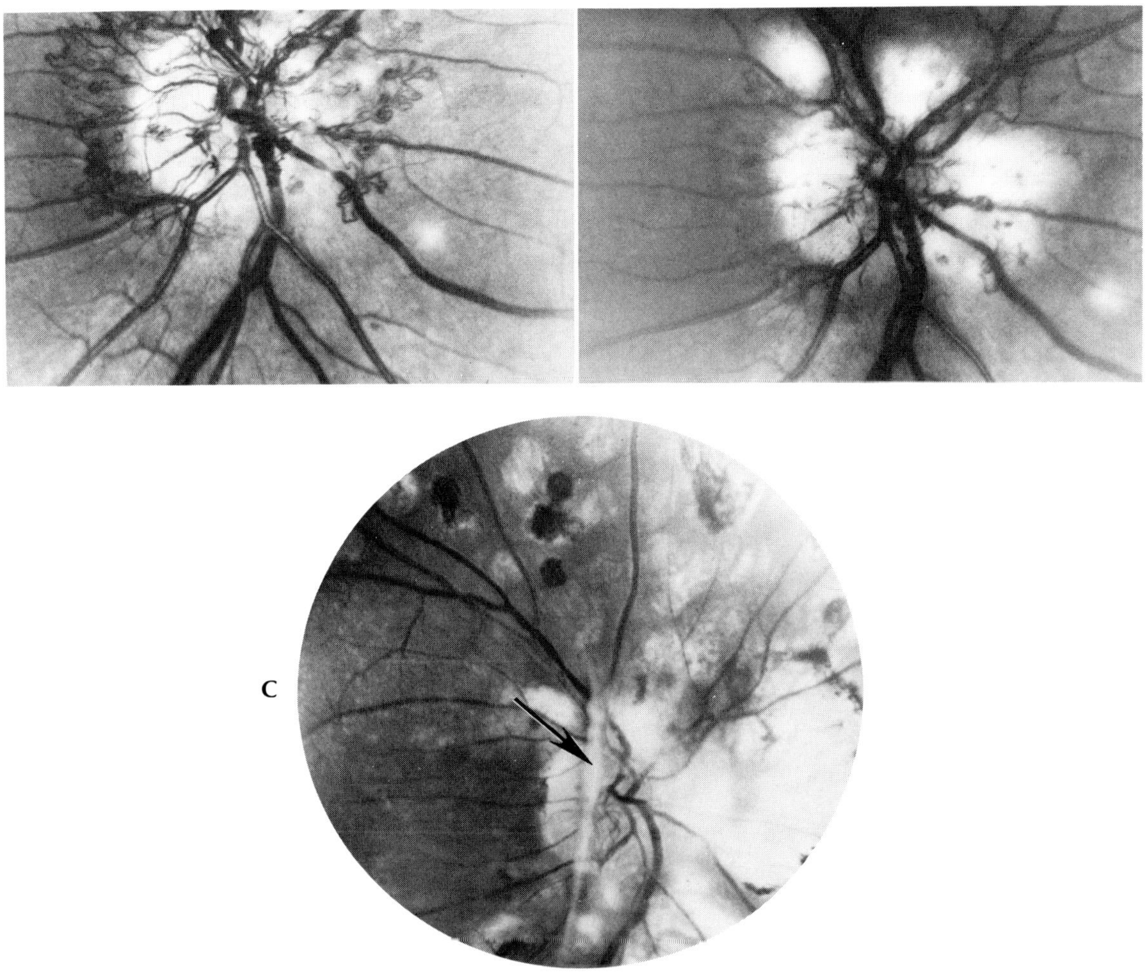

Fig. 7-25. A, Moderately advanced peripapillary neovascularization in a 48-year-old man. Marked vascular proliferation has occurred along the shallowly detached posterior hyaloid. **B,** Radial photocoagulations through all aspects of the peripapillary neovascularization, resulting in disruption of the vascular channels. **C,** Optic disc region 3 months after argon laser photocoagulation, showing complete disappearance of the peripapillary neovascularization and some overgrowth of glial tissue on the central optic nerve region (arrow).

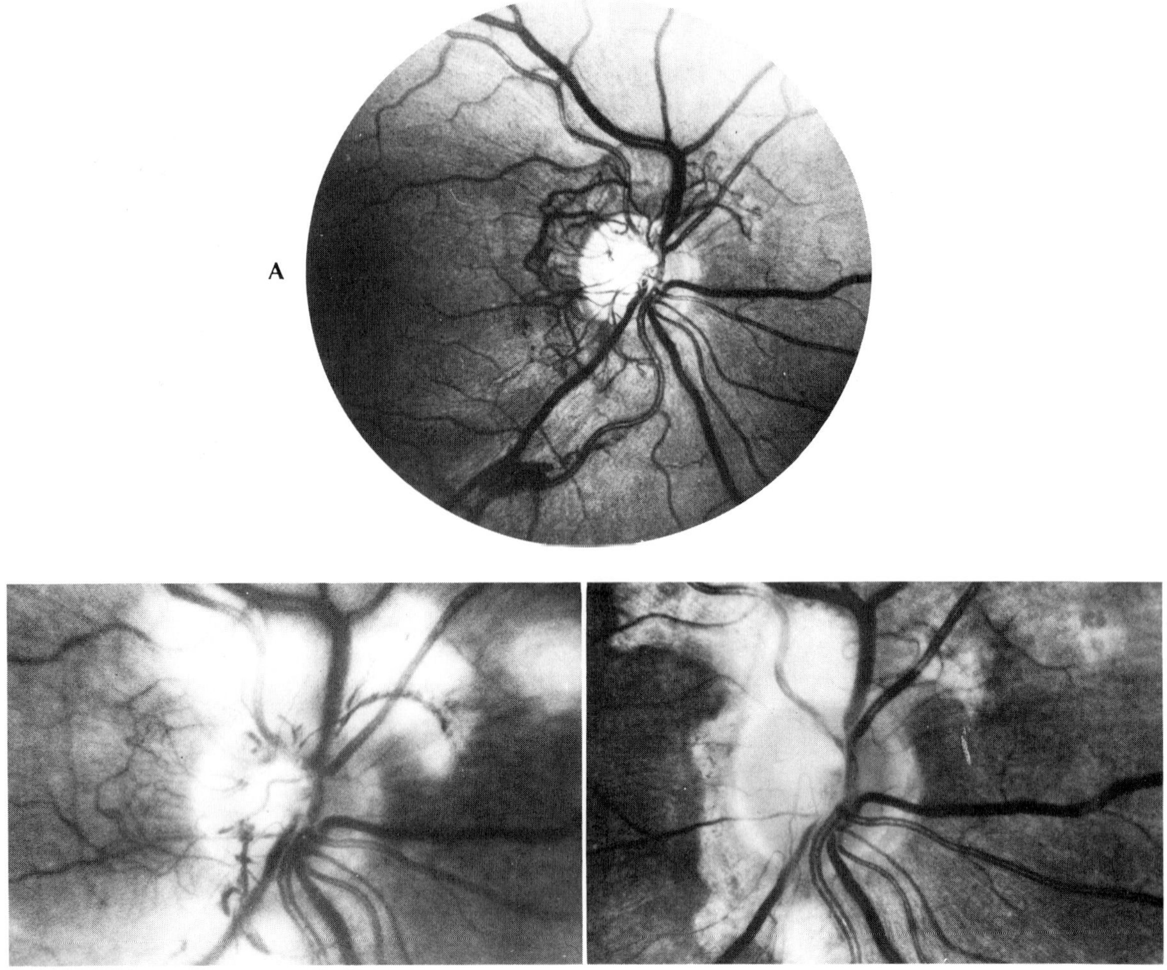

V-6

Fig. 7-26. A, Moderately advanced peripapillary neovascularization along the superior and temporal optic disc area in a 27-year-old woman with diabetes who had experienced multiple vitreous hemorrhages from this zone of neovascularization. **B,** Radial photocoagulations extending outward from the inner rim of the optic disc, producing segmentation and coagulation of the areas of neovascularization. **C,** Optic nerve area after eight focal argon laser photocoagulation treatments to the peripapillary neovascularization. The neovascular tissue has been obliterated and the ocular condition stabilized.

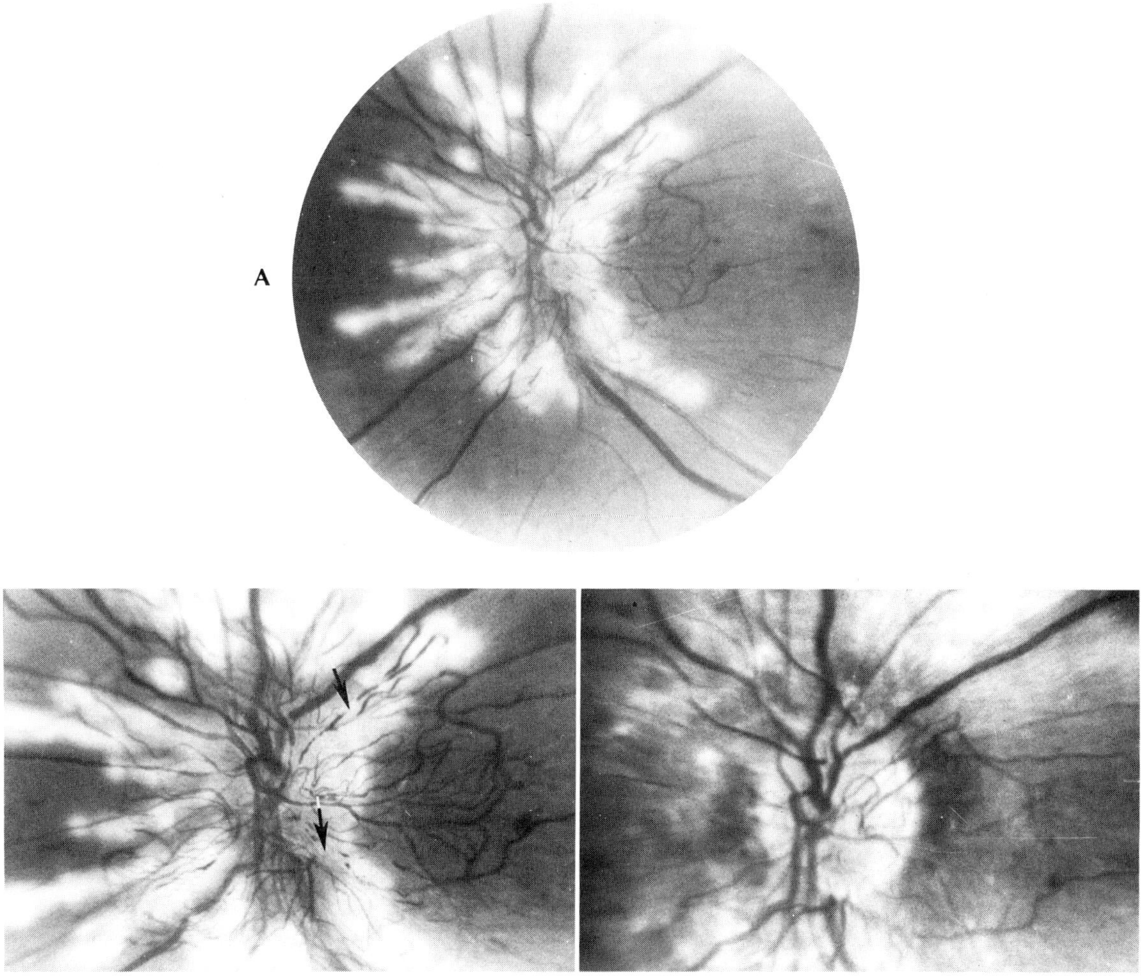

V-7

Fig. 7-27. A, Advanced peripapillary neovascularization extending from the region of the optic disc in a 49-year-old diabetic woman after radial photocoagulation. **B,** Enlarged view of the optic nerve region. Argon laser photocoagulation has produced marked coagulation and segmentation of the blood column in all areas of the peripapillary neovascularization (arrows). **C,** Optic nerve 7 weeks after argon laser photocoagulation to the peripapillary neovascularization. Several stringy inactive new vessels remain on the temporal aspect of the disc.

blood flow through the frond exists, photocoagulation should be performed; the patient should then be reevaluated in approximately 2 weeks. Several sessions may be necessary to create a coagulum that effectively blocks the blood flow through the neovascular tissue.

Papillovitreal neovascularization

Ophthalmoscopic appearance. Papillovitreal neovascularization can be defined as the massive amount of combined neovascular and glial tissue that extends from the head of the optic nerve far into the vitreous body (Fig. 7-28). It may represent the final developmental stage of epipapillary or possibly peripapillary neovascularization and usually has well-developed vascular channels initially. As the papillovitreal frond matures, the glial component is most prominent and becomes closely interdigitated with the vascular channels, which tend to regress to some degree. The neovascular proliferation extends into the vitreous by one of three processes. The most common process of proliferation is the intertwining of neovascular buds along the posterior hyaloid face, which acts as a trelliswork. The next most common proliferation route is along the residue of fibrin from a previous intravitreal hemorrhage. The least common proliferation process is the gradual budding and extension of the vascular channels into the vitreous from a well-established neovascular stalk that has become supported by glial tissue. These papillovitreal stalks are not apt to proliferate a great distance into the vitreous because of their lack of vertical supportive structures.

Three basic types of papillovitreal neovascularization exist: columnar, arcuate, and confluent. The columnar papillovitreal neovascularization extends along the posterior hyaloid in a closely gathered group of vessels and glial tissue proliferation. This extension of neovascular tissue is neither confined by nor closely associated with any of the vascular arcades and appears elongated without much lateral extension. One or more feeder vessels extend from the optic nerve into the frond, and 2 to 6 collector vessels then return the blood to the optic nerve region. Detection of the feeder and collector vessels is easily accomplished, and photocoagulation is usually successful.

The arcuate type of papillovitreal neovascularization originally extends along the

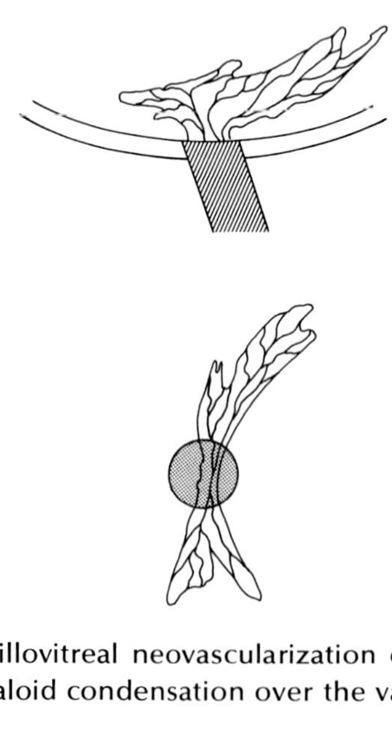

Fig. 7-28. Typical arcuate papillovitreal neovascularization extending from the optic nerve region along the posterior hyaloid condensation over the vascular arcades.

vascular arcades, more frequently to the temporal side, and initially begins with a somewhat higher proportion of glial tissue than does the columnar type. As the arcuate papillovitreal frond matures, a greater degree of lateral and intravitreal extension appears, as well as neovascular proliferation along the distal end of the supportive vascular arcade. In some cases, this type of neovascularization connects horizontally with the opposite arcade to form an interdigitation of neovascular and proliferative tissue, resulting in a large interhemispherical shunting complex. Growth during the initial stages of formation is rapid throughout the central body of the frond, but during the late mature stages it is confined to endothelial budding along the distal aspect and border of the large frond. During the early stages of development, bleeding can occur from any of the vessels and may be disastrous. The later stages are marked by smaller hemorrhagic episodes, which usually emanate from the small endothelial buds that form along the outer margins of the body of the frond. Because of the marked involvement of the posterior hyaloid face by the proliferating glial and vascular tissue, contracture of the frond, the posterior hyaloid or any of the components of the vitreous body will cause great strain on the retina in the posterior pole in the peripapillary region. It is common to find the end stage of this type of neovascularization represented by a central tentlike retinal detachment with marked striae radiating from the central frond to the more peripheral parts of the retina.

The confluent type of papillovitreal neovascularization can be described as neovascular glial tissue that has extended from the optic nerve into the vitreous body without lateral extension or any close association with the vascular arcades. This neovascularization can take the form of either a shallow saucer or a partial, deeper, cuplike configuration and can extend to any size. The feeder vessels are multiple, and without the aid of fluorescein angiography they are difficult to differentiate from the collector vessels, which also may be multiple. Growth may be extremely rapid with this type of neovascularization because of its multidimensional vascularity. Growth is usually oriented toward the nasal side, but large fronds have been seen extending directly over the macular area in a canopy fashion, completely obscuring the central vision. Bleeding into the vitreous is usually from the distal portion of the frond; occasionally, however, massive vitreal hemorrhages occur from the proximal feeder or collector vessels during a period of extreme hypertension.

Photocoagulation approach. The primary treatment procedure involves the occlusion of the feeder vessels in the papillovitreal frond and subsequent painting and coagulation of the hemoglobin trapped within the distal frond.

Attempts should be made in the treatment of any of the three types of papillovitreal

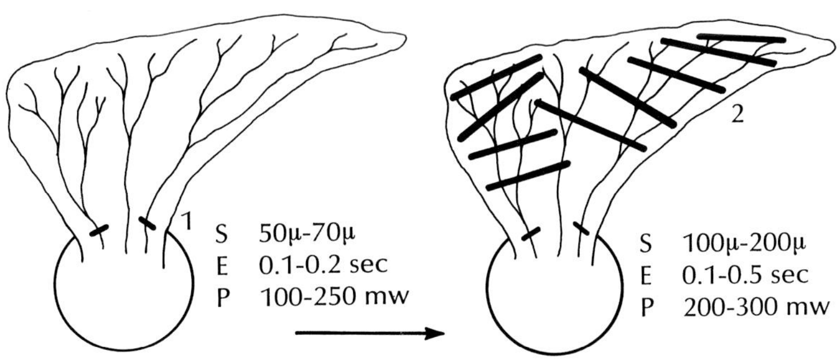

Fig. 7-29. Photocoagulation parameters utilizing the feeder-frond technique wherein the feeder vessels are coagulated initially, *1*, and the more distal aspects of the frond are coagulated with larger coagulations in a streaked fashion, *2*.

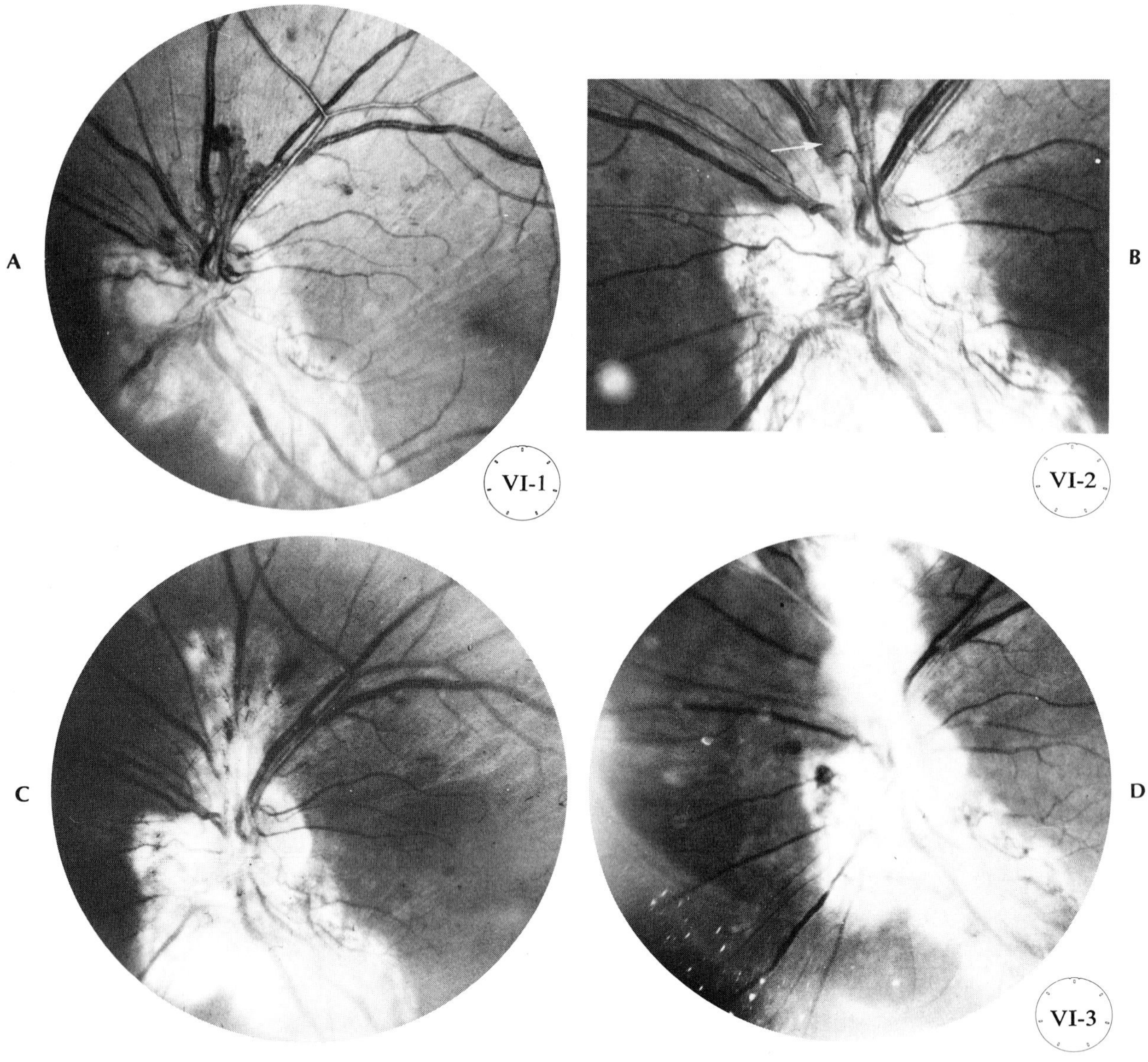

Fig. 7-30. A, A moderately advanced arcuate papillovitreal frond in a 28-year-old man who had experienced repeated vitreous hemorrhages from this area of neovascularization. **B,** Papillovitreal frond immediately after photocoagulation, showing segmentation of the feeder vessels and portions of the more distal frond area (arrow). **C,** Arcuate papillovitreal frond 10 days after photocoagulation, showing complete disruption of the immature vascular channels. **D,** Posterior polar region 2 months after argon laser photocoagulation to the arcuate papillovitreal frond, showing complete obliteration and lack of perfusion of the neovascular tissue.

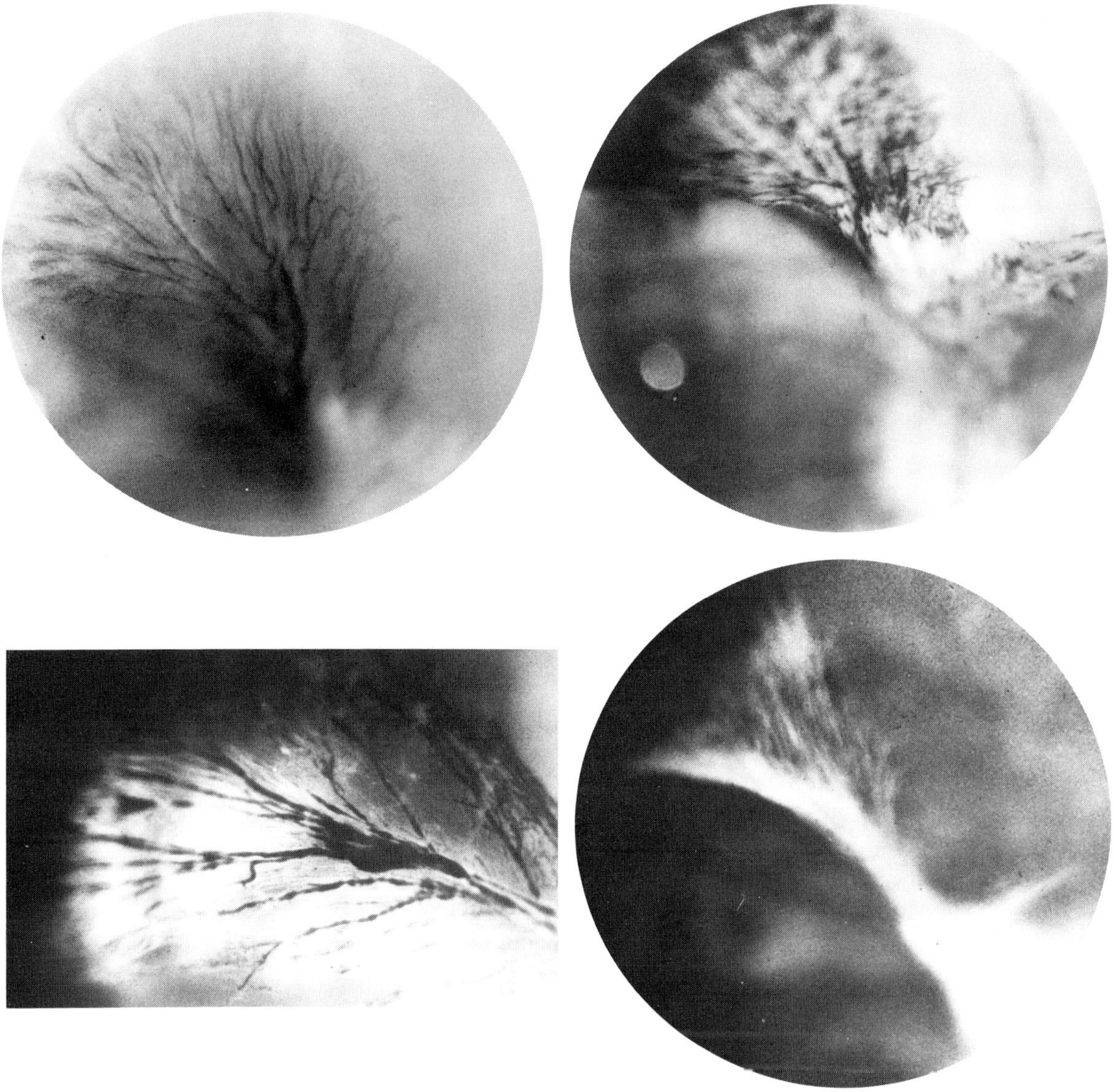

Fig. 7-31. A, An extremely large, mature arcuate papillovitreal frond in a 32-year-old diabetic woman whose vision had been decreased to the level of counting fingers because of repeated vitreous hemorrhages. Note the well-entrenched vascular channels and increased glial supportive tissue. **B,** Large arcuate frond immediately after argon laser photocoagulation to the entire frond. **C,** Magnified view of the segmentation and coagulation of the vascular channels in the frond immediately after argon laser photocoagulation. **D,** Treated arcuate papillovitreal frond 10 weeks after argon laser photocoagulation, showing complete disappearance of the vascular tissue with only glial supportive tissue remaining in the avascular stalk.

neovascularization to isolate the feeder vessels by fluorescein angiography or hemobarometry. The feeder vessels are then treated within the optic nerve region with a coagulation size (**50μ to 70μ**) and power level (**100 to 250 mw**) sufficient to produce spasm (Grade II), or possibly a coagulation of those feeder vessels (Grade III) (Fig. 7-29). Solitary impacts (**0.1 sec**) or short coagulation strokes (**0.2 to 0.5 sec**) across the feeder vessels are advisable and are usually sufficient to produce the appropriate vascular spasm or coagulation. Ideally, all feeder vessels should be coagulated; realistically, however, any decrease in the arteriolar feeder flow into the frond by coagulation of any number of the feeder vessels will result in a decrease in the flow rate of blood through the distal portions of the frond, and a reduced energy requirement for coagulating these distal areas (Figs. 7-30 and 7-31).

Feeder vessels into the columnar type of neovascularization are readily discernible, and coagulation of these vessels at the inner rim of the optic nerve area can be accomplished easily. The arcuate and confluent types of neovascularization incorporate feeding channels that are more intimately combined with glial tissue and, in some instances, are hidden from both fluorescein angiographic and ophthalmoscopic view. Therefore, the search for the feeders and the ultimate coagulation of these feeder vessels may be more difficult and occasionally impossible. Attempts should be made, nevertheless, to decrease the inflow into the large papillovitreal fronds.

Occasionally, segmentation of the blood column can be seen at this point, although a slight pulsatile movement of the blood remains. If the segmented portions of the blood column move slowly through the channels, it must be assumed that one of the feeder vessels is still partially open. This situation is not a great problem if photocoagulation is performed immediately. Serum and protein particles smaller than erythrocytes can pass through a vessel in spasm, however, and clumps of erythrocytes in the distal frond can be pushed through the vessels by this mechanism, eventually evacuating the frond of any hemoglobin content and dramatically reducing the effectiveness of argon laser photocoagulation on these distal regions. Therefore, once segmentation or a reduction in blood flow has taken place, as observed by the use of higher biomicroscopic magnification, photocoagulation of the distal frond should be done immediately.

Photocoagulation of the distal aspects of the papillovitreal frond is then performed with **100μ to 200μ** coagulations at approximately **200 to 300 mw** of power. These power inputs may vary, depending on the clarity of the media and the ratio of vascular to glial proliferation in the frond. More power is usually required if advanced amounts of glial tissue are present. The distal neovascular tissue is treated with interrupted exposures of **0.1 to 0.2 sec** or with short painting strokes (**0.2 to 0.5 sec**). The coagulation endpoint is usually a change in the morphologic configuration and a slight graying of the treated vessels after the photocoagulation procedure (Grade III). The latter usually occurs when a large amount of glial tissue is present in close association with the vascular components. It is usually advisable not to re-treat adequately treated areas with additional argon laser photocoagulation, since these well-treated vessels are extremely fragile; even slight amounts of heat can cause rupture of these particular vessels.

Re-treatment of the feeder and collector vessels can then be performed, since presumably the entire vascular perfusion system has been occluded and there is no longer any fear that blockage of the collector channels will lead to ballooning or rupture of the vessels in the frond. More permanent occlusion of these vessels is important for preventing reperfusion of the more distal areas after treatment.

The treated frond is then evaluated after an interval of 3 hours to 3 days so that any

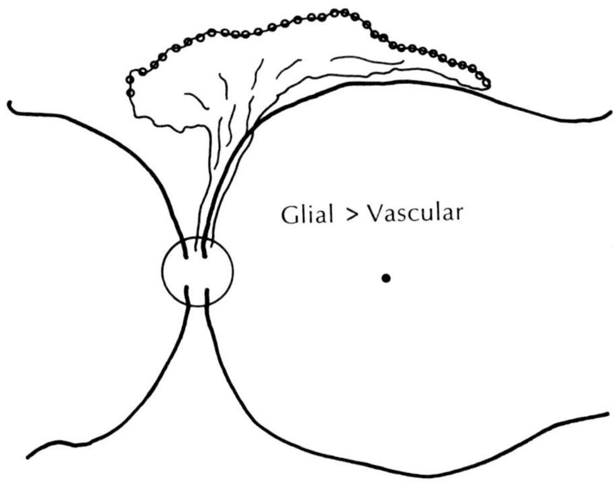

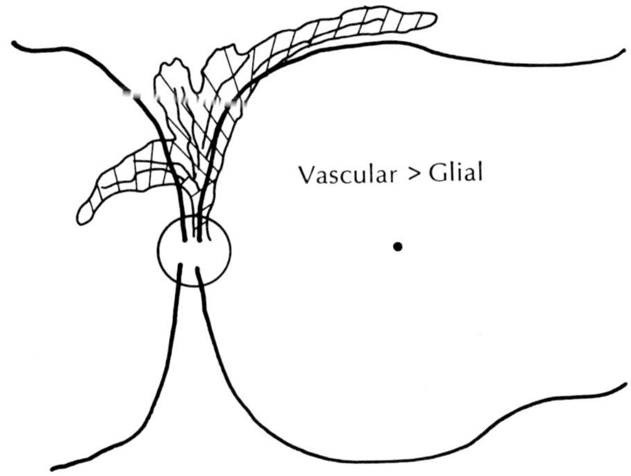

Fig. 7-32. Photocoagulation approach to immature (vascular content greater than glial) papillovitreal fronds, as illustrated in Fig. 7-29, and mature fronds (glial content greater than vascular), as noted in Fig. 7-33.

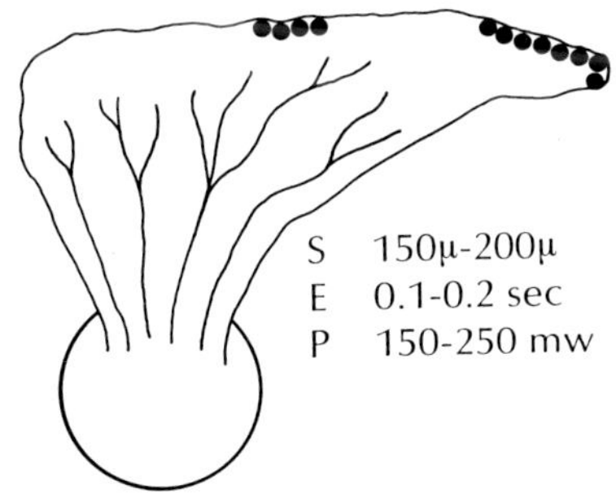

Fig. 7-33. Photocoagulation should be directed to vascular proliferation on the border of a mature frond rather than to the well-entrenched vessels in the body of the highly glial arcuate frond.

vessels still perfused in the region of the treated frond can be detected. Treatment is then repeated on the patent vessels with coagulation spot sizes of **100μ to 200μ** at an exposure interval of **0.2 sec,** and with lower power levels in the range of **50 to 150 mw.** It can be considered that coagulation has been accomplished when a slight graying and constriction of the impact area is observed (Grade III). At this stage fluorescein angiography may be required for the demonstration of any channels with vascular flow, since ophthalmoscopic visualization alone may not prove adequate.

The patient is reexamined in approximately 1 week, and another fluorescein angiogram may be necessary for the identification of any channels that are still patent. These channels are treated in a manner similar to that demonstrated in Fig. 7-29, and the patient is asked to return at 2-week intervals for repeated evaluations. This routine is followed until total obliteration or glial reinforcement of the frond has been accomplished.

As the papillovitreal frond matures, becoming less vascular and more gliotic, areas of neovascularization develop along the border of the frond tissue. These endothelial buds and more well formed neovascular channels at the distal edge of the frond can proliferate rapidly and extend along the posterior hyaloid or other supportive structures. Treatment is directed toward obliteration of the fragile distal areas of neovascularization, since they have a tendency to rupture easily because of hypertensive episodes or excessive traction on the neovascular tufts.

Photocoagulation therapy for these neovascular areas consists of individual impacts directed along the border of the neovascularization. Coagulation sizes of **150μ to 200μ**, exposures of **0.1 to 0.2 sec,** and powers of **150 to 250 mw** have proved sufficient for obliteration (Grade 4) (Figs. 7-32 and 7-33). Treatment sessions may have to be repeated at

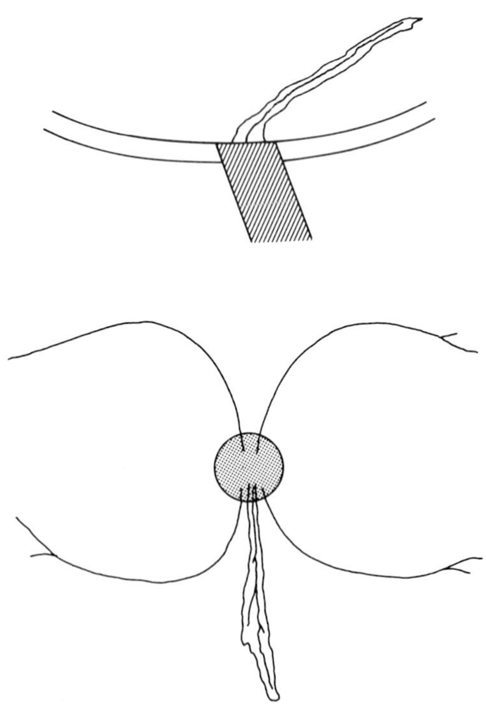

Fig. 7-34. A columnar papillovitreal frond extending in a narrow and direct fashion from the optic disc along the posterior hyaloid into the vitreous cavity.

intervals of 3 to 7 days for the optimal coagulative effect. The coagulation endpoint is a graying of the neovascular tissue; this graying usually results in obliteration. Patients must be followed closely at 3- to 6-week intervals in order to assess the effect of therapy. Excessive coagulation of the distal frond should be avoided, since shrinkage of the frond or hyaloid tissue will result in the occurrence of stress hemorrhages. Furthermore, the stalk or more proximal frond tissue need not be treated, since neovascularization occurs less frequently in this area, and the proximal glial overgrowth tends to scatter the coagulation beam, thereby decreasing the effectiveness of the coagulation therapy (Figs. 7-34 to 7-36).

A

B

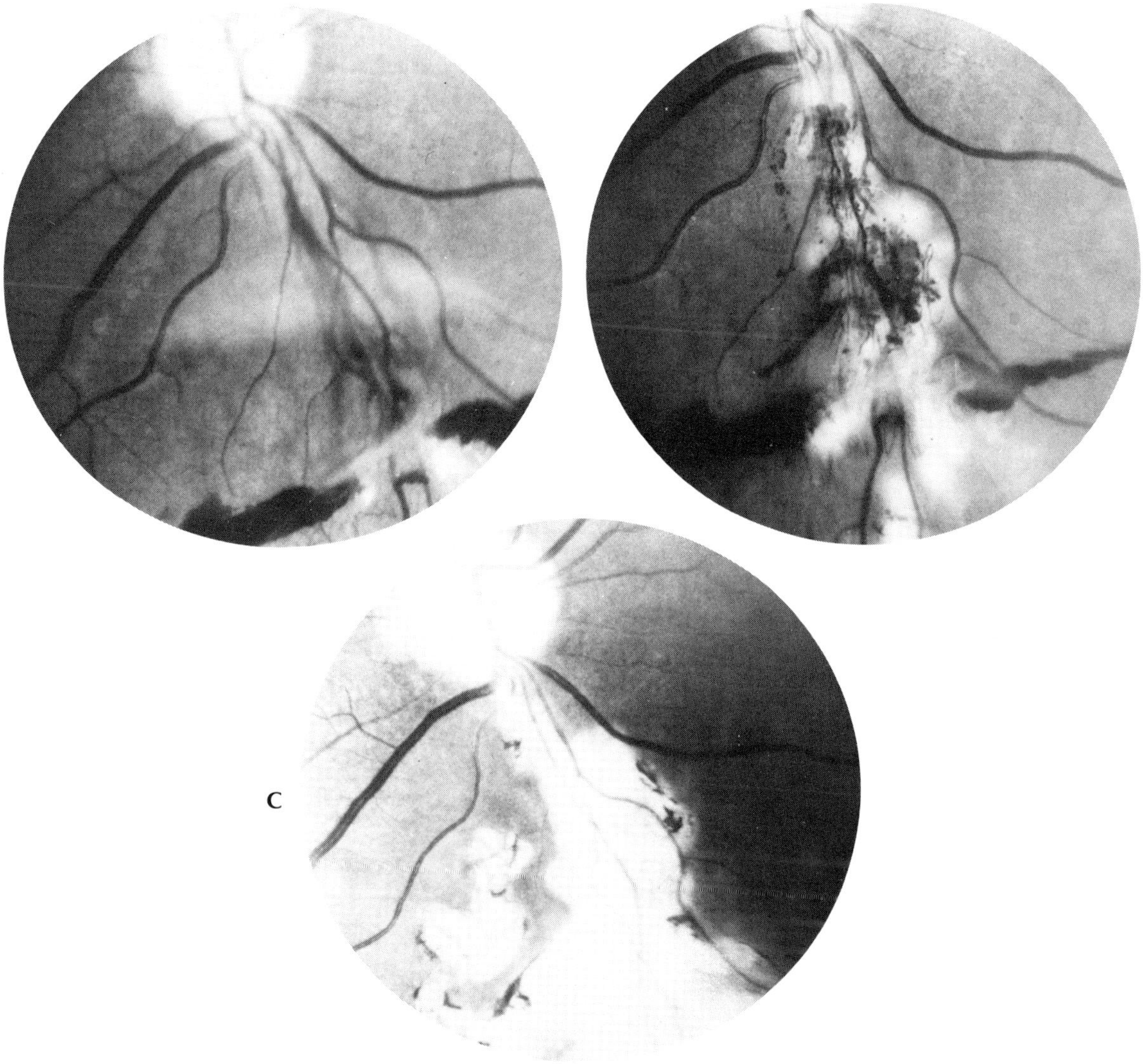

C

Fig. 7-35. A, A typical columnar papillovitreal frond in a 36-year-old woman. There is obvious hemorrhaging from the distal aspects of the frond into the vitreous. **B,** Complete disruption and segmentation of the columnar papillovitreal frond by krypton laser photocoagulation (argon laser photocoagulation would produce the same results) along the extent of the linear, stringy neovascularization. **C,** Posterior polar area 2 months after krypton laser photocoagulation, showing complete obliteration of the neovascularization and an adequate healing response.

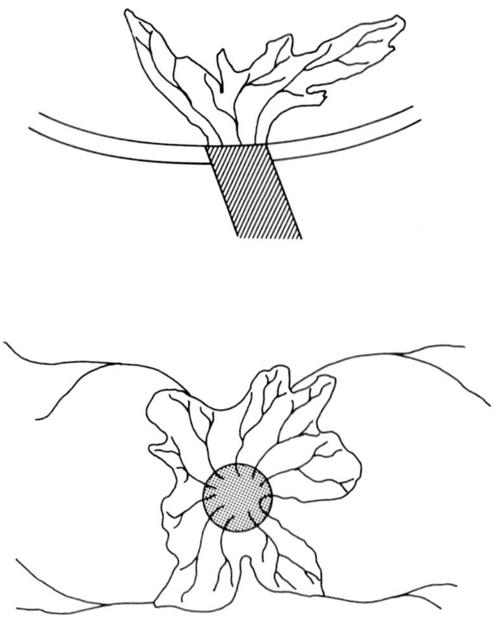

Fig. 7-36. Confluent papillovitreal neovascularization extending from the optic nerve region into the vitreous along the posterior hyaloid membrane, somewhat in the form of a funnel or flower pot. These fronds are best treated by panretinal photocoagulation (see section on Panretinal photocoagulation, p. 146).

Retinovitreal neovascularization

Ophthalmoscopic appearance. Retinovitreal neovascularization may be defined as neovascular tissue extending from the retina toward the central vitreous cavity from any portion of the retina, with the exception of the optic nerve region (Fig. 7-37). Proliferation usually occurs from a larger vessel—in most cases, one of the veins in the vascular arcade. Extension into the vitreous occurs along the latticework provided by an adherent vitreal retinal strand or along fibrin produced by a previous vitreal hemorrhage. Retinovitreal neovascularization can occur from any portion of the vascular tree but usually is found distal to the first bifurcation of the large arcades. It can be arteriolar or venular in distribution, usually growing slowly along the vitreal surface in a well-entrenched, deliberate manner. The retinovitreal frond is primarily vascular during its early stages; it slowly becomes entwined with a large amount of glial proliferation and grows on this proliferation farther into the vitreous body. These fronds usually do not bleed because of increases in blood pressure; rather they bleed because of the shrinkage of the vitreous body and the inevitable stress on the vitreal retinal strand to which the retinovitreal neovascularization is intimately adherent. This type of neovascularization is usually associated with a highly detached posterior hyaloid from which stringy vitreoretinal strands are adherent to the vitreal portion of the neovascularization. In contrast to this moundlike neovascular tuft configuration, retinovitreal neovascularization may occasionally proliferate along the very shallowly detached posterior hyaloid, particularly in the distal arcade areas, and appear as a flat, tablelike area of neovascularization in that particular portion of the fundus.

Photocoagulation approach. Retinovitreal neovascularization can be rather hazardous to treat because these neovascular areas commonly occur at arteriolovenular crossings and coagulations must be placed near vessels containing relatively high blood pressures. In

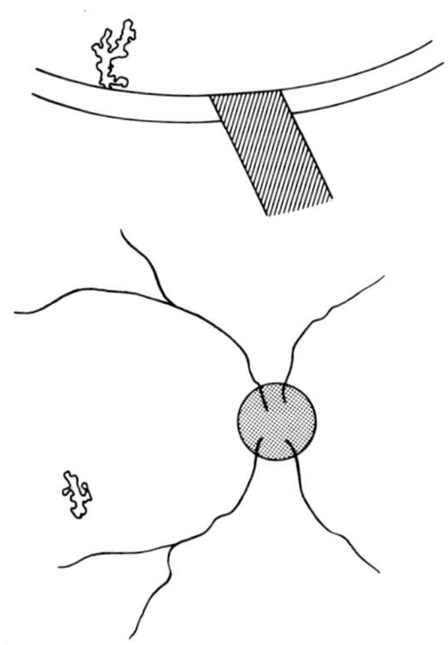

Fig. 7-37. Retinovitreal neovascularization; the fibrovascular proliferation extends from the retina toward the vitreous cavity along a fibrin strand or collapsed collagen attachment of the posterior hyaloid to the retinal surface.

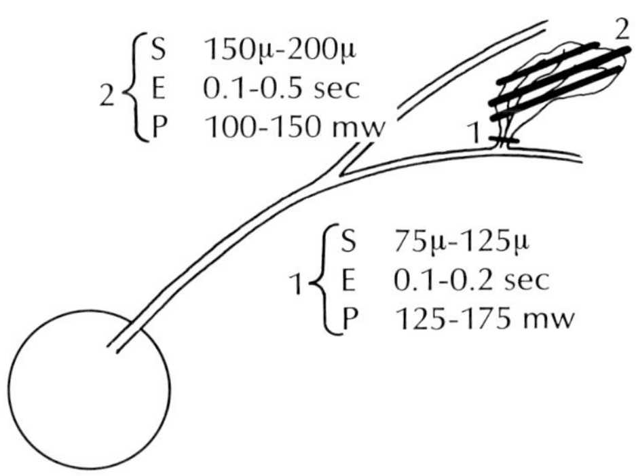

Fig. 7-38. Photocoagulation parameters for retinovitreal neovascularization if a stalklike configuration is present or if the feeder-frond technique can be utilized.

these cases the entire neovascular region is usually treated with low-power coagulations (**100 to 150 mw**) approximately **150μ to 200μ** in diameter, with **0.1- to 0.5-sec** exposures, so that the retinovitreal frond will eventually collapse by virtue of the shrinkage of the glial supportive tissue as well as the coagulative effect. In this manner the danger of rupture of the high-pressure vessels is minimized but not entirely overcome.

If the neovascularization has a distinct feeder vessel from the arteriolar side of the circulation, it is advisable to constrict this particular vessel and to proceed with obliteration of the distal portion of the retinovitreal frond in a manner similar to that previously discussed. That is, a small beam (**75μ to 125μ**) with longer exposures (**0.1- to 0.2-sec**) and lower power levels (**125 to 175 mw**), is employed to cause obliteration of the distal frond (Fig. 7-38).

If the feeder vessel cannot be found with certainty and the area of neovascularization is fairly distal in the arcade tree, it is advisable to obstruct the larger arteriole proximal to the outcropping of the neovascularization with an impact sufficient to cause a spasm of the particular arteriole. Coagulation and obliteration of the distal frond are then performed as previously discussed (Fig. 7-39).

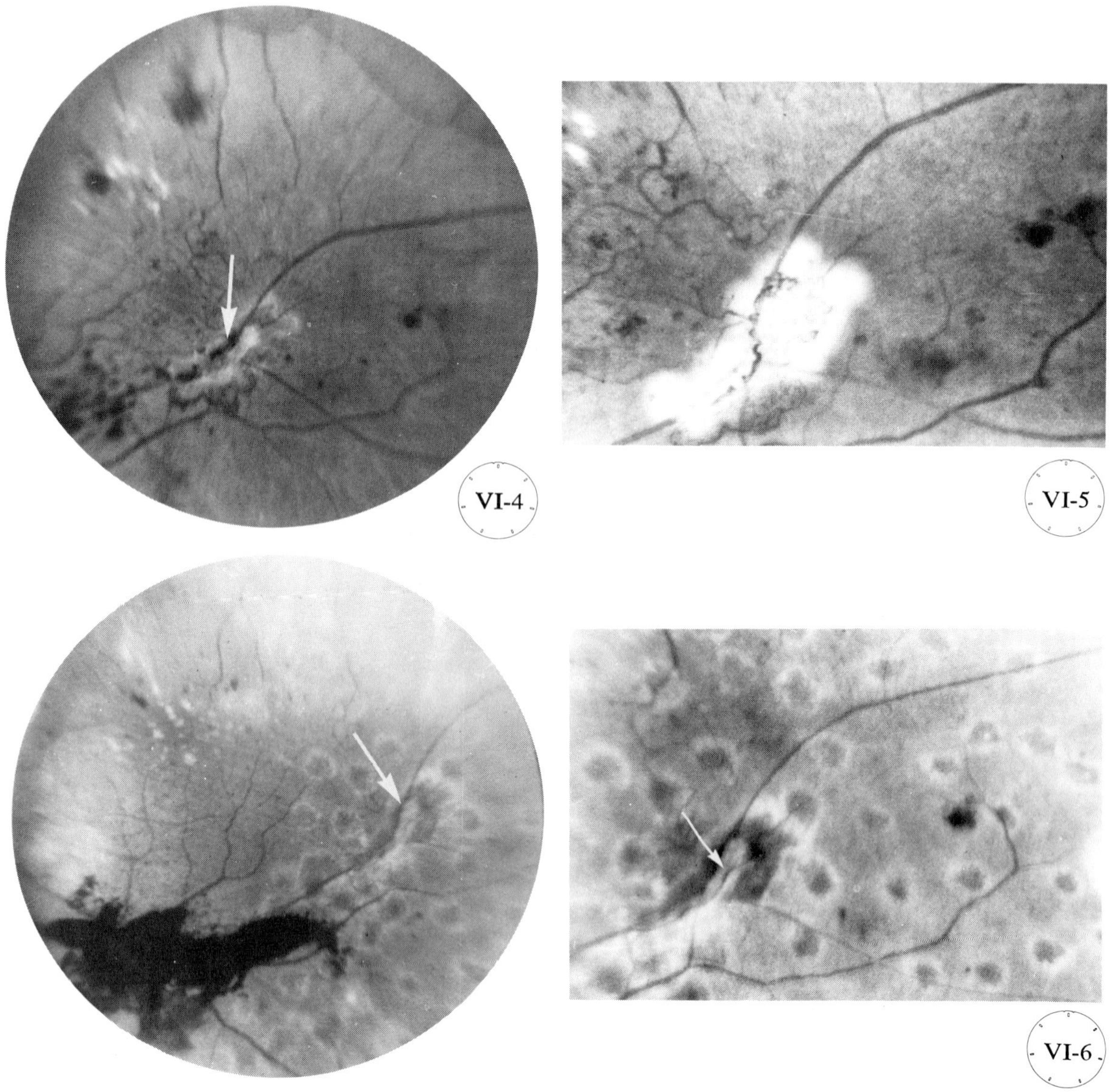

Fig. 7-39. A, An area of retinovitreal neovascularization extending from the superotemporal arcade (arrow) into the vitreous body in a 42-year-old woman who experienced a sudden loss of vision caused by a vitreous hemorrhage from this region. **B,** Argon laser photocoagulation to the retinovitreal neovascularization resulted in obliteration and segmentation of the neovascular channels. Streaked 100μ coagulations were used. **C,** Area of neovascularization (arrow) 2 months after argon laser photocoagulation, showing complete destruction of the neovascular tissue. An old hemorrhage from the neovascular site still remains in the inferior vitreous. **D,** Enlarged view of the area of obliterated neovascularization, showing the pigment response and mild glial proliferation in the area of occlusion (arrow).

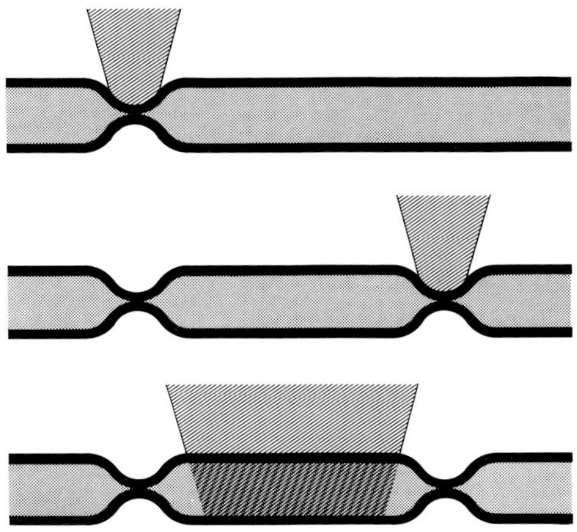

Fig. 7-40. Proper photocoagulation technique for obliteration of a major arteriole to a region of neovascularization. The arteriole is thrown into spasm in two regions approximately 500μ apart, and the blood trapped between the two constricted areas is gently coagulated to obtain a definite occlusion. This "frying the sausage" technique is the only reliable method for obliteration of a large high-flow arteriole.

A

B

C

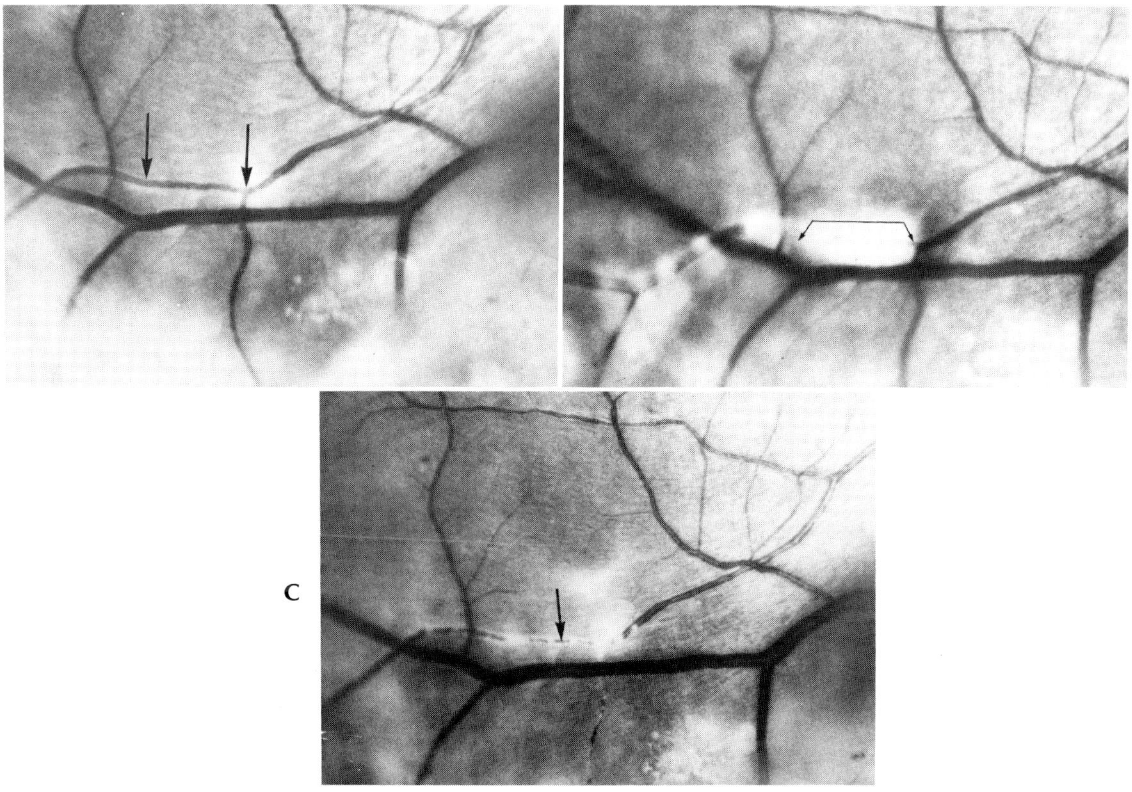

Fig. 7-41. A, Stage 1. A focal constriction is made at two points along an arteriole approximately 500μ apart (arrows). **B,** Stage 2. The blood trapped between the arteriolar constrictions is coagulated by lower-power argon laser photocoagulation (arrows). **C,** The totally occluded arteriole 6 weeks after argon laser photocoagulation, showing glial tissue ingrowth between some residual pockets of intact blood (arrow).

In some cases it is advisable to constrict the arteriolar input alone, since photocoagulation of the distal frond could possibly cause vitreous contraction and increased traction on the retinovitreal frond. In these cases the feeder arteriole is treated with coagulations of **125μ to 175μ** at power levels of **150 to 250 mw** for **0.2- to 0.5-sec** exposures to create spasm (Grade III) in two focal areas approximately 300μ to 500μ apart. The intervening trapped blood is then coagulated in a continuous painting fashion with a slightly lower power (**125 to 175 mw**) until a distinct, white coagulum is produced (Grade 4). This procedure can be done repeatedly along certain areas of the feeder vessel and appears to have the best chance of producing a permanent occlusion of these larger arteriolar feeder vessels. This particular technique may be preferred in many cases where vitreoretinal attachment to the frond is extensive and the danger of vitreous shrinkage is considerable. In these cases the blood in the retinovitreal frond is slowly absorbed, and the frond is rendered avascular by virtue of the occlusion of the feeder arteriole (Figs. 7-40 and 7-41).

The patient should be reevaluated 3 hours to 3 days after treatment, and photocoagulation should be performed again if the nutrient vessel has not been occluded or if the frond has not been rendered avascular. Several monthly observation periods should then be scheduled so that it can be assured that the retinovitreal frond has been permanently obliterated.

In these cases evaluation of the position of the posterior hyaloid face or condensation should be carried out carefully. If the posterior hyaloid is highly detached into the vitreous and there are long footplates to the retina, it is usually easier to isolate the feeder vessels and to coagulate the distal frond. If the posterior hyaloid is shallowly detached from the retinal surface and the neovascularization is growing in a mushroom fashion along the posterior hyaloid, it is more difficult to isolate the feeder vessels and to coagulate all portions of the frond without affecting the physical state of the posterior hyaloid itself. Shorter exposure times and slightly higher power levels should be used in these cases to minimize thermal diffusion outside the impact area. If the frond is extensive, it may not be advisable in some cases to consider photocoagulation as a useful therapy.

Preretinal neovascularization

Ophthalmoscopic appearance. Preretinal neovascularization may be defined as that type of neovascular tissue that extends onto or a short distance into the internal limiting membrane; it is usually derived from the retinal vessels apart from the vascular tissues on the optic nerve (Fig. 7-42). These areas of neovascularization may be fan shaped or threadlike. They may be extremely tortuous, or they may form clusters or vinelike configurations. The neovascularization may be intermeshed with small or large amounts of glial tissue, depending on the maturity of the vascular process. This type of neovascularization can be found anywhere in the posterior pole, although there seems to be a predilection for the distal ends of the vascular arcades, the macular and paramacular areas, and the area between the arteriole and venule in the main vascular arcades. In many cases the vitreous face or posterior hyaloid is intimately approximated to the neovascularization and sometimes provides a latticework on which the neovascularization converts from the surface variety to the retinovitreal or peripapillary type. In these cases evaluation of the vitreous and the state and position of the posterior hyaloid before photocoagulation is most important.

Photocoagulation approach. If the neovascularization is closely approximated to the internal limiting membrane, the proper treatment by argon laser photocoagulation depends on the type of surface neovascularization encountered. The three main types of surface neovascularization should be approached in the following different manners.

Arborescent surface neovascularization. Arborescent surface neovascularization is seen as a relatively large proliferation distal to a small pedicle of feeder and collector vessels. This treelike or shrublike proliferation from a more proximal feeder stalk can best be coagulated by occluding the arteriolar feeder vessel proceeding to the outlying arcade vessels. Spot sizes of **50μ to 100μ**, intensities of **100 to 200 mw**, and **0.1- to 0.2-sec** exposures are employed in short painting strokes across the body of the stalk and proximal arborization (Fig. 7-43). This procedure produces a segmentation of the distal vessels, as well as coagulation of the intervening blood column by direct absorption of the argon laser beam and by heat produced in the pigment epithelium and conducted internally through the retinal layers to the treated vessels. Because of the marked absorption of the beam (and conversion to heat) by the pigment epithelium and by hemoglobin in the overlying vessels, it is not uncommon to find lower power levels adequate for coagulation. Occasionally, only

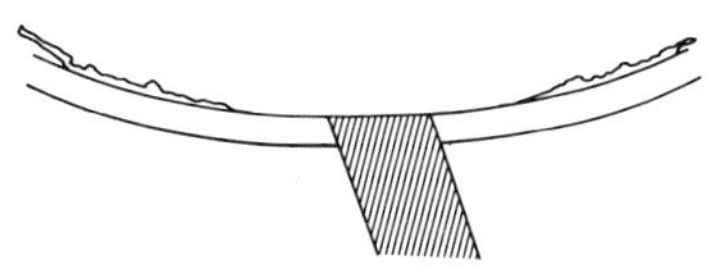

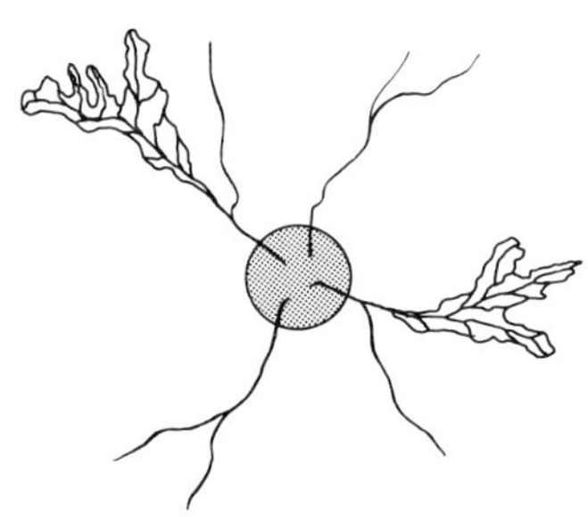

Fig. 7-42. Preretinal (surface) neovascularization. The newly formed vessels tend to grow along the internal limiting membrane or a shallowly detached posterior hyaloid, particularly in the region of the vascular arcades.

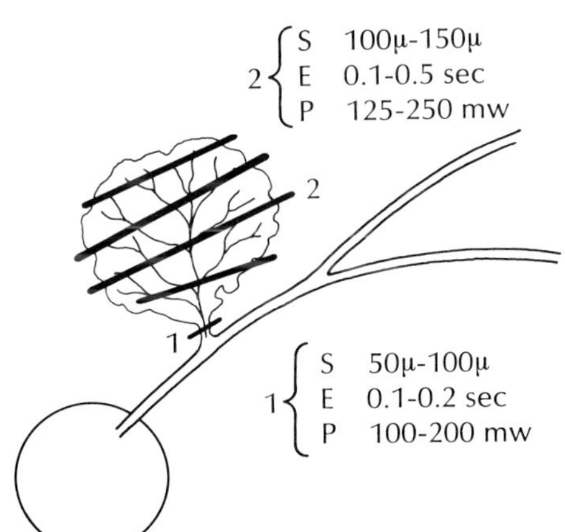

Fig. 7-43. Photocoagulation parameters for the coagulation of surface neovascularization, particularly of the arborescent type. Stage 1 illustrates coagulation of the proximal feeder stalk; Stage 2 shows longer linear coagulations to the body of the distal surface neovascularization.

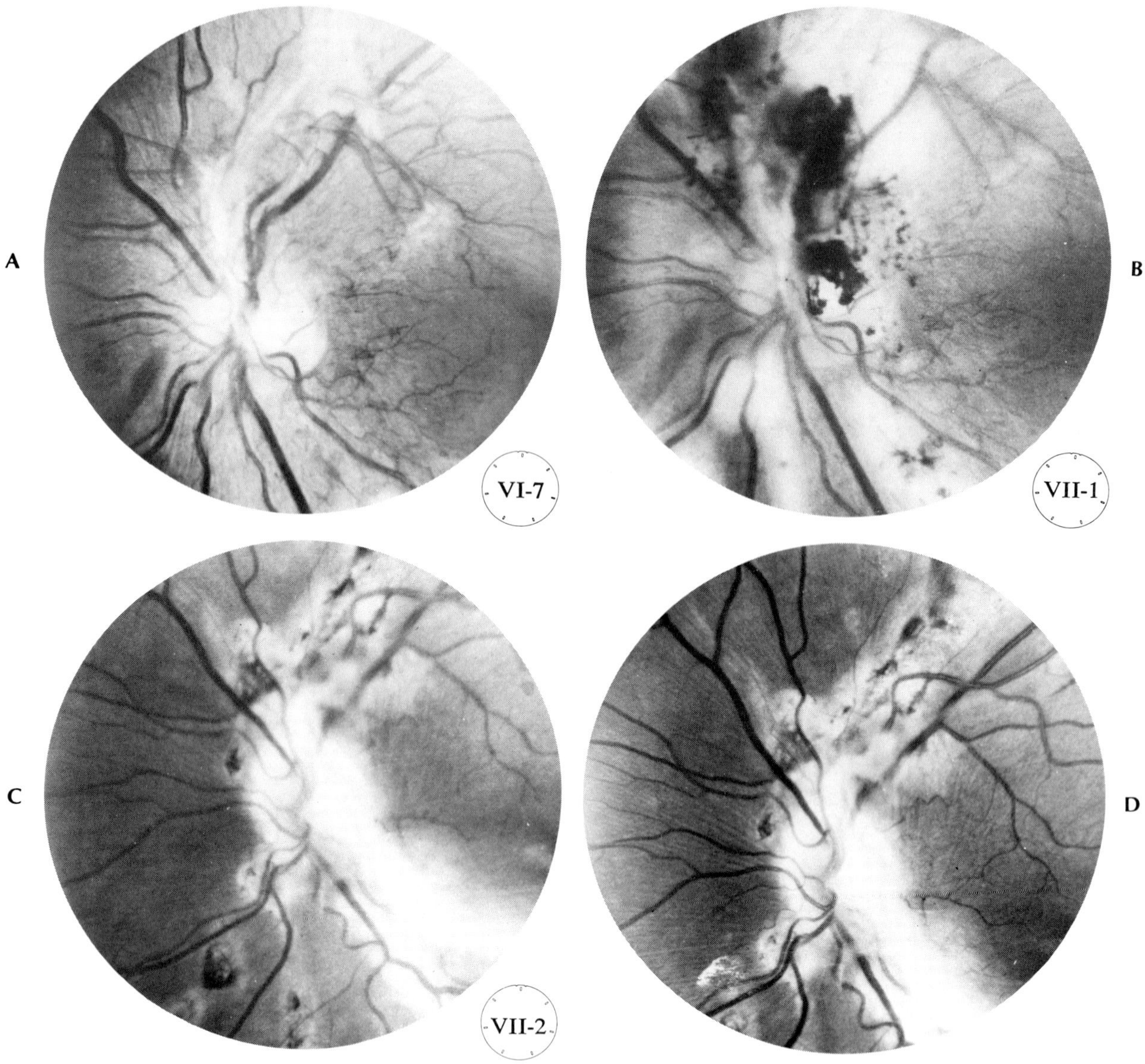

Fig. 7-44. A, Left eye of a 19-year-old diabetic woman who complained of having blurring and distortion of vision for 2 months before ophthalmoscopic examination. Considerable surface and peripapillary neovascularization were observed. **B,** Radial and streaked linear coagulations through the surface neovascularization were attempted, resulting in segmentation and occlusion of most of the neovascularization and inadvertent rupture of nests of small neovascularization. **C,** Posterior polar region 3 months after photocoagulation, showing early glial and pigment proliferation and complete disappearance of the neovascularization. **D,** Posterior polar region 5 years after argon laser photocoagulation to the surface and peripapillary neovascularization. There has been no recurrence of the neovascularization, and the patient has retained 20/20 vision in that eye.

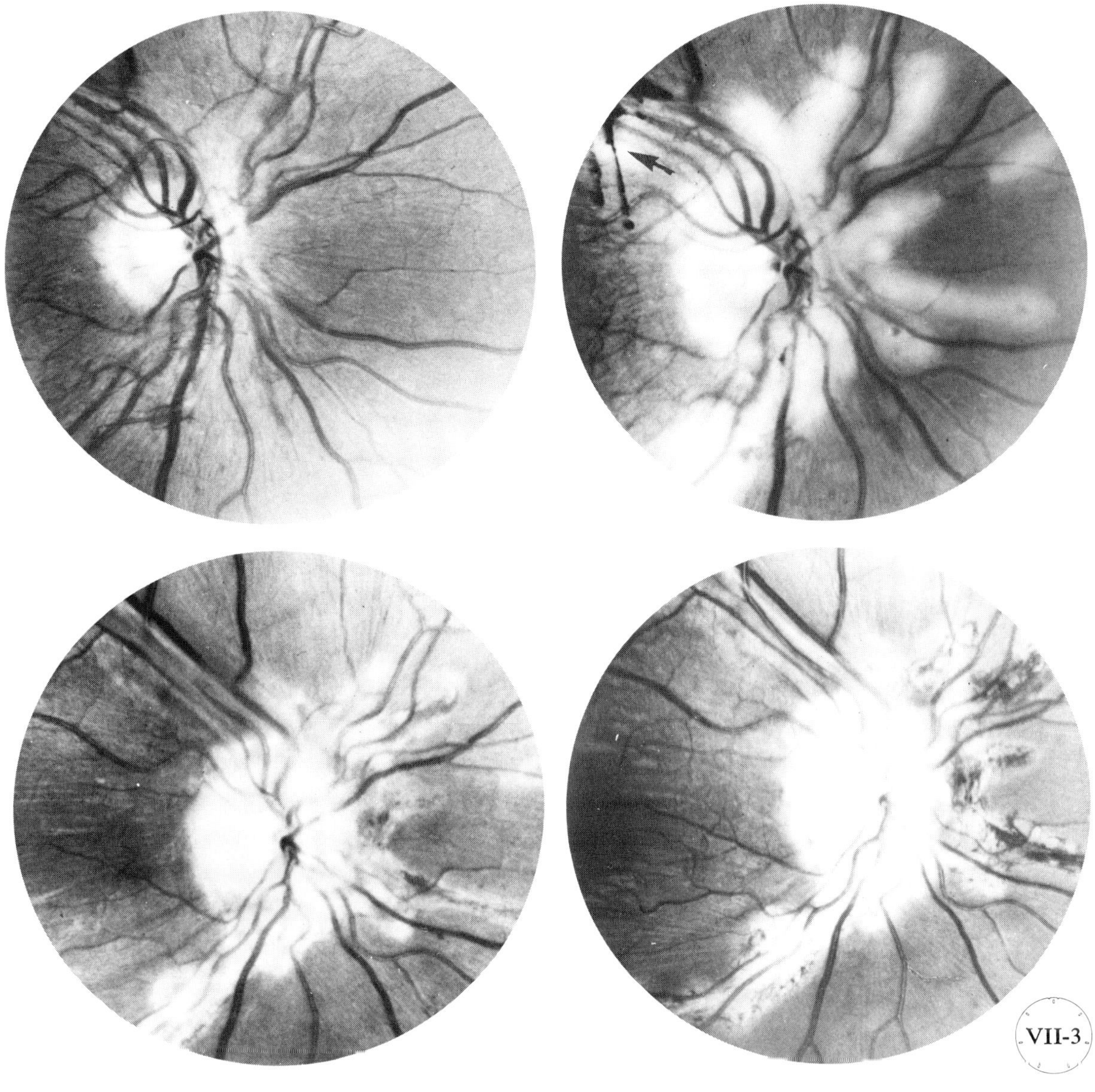

Fig. 7-45. A, Moderately advanced surface neovascularization and early gliosis in the region of the optic nerve in a 29-year-old diabetic woman who had noted occasional blurred vision and metamorphopsia. **B,** Multiple, streaked, linear 150μ to 200μ photocoagulations were applied through the areas of neovascularization to segment and occlude these neovascular channels permanently. A small hemorrhage occurred from the superotemporal nest of extremely small neovascular tufts (arrow). **C,** Optic nerve region 10 weeks after argon laser photocoagulation, showing some gliosis and chorioretinal atrophy and complete obliteration of the neovascularization. Mild macular striae can be seen. **D,** Posterior polar region 6 years after argon laser photocoagulation; there has been no recurrence of the neovascularization. Slight hyperpigmentation of the photocoagulation areas is present, and the patient has retained 20/20 vision despite mild macular striae.

the feeder vessels and collectors need be coagulated for complete obliteration of the frond during a period of 3 to 6 weeks. Experience has shown, however, that the linear coagulations through the body of the neovascularization are more satisfactory, and the feeder coagulative technique is reserved only for those areas of surface neovascularization extending into the macular area, where linear coagulations would not be advisable (Figs. 7-44 and 7-45).

Filamentous surface neovascularization. The filamentous type of surface neovascularization can be seen in any portion of the fundus, although it is seen more commonly near the main vascular arcades or radiating from the optic nerve toward the macular region or the nasal retina. These vessels are not tortuous and have the appearance of tiny sea urchin bristles coming from a normal or neovascular vessel in the region of the posterior pole. These echinoform vessels are treated most appropriately by linear paravascular coagulations along the sides of the nutrient vessel. This form of coagulation usually destroys or shrinks the filamentous vessels extending from the main channels without extensively damaging the involved retinal area. Coagulations with a **50μ to 75μ** spot size, power levels of **100 to 175 mw,** and exposures of **0.5 to 1.0 sec** are created in a painting linear fashion. In this manner coagulations can be made along the main vessel as far as necessary into the midperipheral retina. Obliteration or shrinkage of the echinoform vessels usually occurs within 4 to 6 weeks.

Vinelike surface neovascularization. Vinelike neovascularization is commonly seen extending along the surface of the retina and, in some areas, a short distance into the vitreous. This type of neovascularization is observed at any area in the posterior pole but is most commonly seen between the major vessels of a large vascular arcade or between individual major arcades. The vessels are extremely tortuous, vary greatly in diameter and in the number of individual vascular segments, proliferate rapidly, and rupture easily. The feeder vessels to a clump of vinelike surface neovascularization can be found by careful fluorescein angiography, and it is not uncommon that several feeder vessels will enter an area of marked neovascularization at various points and levels within the meshwork. My experience has shown that it is extremely difficult to occlude all the arteriolar feeder vessels; therefore, the entire patch of neovascularization must be treated with linear coagulations. When feasible, the arteriolar feeder vessels are coagulated as a first step toward reducing the overall flow through the neovascular patch. The entire area of surface neovascularization is then broken into segments approximately 400μ to 600μ in width by long, linear **75μ to 125μ** coagulations utilizing exposures of **0.2 to 0.5 sec.** A power intensity in the range of **175 to 275 mw** ensures permanent coagulation of the vessels. If the neovascular area occupies a region other than the macular, paramacular, or peripapillary zones, the beam is enlarged to **150μ to 175μ** with exposures of **0.2 to 0.5 sec** and power levels of **275 to 400 mw.** Additional coagulations are placed on the budding or leading edge of the neovascularization to prevent any further development of the neovascular process. This combined technique has proved most effective for the total obliteration of surface neovascularization of this particular type.

Panretinal photocoagulation

Indications for panretinal photocoagulation

Epipapillary neovascularization should be treated initially by focal argon laser photocoagulation if the frond is not complex and involves only several feeder and collector vessels. If the frond cannot be obliterated after multiple focal treatments and it has been documented that the frond is increasing in size and vascularity or has hemorrhaged into the vitreous, panretinal photocoagulation should be considered to control the neovascular process.

Peripapillary neovascularization should be treated initially by focal photocoagulation if the vascularity is not extensive and if the neovascularization does not extend more than 1 DD from the margin of the optic nerve. If these conditions are superseded or if multiple focal photocoagulation sessions are unsuccessful in obliterating the peripapillary neovascularization, panretinal photocoagulation should be performed.

Arcuate and confluent papillovitreal neovascularization should be treated initially by the panretinal photocoagulation technique. Immature fronds (those with a greater amount of vascularity than gliosis) will respond more dramatically than will mature fronds (those with a greater amount of gliosis than vascularity) when the surrounding retina is treated by the ablation technique. Columnar papillovitreal fronds should be treated initially by focal photocoagulation because of the paucity of glial tissue and the vulnerability of the stringlike, exposed vessels to direct photocoagulation. If focal photocoagulation for columnar papillovitreal neovascularization fails, the panretinal photocoagulation technique can be employed.

Retinovitreal neovascularization should be treated initially by focal argon laser photocoagulation if the patch of neovascularization is less than 1 DD in extent, is under minimal vitreoretinal traction, and does not extend a great distance into the vitreous. Otherwise, quadratic or hemispherical panretinal photocoagulation can be attempted in the area of neovascularization.

Surface neovascularization should be treated initially by focal photocoagulation if the area of neovascular tissue is less than 2 DD in extent and is under minimal vitreous traction. If the area of surface neovascularization is greater than 3 DD in extent, panretinal photocoagulation combined with focal argon laser photocoagulation should be considered as the treatment of choice.

Panretinal photocoagulation should not be employed when there is Grade 2 to 4 vitreoretinal traction. Since less energy is transmitted through the ocular media, focal photocoagulation can be used with Grade 2, but not Grade 3 or 4, vitreoretinal traction. If diffuse or clotted blood is present in the vitreous or if the vitreous situation is an obviously unstable one that could lead to massive contraction and retinal detachment, photocoagulation should not be considered. Panretinal photocoagulation necessitates the transmission of large amounts of laser energy through the ocular media during the procedure; the vitreoretinal condition should be stable and relatively free from the potential risk of vitreoretinal contraction.

Focal and ablative photocoagulation techniques should not be attempted if gliosis of the vitreoretinal interface is greater than Grade 2 (early vascular arcade glial proliferation), since these procedures would contribute to the extension of the vitreoretinal traction and the possibility of a retinal detachment.

Photocoagulation approach

An anesthetic administered topically is placed in the cul-de-sac of both eyes before the contact lens is inserted. The panretinal photocoagulation (retinal ablation) procedure is conducted in 3 stages approximately 2 to 7 days apart (Fig. 7-46). The central portion of a Goldmann three-mirror contact lens or the plano–low-vacuum contact lens is used for photocoagulation of the posterior polar region (Stage 1). The three-mirror lens or the Jungner contact lens is used for the Stage 2 and Stage 3 treatments that involve photocoagulation of the midperipheral and peripheral superior (Stage 2) and inferior (Stage

3) regions of the fundus (Fig. 7-47). A retrobulbar anesthetic is usually not necessary but can be employed at any time for the relief of discomfort or photophobia.

The entire posterior polar region is photocoagulated with coagulations that routinely extend from the paramacular area to the midperiphery (Fig. 7-48). These coagulations are placed approximately 0.5 to 1 coagulation diameter away from one another and extend up to the optic disc margin on the superior, inferior, and nasal portion of the optic nerve.

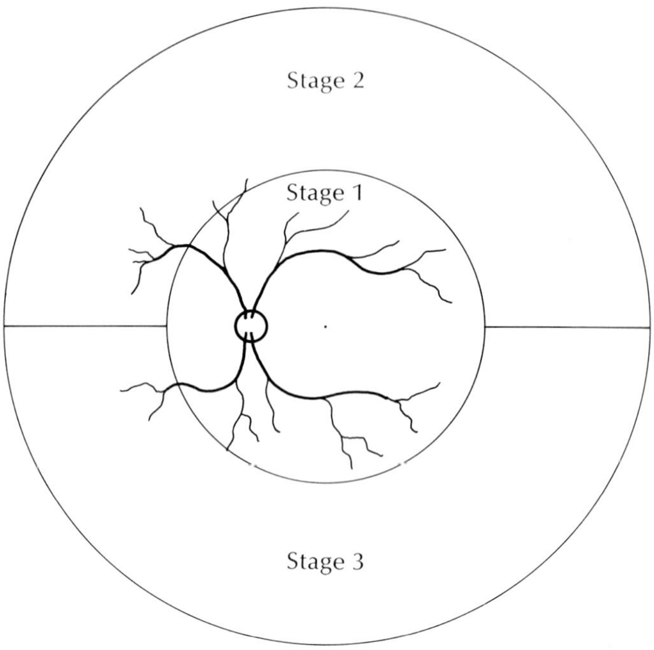

Fig. 7-46. Retinal areas treated during Stage 1 (posterior polar region), Stage 2 (superior hemisphere), and Stage 3 (inferior hemisphere) photocoagulation. Each stage is separated by 2 to 7 days.

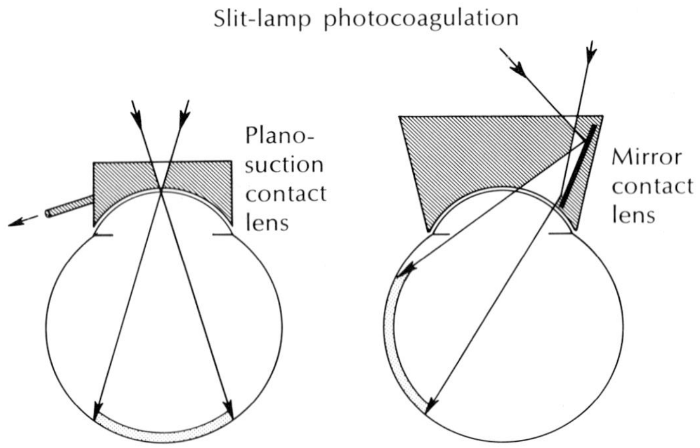

Fig. 7-47. Utilization of the proper contact lens for the three stages of panretinal photocoagulation: the plano-suction contact lens for photocoagulation of the posterior pole during Stage 1 and the Goldmann three-mirror contact lens for photocoagulation of the superior hemisphere (Stage 2) and the inferior hemisphere (Stage 3).

Coagulations of **50μ to 200μ** in diameter with power intensities of **100 to 300 mw** and an exposure of **0.1 sec** are placed in the outer macular and paramacular region (Fig. 7-49). The coagulations near the temporal or nasal vascular arcades and in the most posterior regions of the fundus are **200μ to 500μ**, have power intensities of **200 to 500 mw,** and are delivered at an exposure of **0.1 sec.** The retinal vessels should not be coagulated directly; nor should there be a layering or superimposition of the coagulations. Areas of intraretinal hemorrhage or pigment accumulation should also be avoided.

The second photocoagulation session should be conducted 2 to 7 days after the posterior polar treatment. During this session the coagulations are extended from the

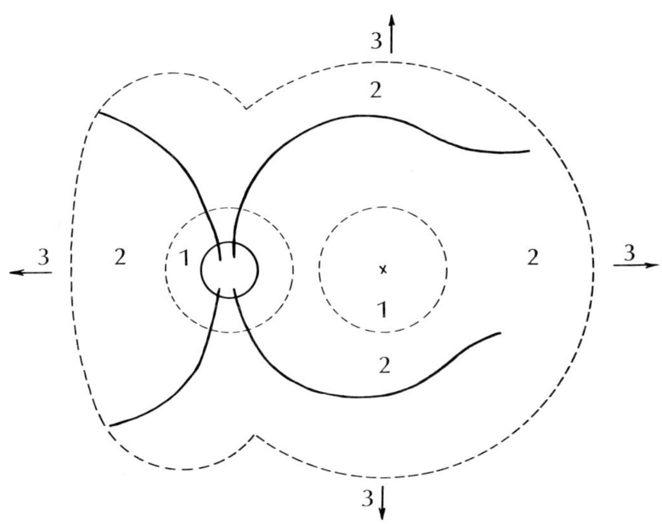

Fig. 7-48. Various chorioretinal zones requiring different coagulation sizes and power intensities: *1,* the macular, paramacular, and peripapillary area; *2,* the vascular arcade area; and *3,* the midperipheral and peripheral chorioretinal area.

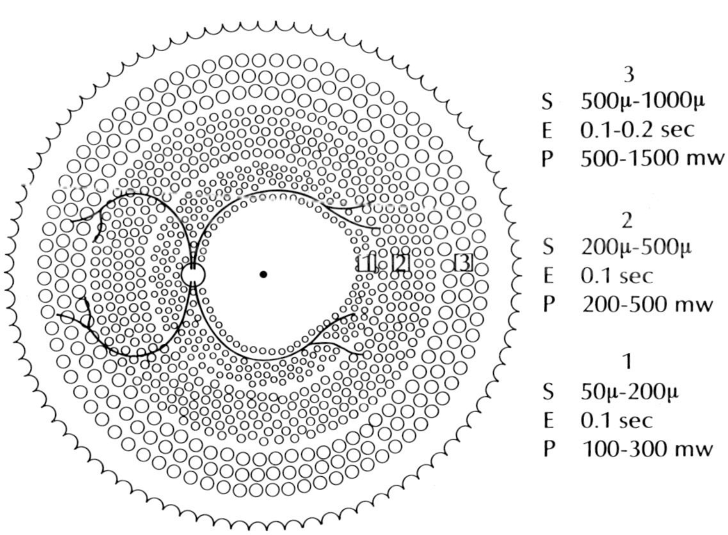

Fig. 7-49. Placement of differently sized coagulations with representative photocoagulation dosages for the three chorioretinal areas.

midperipheral region, as performed during Stage 1, to the anterior equatorial region or as far anterior as possible with the three-mirror lens. These coagulations are confined to the superior hemisphere of the eye during this Stage 2 photocoagulation procedure. The coagulations are **500μ to 1,000μ** in diameter with power intensities of **500 to 1,500 mw** at exposures of **0.1 to 0.2 sec.** An interval of 2 to 7 days is then allowed to elapse before the Stage 3 treatment is conducted. These intervals between treatments appear necessary for the eye to become adjusted to the thermal insult and hemodynamic change.

The inferior hemisphere is then treated with doses of argon laser energy similar to those used in the Stage 2 treatment. Coagulations are extended as far anteriorly as possible. During this three-stage panretinal photocoagulation procedure, approximately 1,000 to 1,500 coagulations are produced, resulting in destruction of 20% to 30% of the retinal surface (Figs. 7-50 to 7-54).

The patient is given cycloplegics and steroid medications topically throughout the duration of the three-stage procedure and for a period of 2 weeks following the last treatment. Acetazolamide (Diamox) or another carbonic anhydrase inhibitor can be given if the patient's intraocular pressure rises.

Approximately 2 weeks following the last treatment session, the patient should be examined for evaluation of the healing response. Atrophy of the retina and partial pigmentation at the coagulation site should be noted at this time. The vitreous, lens, and cornea should be clear, and there should be no evidence of anterior chamber reaction. If cells or flare is noted in the anterior chamber, the cycloplegic and steroid medications should be continued for 1 to 2 weeks.

The patient is observed closely at 2-week intervals, and the areas of neovascularization are photographed during each visit. No further treatment is considered for a period of at least 3 months so that the complete effect of the ablation technique can be appreciated.

A

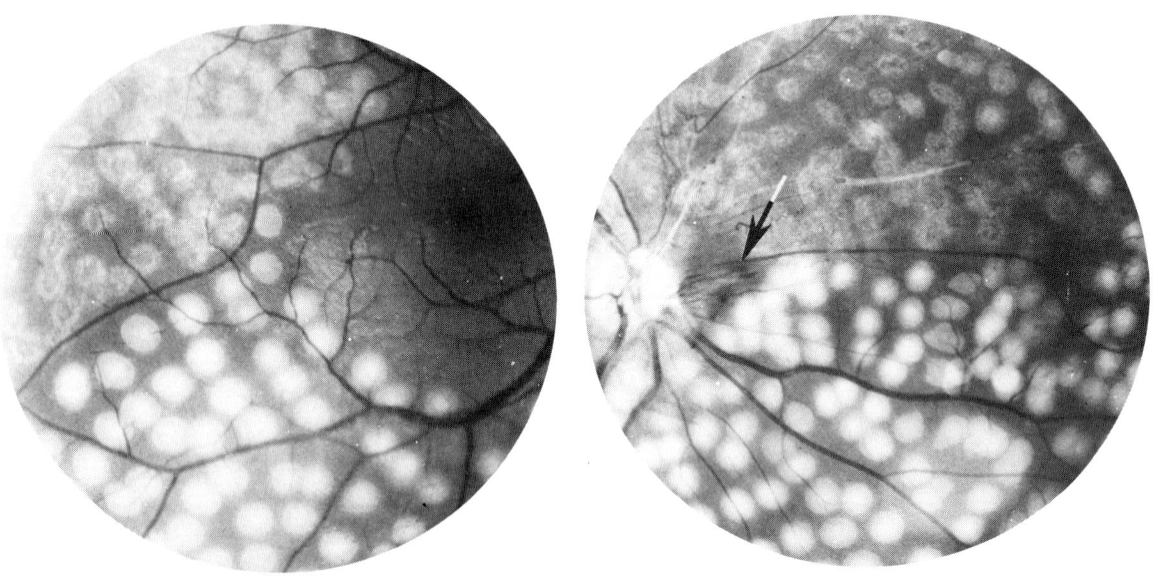

B

Fig. 7-50. A, Temporal macular region of a diabetic eye immediately after argon laser photocoagulation of the inferior hemisphere (Stage 3) and 1 week after previous photocoagulation of the superior hemisphere (Stage 2). **B,** Nasal retina and optic disc, showing a photocoagulation configuration similar to that of **A,** for a moderately advanced papillovitreal frond extending from the optic disc (arrow).

If neovascularization, which is considered dangerous because it leads to further vascular proliferation, hemorrhagic activity, or fibrovascular response, is still present 3 months after panretinal photocoagulation, further ablation of the retina can be considered. A less extensive course of panretinal photocoagulation can be administered to the involved eye, and the eye is then allowed to stabilize for a period of 2 months. If the neovascularization is not affected by this second course of panretinal photocoagulation, focal argon laser photocoagulation should be considered if the visual health of the eye is threatened from the obviously progressing neovascularization.

A

B

C

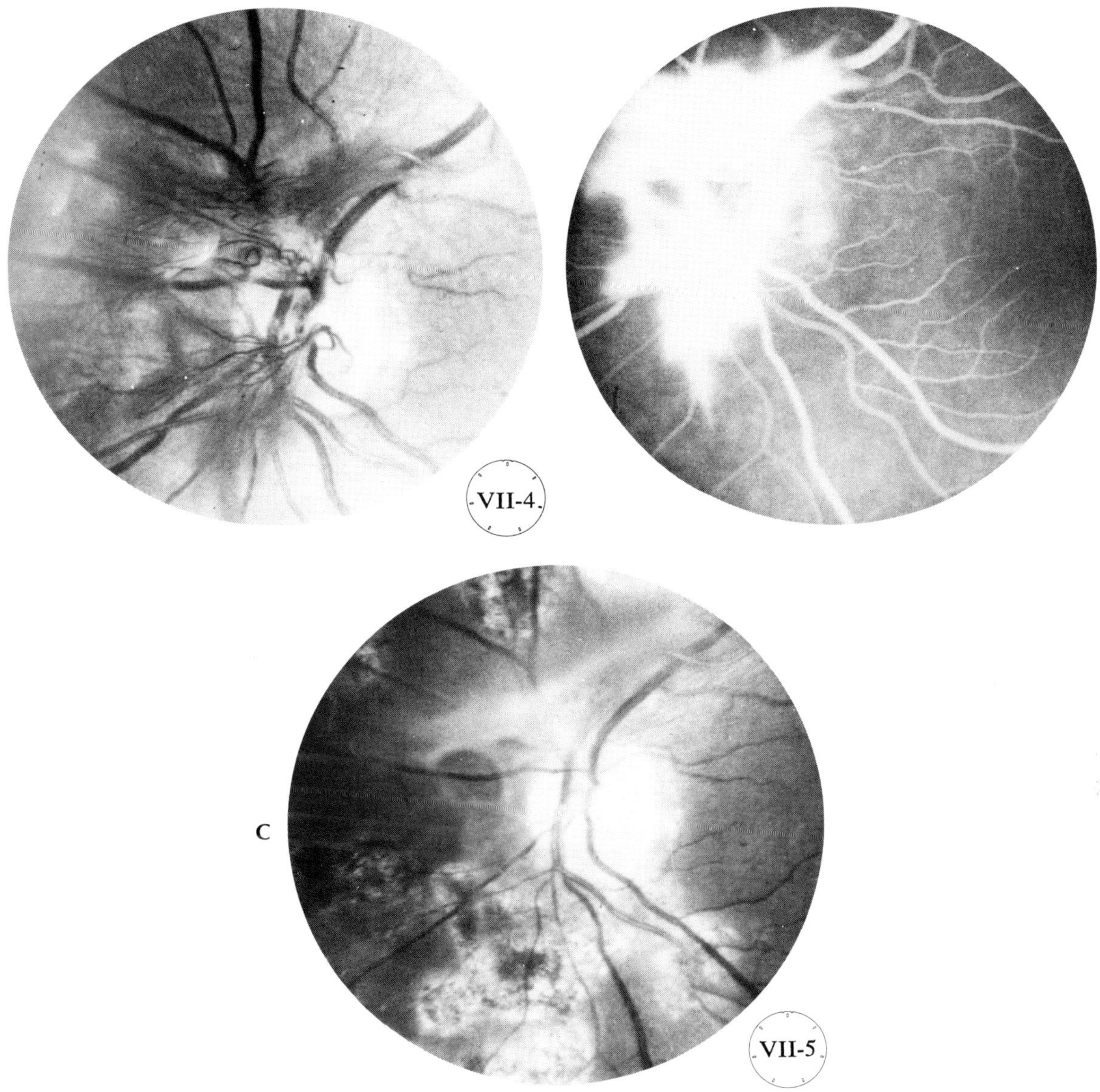

Fig. 7-51. A, A confluent papillovitreal frond in a diabetic 38-year-old woman before photocoagulation. **B,** Fluorogram of the papillovitreal frond, showing intense leakage of the dye into the vitreous body. **C,** Complete obliteration of the confluent papillovitreal neovascularization 6 weeks after panretinal photocoagulation therapy.

A

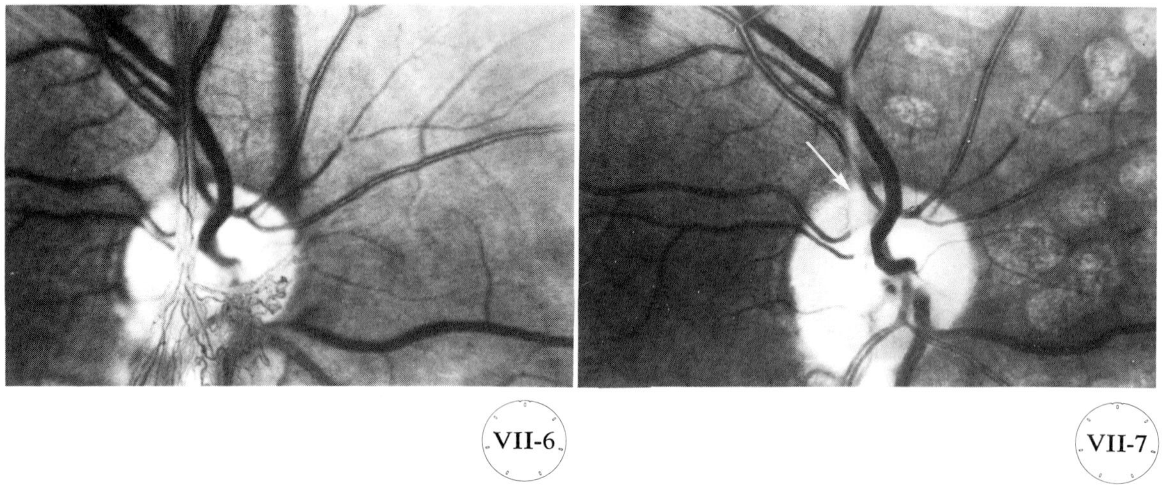

B

Fig. 7-52. A, A rapidly progressing papillovitreal frond extending from the optic nerve into the vitreous in a 39-year-old diabetic man before photocoagulation. **B,** Retention of the glial supportive tissue (arrow) and disappearance of the papillovitreal neovascularization 7 weeks after argon laser photocoagulation utilizing the panretinal photocoagulation technique.

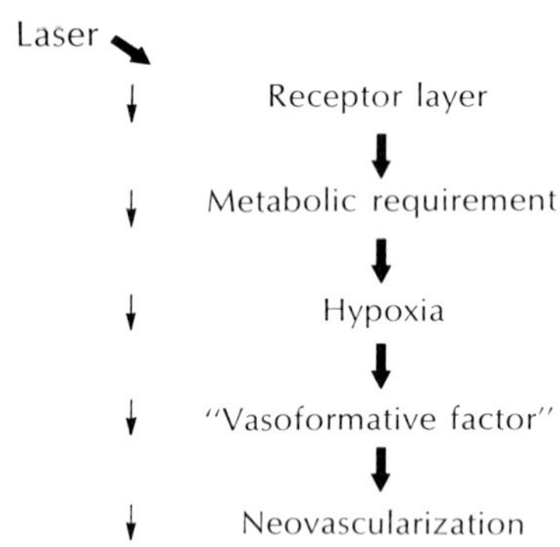

Fig. 7-53. Theory that a decrease in the receptor layer of the retina caused by photocoagulation may ultimately lead to a decrease in neovascularization.

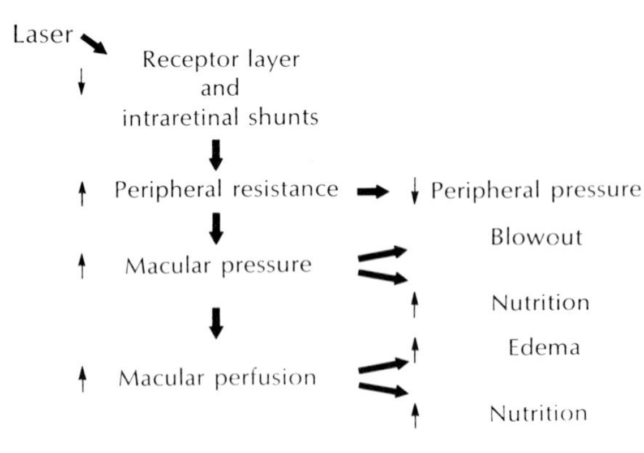

Fig. 7-54. Alternate theory that destruction of portions of the receptor layer and intraretinal shunts leads to an increase in peripheral vascular resistance and an increase in macular perfusion. These alterations can result in an increase in macular nutrition or unfortunately, on occasion, to blow out, edema, and macular decompensation.

When the neovascularization has been obliterated and the eye rendered stable, the patient should be examined at 3-month intervals with wide-angle fundus photography and fluorescein angiography.

Complications

The most common complication of panretinal photocoagulation is a blowout hemorrhage from the optic disc region. This hemorrhage may be caused by an increase in peripheral resistance secondary to photocoagulation or by an inadvertent Valsalva maneuver made by the patient. For this reason the patient is advised to observe the listed regulations during the postphotocoagulation interval.

Complications such as macular striae, increased vitreal traction, central retinal artery occlusion, clouding of the vitreous, and increased hemorrhagic activity in the retina have been observed, although rarely. Panretinal photocoagulation should not be attempted in an eye with Grade 2 to 4 vitreoretinal traction, because the transmitted energy required for the procedure might lead to further contraction of the vitreous body.

Chapter 8

Peripheral chorioretinal tumors

RETINOBLASTOMA

Clinical symptoms. The young child with retinoblastoma may have bilateral blindness, or the parents may note a monocular visual defect. Classically, a white pupil or strabismus is observed. Complaints of blurred vision and distortion can sometimes, but not usually, be elicited from these children.

Ophthalmoscopic appearance. Retinoblastoma can appear as large, contiguous, elevated, nodular growths in the posterior pole, with multiple seedings of tumor tissue present throughout the vitreous body. The tumor can also appear as a solitary white nodule in various areas of the fundus, causing considerable consternation in regard to its differential diagnosis. Classically, the tumor can appear as a slightly elevated white mass or as an exophytic mulberry tumor with several white projections on its surface. Seeding of the small tumor fragments from the original tumor mass is a frequent occurrence. Calcium deposits following tumor necrosis are present in almost every case. Inflammatory signs of vitreous clouding and retinal edema are not usually associated with retinoblastoma.

Ancillary diagnostic examinations. Thorough examination by indirect ophthalmoscopy, usually with the patient under general anesthesia, should be done with complete retinal drawings of the fundi on all patients at intervals of several months.

Stereoscopic Kodachrome fundus photography, particularly with a vertically mounted fundus camera and the patient under general anesthesia, is useful for evaluating and following these tumors in young children.

Fluorescein angiography is not of value in retinoblastoma, since there usually is no change in the basic fluorescent pattern. There appears to be no increase in tumor fluorescence following injection of fluorescein, even at later stages.

^{32}P uptake is not significantly useful for examination of these particular tumors.

Indications for photocoagulation. If the patient is affected bilaterally, photocoagulation of the less severely affected eye is more desirable than the alternative, bilateral enucleation. Usually, the most severely affected eye is enucleated, and the tumor mass of the less-affected eye is photocoagulated directly with xenon-arc or argon laser photocoagulation.

If the process is extensive, photocoagulation is probably not indicated. Photocoagulation should be reserved for those cases when the tumor is isolated from the optic disc and accessible visually for photocoagulation purposes.

Photocoagulation approach. Photocoagulation, preferably with the xenon-arc source, should be applied directly to the tumor mass with high powers sufficient to interrupt the blood supply to the tumor as well as to cause necrosis of the tumor itself. Argon laser photocoagulation does not seem to be as effective as the xenon-arc method for direct impact on the tumor tissue itself. Argon laser photocoagulation may be beneficial in obliterating the feeder vessels to the retinoblastoma tissue, but xenon-arc photocoagulation still appears to offer significant advantages for treating this tumor. The tumor tissue should be treated until an obvious coagulation is apparent on its surface and the blood supply is interrupted. Coagulations around the base of the tumor should also be attempted to limit the vascular supply from the surrounding retina.

Six-degree spots with power intensities of **Red I or II** should be employed at exposures of **0.5 to 1.0 sec** for most peripherally placed tumor sites. Tumors located more posteriorly near the macular or optic disc region can be treated with smaller spot sizes to diminish the amount of surrounding retinal destruction. Energy dosages higher than those indicated should be avoided to obviate the possibility of explosion and subsequent seeding of the tumor tissue.

Argon laser photocoagulation to the retina peripheral to the tumor can be beneficial by obliterating the vascular supply entering the tumor from the nearby retina. Coagulations with spot sizes of **200μ** are usually employed with a **0.5-sec** exposure and power levels in the range of **400 to 600 mw** (Figs. 8-1 and 8-2). A Grade 4 coagulation should be created in

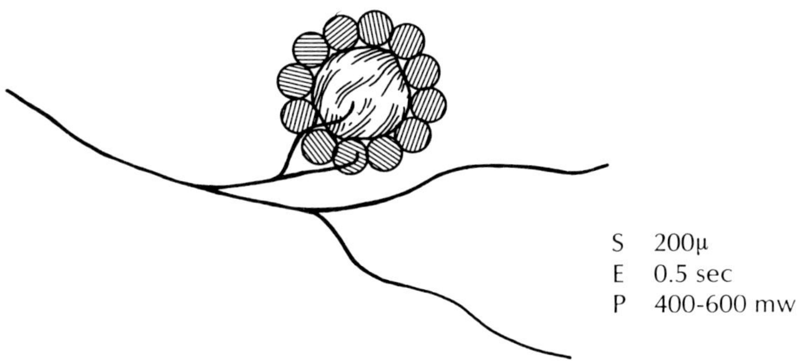

Fig. 8-1. Placement of punctate, linear, contiguous 200μ argon laser coagulations around the border of the retinoblastoma mass to restrict or obliterate the blood supply to the tumor.

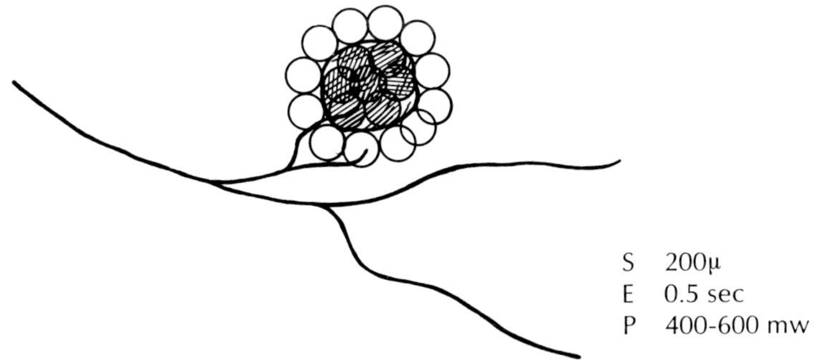

Fig. 8-2. Application of relatively high doses of photocoagulation directly to the retinoblastoma tumor mass to destroy vessels within the tumor itself.

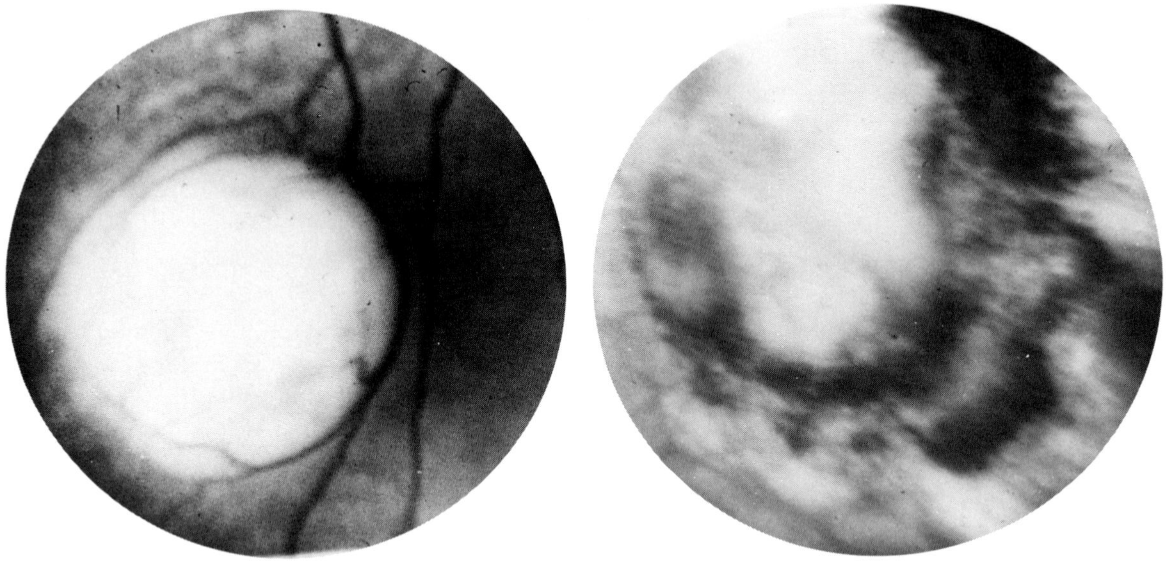

A B

Fig. 8-3. A, A 3-DD retinoblastoma located in the midperiphery of an 11-month-old boy; it appeared to be solitary and well visualized. **B,** Destroyed retinoblastoma lesion 3 months after photocoagulation, showing pigment and glial proliferation but no evidence of tumor tissue. (Courtesy Robert Ellsworth, M.D.)

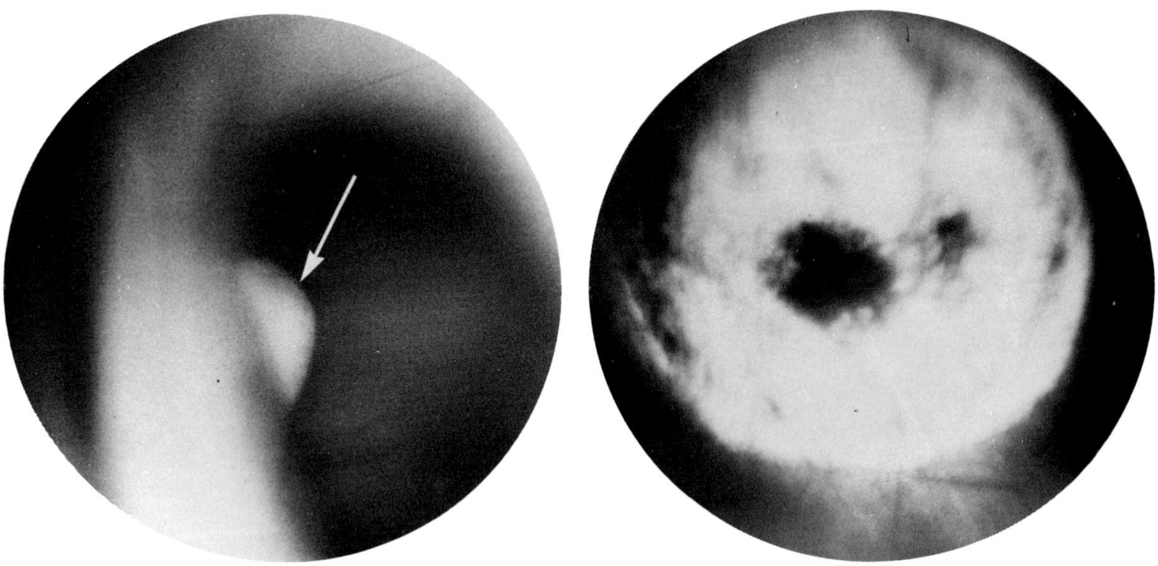

A B

Fig. 8-4. A, Edge of a 4-DD retinoblastoma as seen through the pupil in a 13-month-old boy (arrow). There was no evidence of other tumor seedings in the eye, and its accessibility warranted photocoagulation therapy. **B,** Completely obliterated retinoblastoma tumor mass, showing secondary scarring and hypertrophy of the pigment and glial tissues. (Courtesy Robert Ellsworth, M.D.)

the surrounding retina and on the tumor mass when direct impacts are employed secondarily (Figs. 8-3 and 8-4).

Complications. The most common complication is hemorrhage from the feeder supply to the tumor. These hemorrhages can be moderately extensive; however, they do disappear during the course of 4 to 6 weeks, and usually photocoagulation can be continued at that time to that particular tumor site.

Iris damage and opacification and shrinkage of the vitreous body have also been noted with photocoagulation therapy of this type. Using short exposures and centering the xenon-arc beam in the pupillary aperture will help decrease these problems.

Follow-up. The patients are treated at 4- to 8-week intervals, depending on the degree of vitreous hemorrhage and surrounding retinal damage. Since these photocoagulation treatments must be done with the patient under general anesthesia because of the age of the patient, photocoagulation interventions should probably not be attempted within several weeks of one another. As with the treatment of any other malignant process, long-term follow-up must be considered as extending over a period of several years.

MALIGNANT MELANOMA

Clinical symptoms. Malignant melanoma may reveal no symptoms that the patient may notice, and it may be uncovered only during routine examination. On the other hand, distortion and blurring of vision caused by the actual tumor or the secondary retinal detachment may be noted. Spots, floaters, lightning flashes, and photopsia have been noted along with a host of other vague symptoms.

Ophthalmoscopic appearance. The appearance of a malignant melanoma of the choroid can be quite varied, although it is usually seen as a brownish black, stippled, elevated growth at the choroidal level. In its early stages it is relatively smooth, without eruptions or nodules extending from the surface. The overlying retina may be relatively unchanged or show atrophy, gliosis, and some exudative changes during the later stages. The tumor can be seen in any portion of the choroid, although there seems to be a preponderance of tumor activity in the temporal portion of the eye.

Ancillary diagnostic examinations. Fluorescein angiograms usually demonstrate a pattern showing early fluorescence in the arterial phase and late staining of the tumor mass in the venous phase. The extent of fluorescence may range from mild staining in the venous phase to fluorescence of the entire tumor mass and accumulation of the dye in the overlying subretinal fluid. Lacunas and staining of interstitial tissue can also be observed in more developed tumors.

Kodachrome sequential photographs taken at intervals of 3 to 6 weeks will show the rate of growth of the tumor, especially if the photographs are taken stereoscopically.

A ^{32}P test showing a greater than 100% increase in accumulation of the isotope (as compared with a nonaffected area of the choroid), taken 48 hours after administration of the radioisotope, indicates the presence of a malignant melanoma of the choroid.

The lack of blanching of the tumor with increased intraocular pressure by digital manipulation or suction ophthalmodynamometry usually indicates the presence of a malignant melanoma rather than a choroidal hemangioma.

If it is sufficiently bright, ocular illumination through the pupil will demonstrate a dense area that does not transmit the light through the sclera in the region of the malignant melanoma.

Indications for photocoagulation. If the malignant melanoma process is at least 2 DD from the optic nerve head, occupies a zone of less than 6 DD in lateral extension, and protrudes less than 1.5 mm into the vitreous, photocoagulation can be considered as a possible therapy. For photocoagulation to be considered, these tumors must be visible in their entirety and therefore are usually located in the posterior pole behind the equator in a position eccentric to the optic disc. Any tumors larger than these dimensions, too anteriorly placed, or impinging on the optic disc cannot be considered for photocoagulation intervention.

Photocoagulation approach. Either the xenon-arc source or the argon laser can be used

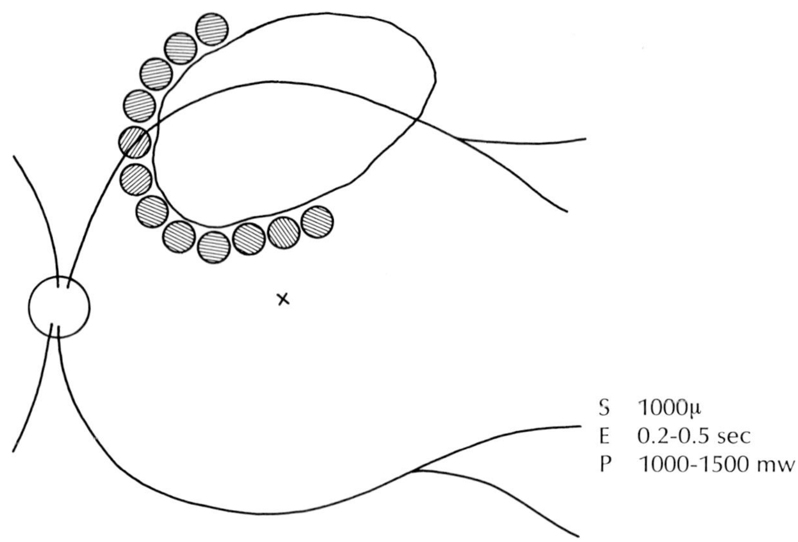

Fig. 8-5. Stage 1: placement of 1,000μ argon laser coagulations or 6° xenon-arc coagulations around the proximal border of the malignant melanoma in the area of normal choroid and retina to decrease the retinal and choroidal blood supply to the tumor mass.

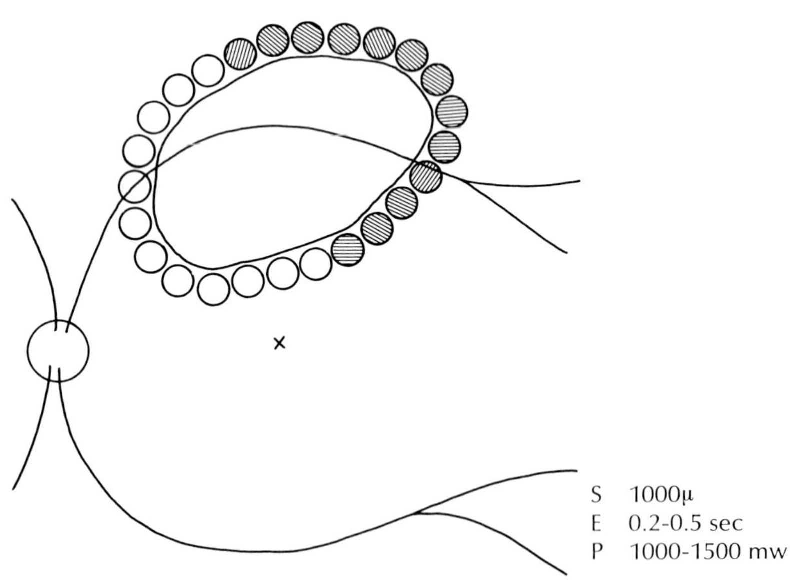

Fig. 8-6. Stage 2: argon laser or xenon-arc photocoagulation 1 month after the previous stage, as shown in Fig. 8-5. Placement of the coagulations is around the distal half of the border of the malignant melanoma in areas of normal retina.

with large coagulations (**6°** spot size for the xenon-arc source and **1,000μ** spot size for the argon laser), which are placed around the circumference of the outer half of the tumor in the region away from the optic disc. These coagulations should be extremely intense, in the range of **1,000 to 1,500 mw** for the argon laser or **Red II or III** for the xenon-arc source, at exposures of **0.2 to 0.5 sec.** They should be placed along the proximal tumor margin for approximately 180° as a Stage 1 procedure (Fig. 8-5).

The area is allowed to heal and scar for 3 to 4 weeks, and a single or double row of

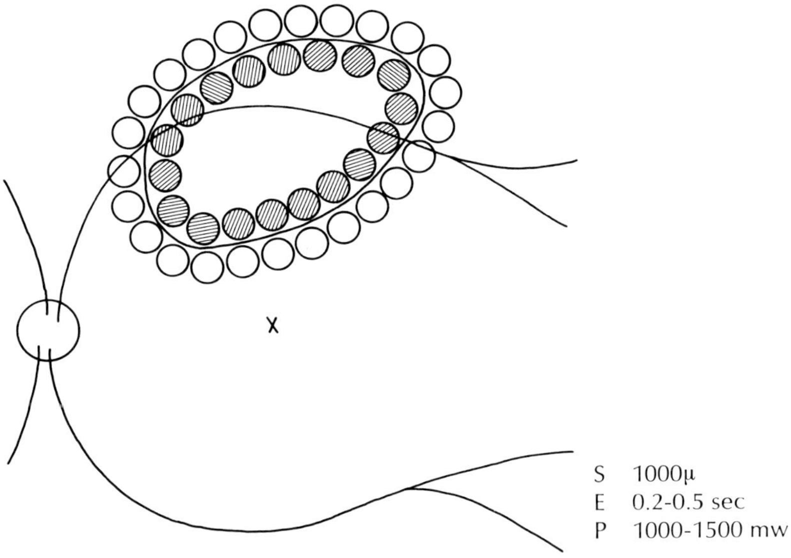

Fig. 8-7. Stage 3: dense Grades 3 to 4 argon laser or xenon-arc photocoagulations to the peripheral body of the tumor mass in a contiguous or overlapping manner.

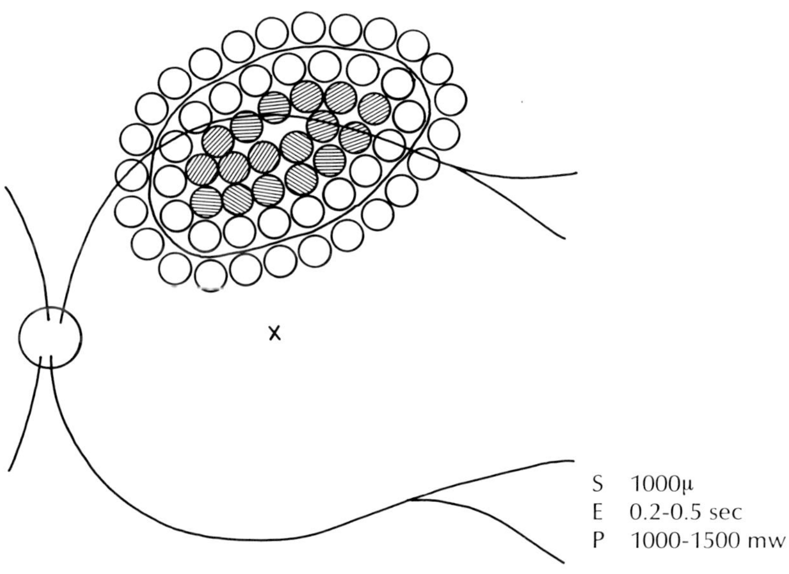

Fig. 8-8. Stage 4: barrage-type, Grade 4 photocoagulations to the central tumor approximately 1 month after the previous stage, as shown in Fig. 8-7. Rephotocoagulation to the periphery of the tumor or to isolated areas of pigmented tissue is usually needed to destroy the malignant tissue effectively and to obliterate the blood supply to the neoplasm.

coagulations of similar dosage is then placed along the tumor's remaining perimeter, which is the area away from the optic disc (Fig. 8-6).

The area is allowed to scar and heal for an additional 3 to 4 weeks, and the coagulations are created centrally toward the apex of the tumor with a single or double coagulation barrage (Fig. 8-7). The coagulations must be of high power, but the coagulation process must not be extensive during each photocoagulation session because of the possible problem of excessive necrosis of the tumor tissue. As the coagulation process moves centrally into the tumor mass, the blood supply of the tumor should be markedly decreased, and most of the possible exits of tumor proliferation should be obliterated (Figs. 8-8 and 8-9). The process of destroying the tumor may require 8 to 12 photocoagulation sessions, and the patient is given cycloplegic and steroid drops throughout this period.

Complications. If a soft coagulation is not produced, an explosion of the tumor tissue can take place, seeding the tumor cells throughout the vitreous body. A longer exposure with a slightly lower power level is needed to obviate this particular complication.

Hemorrhage from the tumor mass can take place, but this complication can be minimized by the production of an effective barrier around the tumor; most of the choroidal vascular input to the tumor itself is thereby occluded.

A

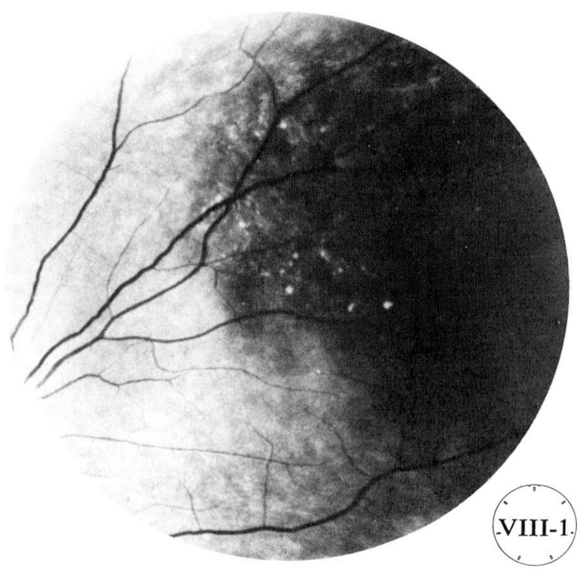

Fig. 8-9. A, A choroidal malignant melanoma in a 56-year-old man who complained of blurred vision and was observed to have a progressively enlarging tumor mass in the superonasal quadrant of his right eye. The malignancy potential was confirmed by the ^{32}P isotope examination. **B,** Capillary phase of the fluorescein angiogram, showing early staining and pooling of the fluorescein dye in the malignant melanoma tissue mass. **C,** Late venular phase of the fluorescein angiogram, showing more extensive pooling and staining of the tumor tissue. **D,** Punctate, linear, contiguous or overlapping $1{,}000\mu$ coagulations were placed around the border of the tumor and extended approximately ½ DD into normal retinal tissue. **E,** Photocoagulated tumor 1 month after the entire circumference of the tumor mass had been heavily photocoagulated to diminish the choroidal blood supply to the neoplasm. **F,** Overlapping $1{,}000\mu$ Grade 4 argon laser photocoagulations were applied to the central portion of the tumor mass to destroy the blood supply and tumor tissue in this region. **G,** Healed tumor mass 4 months after photocoagulation, showing complete destruction of viable tumor tissue and proliferation of glial and pigment elements in the photocoagulated zone.

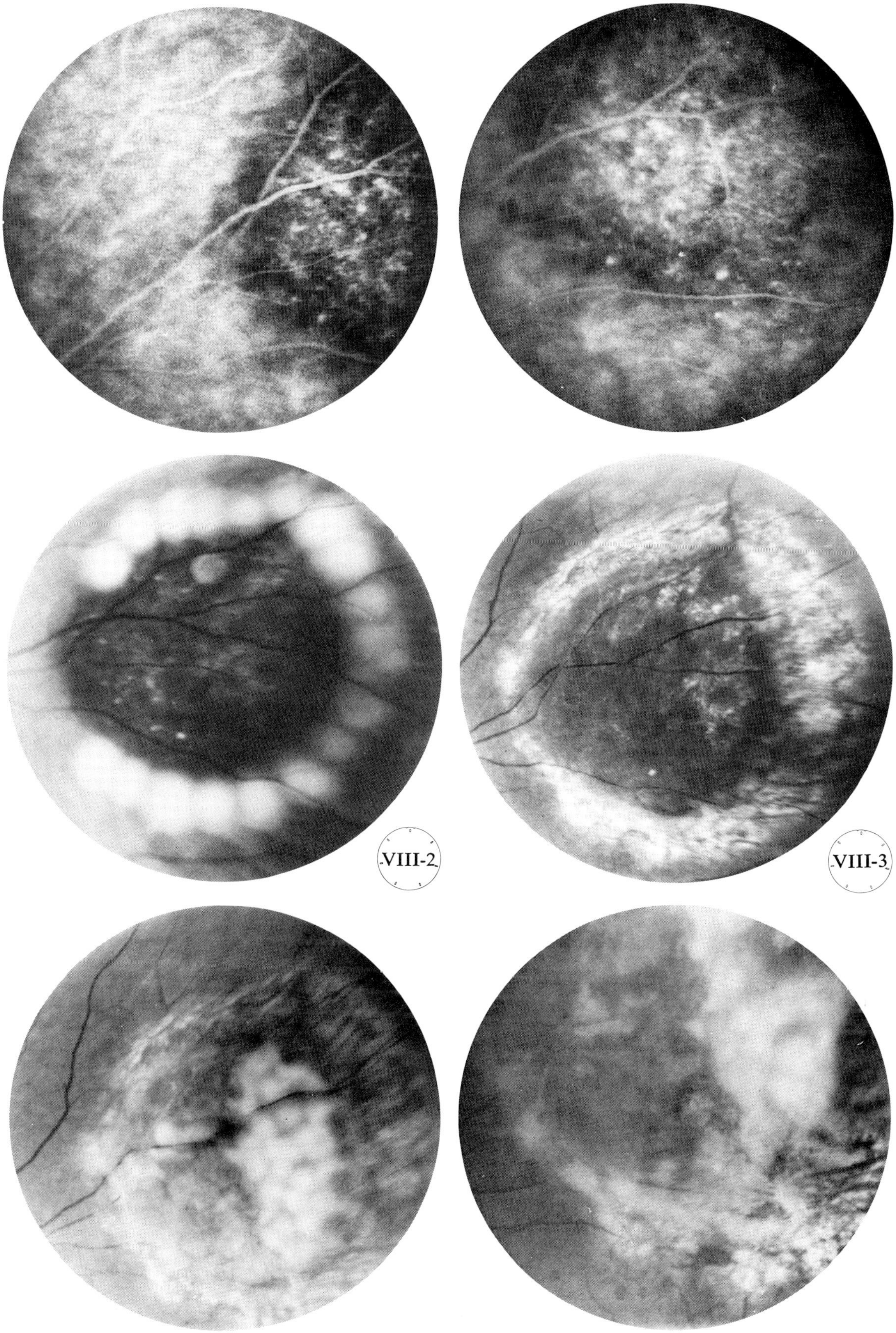

Fig. 8-9, cont'd. For legend see opposite page.

Vitreous contraction can occur but should not be a problem if the energy is properly allocated to the tumor and is not excessive.

Permanent dilation of the pupil because of photocoagulative sphincter damage can occur, but this complication is not as likely to occur with argon laser photocoagulation as it is with xenon-arc photocoagulation, because of the delivery system design and the smaller diameter of the laser beam.

Regrowth of the tumor in an area of previous photocoagulation can occur but can usually be remedied by adequate photocoagulation of the zone of reactivation.

Follow-up. The patient is followed at 3- to 4-week intervals, at which time photocoagulation is usually continued in a manner designed to destroy a particular amount of tumor tissue during each photocoagulation session. Patients may experience moderate amounts of discomfort, and analgesics should be prescribed along with the cycloplegic and steroid drops. All patients must be apprised of their condition during the treatment sessions. (Of course, the entire situation and therapeutic approach must be explained in great detail before treatment is initiated.) Once the tumor tissue has been obliterated, the patient should be followed at 3-month intervals for at least 2 to 3 years. Fluorescein angiograms taken at 6-month intervals will be helpful for detecting new vascular formations or areas of regrowth.

ANGIOMATOSIS RETINAE

Clinical symptoms. The symptoms of angiomatosis retinae usually are those of gradually decreasing vision in one eye as a result of massive exudation and retinal detachment, rather than sudden visual loss because of vitreous hemorrhage. Serous accumulations beneath the sensory retina can cause artificial hypermetropia similar to that seen in central serous choroidopathy. Metamorphopsia and micropsia can be seen, although the micropsia appears less often than it does with central serous choroidopathy. Extensive intraretinal edema and exudate formation can produce an incorrectable decrease in vision. Lightning flashes, an increasing number of scotomas, and decreased sensitivity under poor lighting conditions can be some of the initial complaints of the affected individuals.

Ophthalmoscopic appearance. The ophthalmoscopic picture of von Hippel's angiomatosis of the retina is not difficult to recognize except in its incipient stages and occasionally in its very late stages. During the early stages of its development, minimal widening and slight tortuosity of the nearby artery and vein along the vascular arcades can be seen in conjunction with a tiny arteriovenous anastomosis in the periphery. These early lesions show an area of dilated, small vascular channels with associated retinal edema, microaneurysms, a few minute fatty exudates, and often, small arteriovenous communications most commonly located in the temporal periphery. Occasionally, intraretinal hemorrhages can be seen at this stage.

Much later, when the disease process has become extensive, widespread areas of hard white exudates appear underneath the retina, accompanied by a serous elevation of the retina; these developments may obscure the causative tumor. As the lesion becomes more mature, the angioma with its arteriovenous shunt becomes apparent, and the draining vein enlarges, and the feeding artery enlarges. The tumor itself may be red or yellowish white, oval or round, and have adjacent lateral or peripheral cystic retinal degeneration. It is uncommon to find retinal vessels peripheral to the angioma, although they may exist as threadlike structures in the cystic retina. Usually extending peripherally on either side, a large accumulation of heavy, fatty exudation is commonly seen posterior to the angioma.

Microaneurysms and small retinal hemorrhages are most common, and it may be difficult to differentiate the feeding artery from the draining vein because of the arteriolar nature of the blood now coursing through both vessels. The pigment epithelium posterior to the angioma may be disorganized and disturbed; migrated clumps of proliferative pigment may be noted in the vicinity.

As the angioma enlarges, the paired feeding and draining vessels will be grossly enlarged far into the posterior retina. The arteries appear highly burnished, and both the draining and the feeding vessels become tortuous and markedly dilated in other sectors surrounding the angiomatous lesion. It is quite common to find a large amount of involvement of the macular region. This involvement usually starts as a star figure of exudate formation but progresses to an oval, elevated yellowish mass with smoothly rounded borders. The fatty exudates can extend throughout the macular and paramacular region, and such a lesion can be mistaken for disciform macular degeneration as well as extensive Coats' disease. Progressively, cystic changes and exudation can lead to retinal detachment, retinal and subretinal hemorrhage, vitreous hemorrhage, rubeosis iridis, secondary glaucoma, and eventual loss of the globe.

Ancillary diagnostic examinations. Fluorescein angiography can be useful for demonstrating the high flow pattern of the fluorescein as it passes through the feeder and drainage vessels. The tumor itself stains and leaks fluorescein markedly, regardless of size or maturity. Small angiomatous lesions can be easily detected if they are located in the

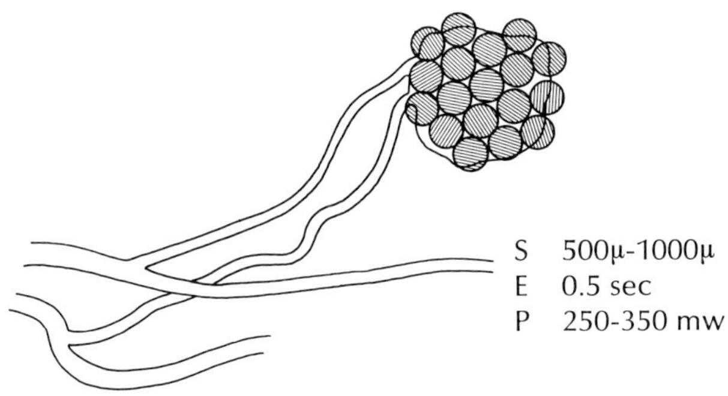

Fig. 8-10. Placement of 1,000μ argon laser photocoagulations or 6° xenon-arc photocoagulations on the body of the angioma in a contiguous or overlapping manner with power levels sufficient to produce obvious shrinkage of tumor tissue at the time of photocoagulation.

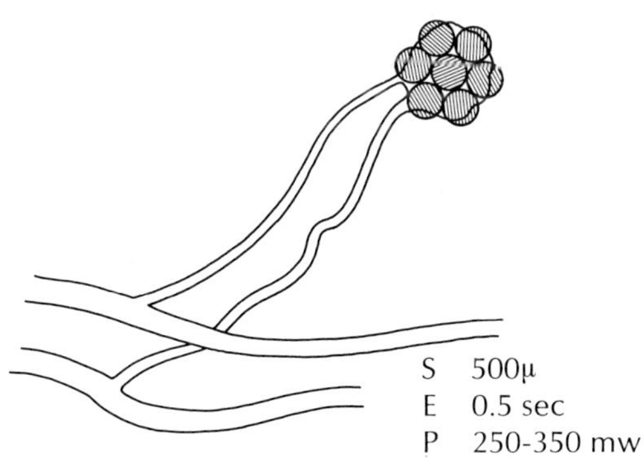

Fig. 8-11. As the angioma decreases in size following photocoagulation treatments at monthly intervals, the remainder of the tumor tissue can be photocoagulated directly, with slightly smaller coagulations, in an attempt to obliterate the vascular channels in the neoplasm.

posterior fundus. In many cases the angioma is far peripheral and does not lend itself to accurate fluorescein photography.

The high-flow system in the feeder and collector vessels does not perfuse well at right angles to these vessels and therefore deprives the macula and surrounding tissues of their nutrient blood supply. The macular region can be shown to be ischemic in many instances, and recognition of this defect, in association with an enlarged artery and vein in one quadrant, should increase the suspicion of the existence of a peripheral angiomatous or telangiectatic lesion. A fluorescein angiogram taken with a wide-field camera, such as the Nikon fundus camera, can be helpful in uncovering early angiomatous formations in the midperiphery of the fundus; this test should be conducted at 6-month intervals for all eyes being evaluated.

Stereo or regular fundus color photography should be done on the treated eye and the fellow eye routinely at 6-month intervals to detect any change in the retinal vessel configuration.

Photocoagulation approach. The photocoagulation approach should consist of a sufficient number of photocoagulation impacts on the tumor to completely cover it by coagulations. Spot sizes of **500μ to 1,000μ** in diameter, power levels of **250 to 350 mw,** and exposures of at least **0.5 sec** are required for the proper photocoagulation intensity (Figs. 8-10 and 8-11). The power should be raised to a level sufficient to cause actual obliteration and blanching of the tumor tissue, as well as a visible crimping or shriveling of the impact site. All visible tumor tissue should be treated with this intensity during the first photocoagulation session.

The patient is then reevaluated approximately 10 days later and observed closely for any signs of extensive hemorrhage or serous elevation of the adjacent retina. It is not uncommon that hemorrhages occur over the face of the tumor in the photocoagulation zone and that the surrounding retina becomes markedly edematous with some degree of serous detachment of the retinal region. If the hemorrhage is not extensive, the patient is rescheduled for further photocoagulation at a period 4 to 6 weeks following the original photocoagulation session (Figs. 8-12 and 8-13).

The patient is advised that his vision may become much more blurred during the following 2 to 3 weeks, and he is cautioned to avoid excessive bending or lifting of heavy objects or doing anything that would stimulate the Valsalva maneuver. Homatropine hydrobromide 2% and dexamethasone 0.1% drops are prescribed to be given three times a day in the affected eye for at least 14 days or until the next evaluation visit. A combination of acetylsalicylic acid (600 mg) and 30 mg of codeine (Empirin-3), or a similar medication for pain, is prescribed to be given every 4 to 6 hours as necessary. If the pain is unusually severe, the patient is urged to call the surgeon for further instructions.

Fig. 8-12. A, Posterior polar region of a 9-year-old boy who complained of a marked decrease in vision over a 3-month period. He was found to have a 3-DD angioma in the inferior portion of his fundus. Note the marked tortuosity of the vessels and the macular star exudates (arrow). **B,** Large angioma extending into the vitreous body and the swollen, engorged feeder and collector vessels from the tumor mass (arrows). **C,** Angioma immediately after photocoagulation, showing a diffuse coat of coagulum and early hemorrhagic activity in the region of the coagulations. **D,** Shrunken angioma after four argon laser photocoagulation treatments at monthly intervals, showing marked gliosis of the angiomatous mass and the preretinal hemorrhages commonly noted from the angioma after photocoagulation. **E,** Angiomatous lesion after complete destruction by argon laser photocoagulation.

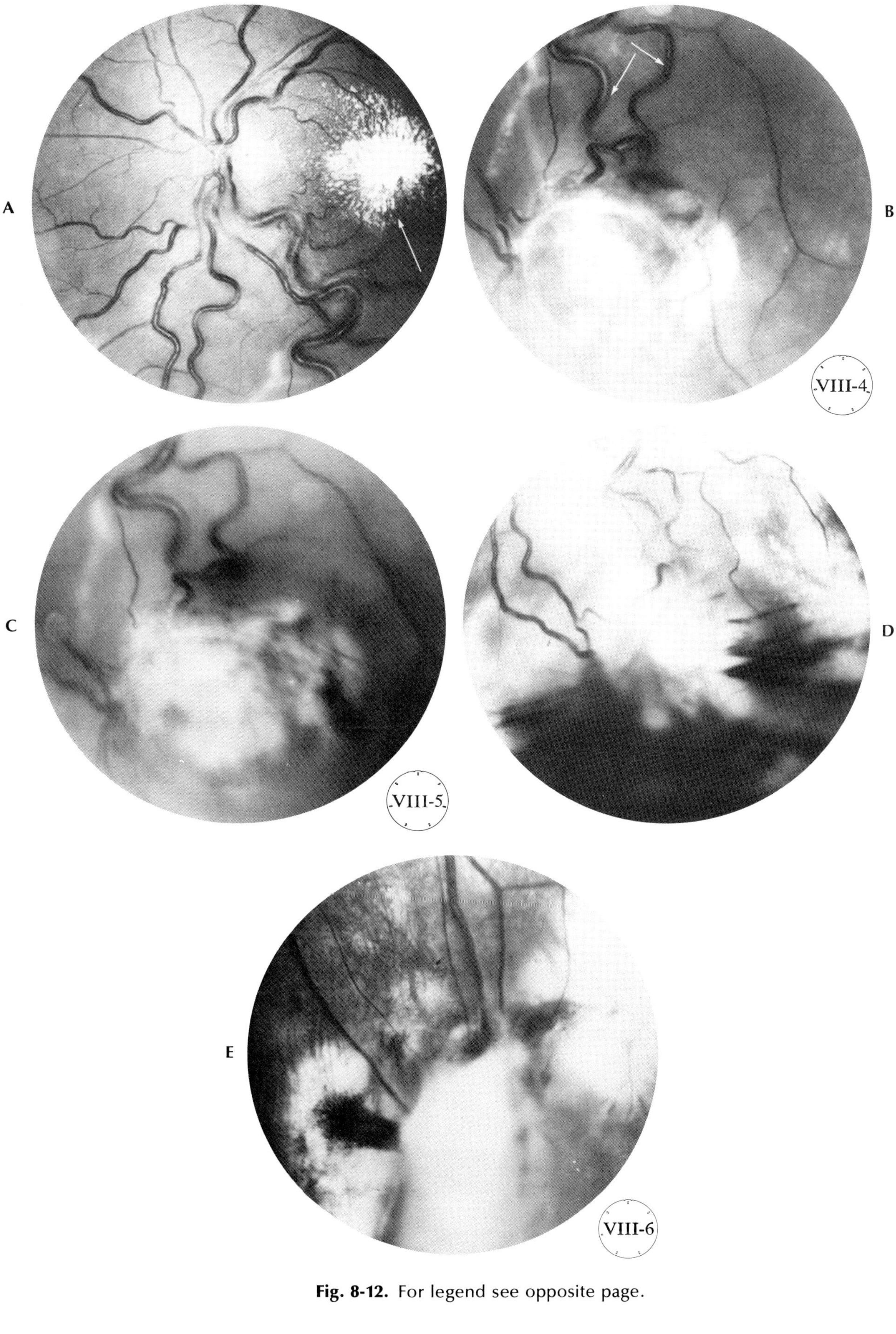

Fig. 8-12. For legend see opposite page.

When the small amount of hemorrhage on the dome of the angioma has cleared sufficiently, photocoagulation is then applied in the manner described during the initial visit. Usually, treating only those pinkish zones of exposed angiomatous tissue is adequate for eventual destruction of the tumor. Three to 8 sessions may be required at approximately 4- to 6-week intervals before the tumor is completely destroyed. Similar postoperative instructions are issued until complete gliosis and obliteration of the tumor have been accomplished.

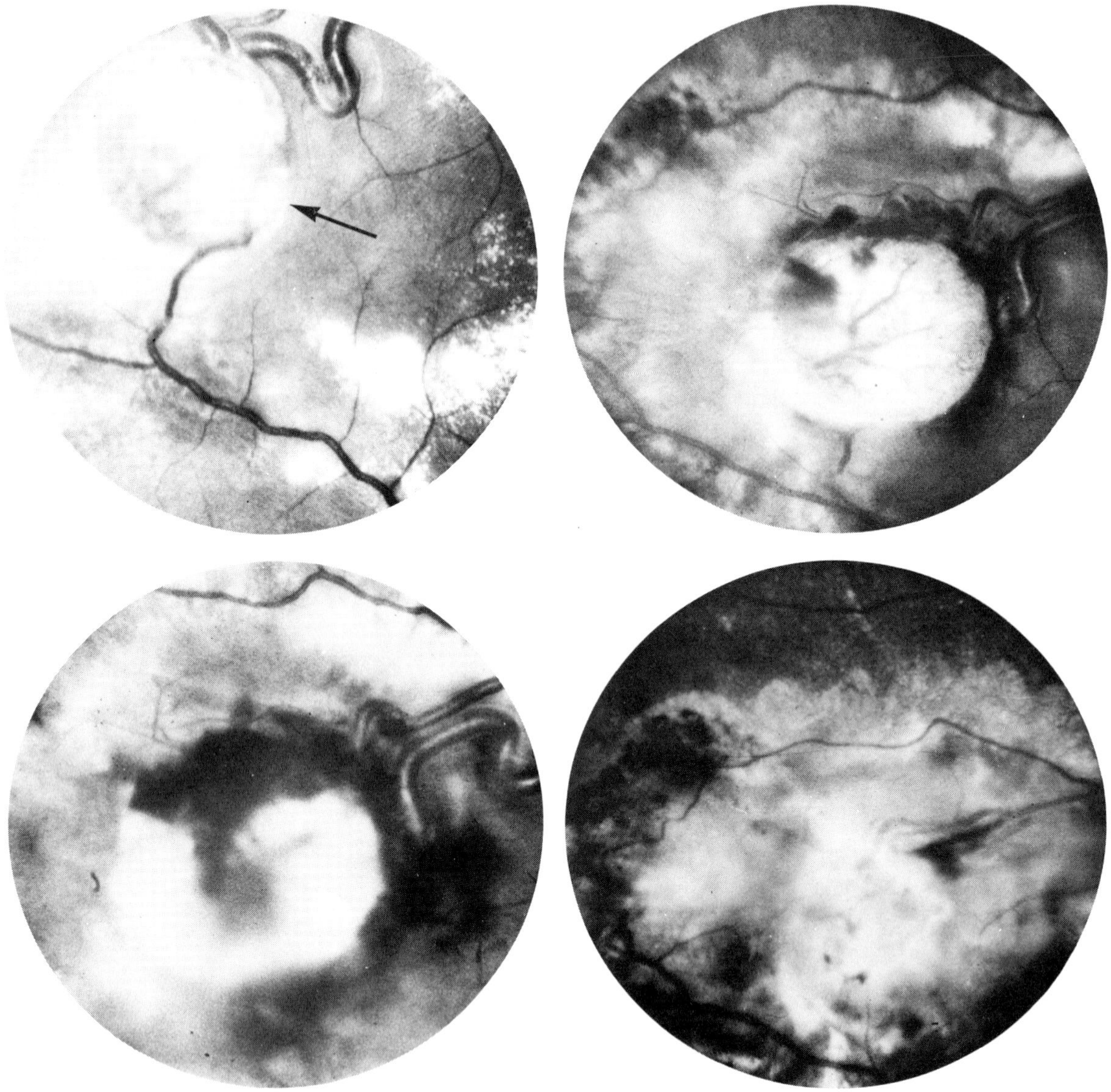

A B

C D

Fig. 8-13. A, A large 3-DD angioma (arrow) in the right eye of a 22-year-old pregnant woman who complained of blurred vision of 6 weeks' duration. **B,** Small hemorrhages from the surface of the angioma after the initial treatment session with xenon-arc photocoagulation. **C,** More extensive hemorrhagic activity after the fourth monthly treatment session with xenon-arc photocoagulation. **D,** Photocoagulated area 6 months after the initiation of photocoagulation therapy, showing complete destruction of the angioma.

If the tumor is larger than 2 DD, a preliminary double linear row of photocoagulations **500μ** in width, **200 mw** in intensity, and at an exposure of approximately **0.2 sec** are placed around the lesion in an area of nearly normal retina. The coagulations actually bridge the zone between the edematous retina near the angiomatous tumor and the normal retina. This ringlike barricade of coagulations around the tumor minimizes an extensive serous detachment of the retina, an occurrence that is quite common after photocoagulation of larger tumors. The initial photocoagulation is delayed 4 to 6 weeks, until the barricade of photocoagulation has healed completely. The routine photocoagulation approach is then employed.

If the tumor is 2 to 4 DD in diameter and partially gliotic, the feeder vessels are treated with argon laser photocoagulation to create a spasm and thereby reduce the amount of blood flowing to the tumor during the actual photocoagulation of the tumor itself (Figs. 8-14 to 8-16). Four to 6 local constrictions of the feeder arteriole can be produced near the angioma, and the tumor can then be attacked directly, as advised. In these cases the spot size must be 50% to 75% larger than the feeder vessel to the tumor, and the photocoagulation intensity is slowly increased (by increasing the power in 25-mw steps) until the spasm has been produced. The intensity should not be short (less than 0.1 sec) and usually ranges in the region of **0.2 to 0.5 sec.** When the flow of blood to the tumor is decreased temporarily, the angiomatous tissue can be more heavily treated, and the results are perhaps more effective. However, when approaching angiomatous tissue with this type of technique, one should consider the hazards of treating an engorged vessel, such as the feeder arteriole, under high pressure.

Complications. The greatest complication following photocoagulation is a large hemorrhage from the tumor. To minimize this problem, patients must be urged not to exert themselves in any way. Hemorrhage around the tumor, regardless of restrictions, is very common and is not serious. Photocoagulation treatment should not be repeated until most of the surrounding hemorrhage has been absorbed.

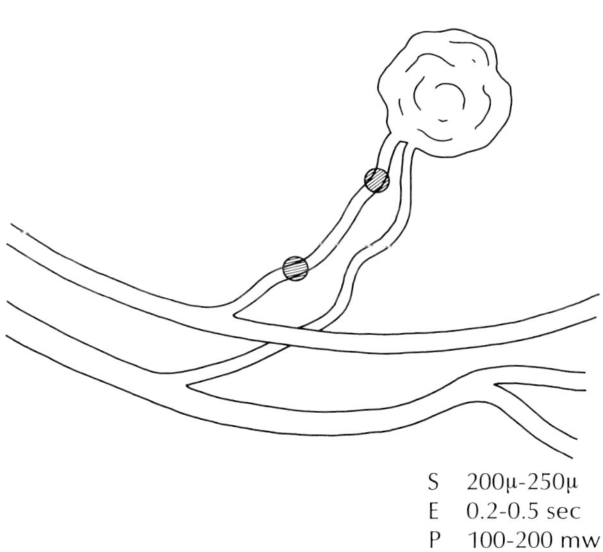

Fig. 8-14. The afferent feeder vessel to a smaller angioma can be treated directly by the production of constrictions in that vessel at 1-DD intervals. Coagulation sizes should be at least 50% larger than the feeder vessel.

A large serous elevation of the adjacent retina can also be commonly observed following photocoagulation. This complication decreases in 3 to 6 weeks. Employing a delimiting row of coagulations before treating the tumor directly helps to minimize this problem.

Follow-up. All patients should be seen at 6-month intervals following successful obliteration of the angiomatous tumor. New angiomas can appear throughout the midperiphery and peripheral regions of either eye, as well as in the region of the optic disc.

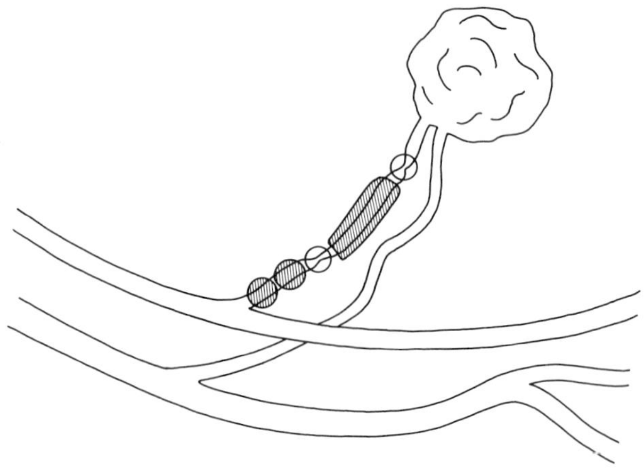

S 250μ-300μ
E 0.5-1.0 sec
P 100-200 mw

Fig. 8-15. After the feeder arteriole has been constricted, the blood trapped between the constriction is coagulated with gentle, continuous, streaked coagulations to produce a complete occlusion of the arteriole.

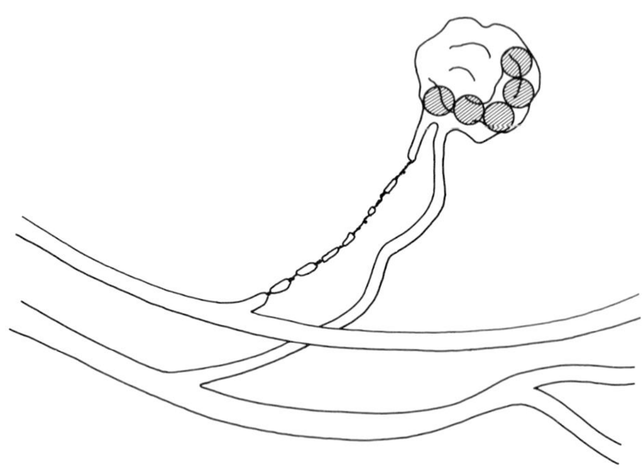

S 500μ-1000μ
E 0.5 sec
P 250-350 mw

Fig. 8-16. When the feeder vessel to the angioma has been constricted or occluded, the main body of the tumor can then be treated with coagulations that are overlapping and Grades 3 to 4 in intensity. Multiple treatment sessions at monthly intervals are usually required for the obliteration of the tumor.

A fluorescein angiogram should be taken (if possible, with a wide-angle fundus camera) and fluorescein ophthalmoscopy employed at least at yearly intervals, particularly in patients during stressful periods such as puberty.

CHOROIDAL HEMANGIOMA

Clinical symptoms. Choroidal hemangioma usually will cause a disturbance of vision that appears as distortion, blurring, or micropsia, especially if the hemangioma occupies the more posterior polar region of the eye, as it usually does. Numerous spots, patterns, progressive hyperopia, and flashes of light can be noted throughout the growth period of the hemangioma. Glaucoma may ensue as the hemangioma grows and may be a presenting sign. This tumor usually occurs in young individuals between the ages of 10 and 20 years, commonly in association with the facial angiomas of the Sturge-Weber syndrome.

Ophthalmoscopic appearance. The appearance of a choroidal hemangioma may vary with the reparative response of the eye to the tumor's continued growth. The hemangioma may appear as an elevation very similar to a malignant melanoma; it is usually located in the posterior pole near the optic nerve but frequently appears without deep pigmentation and clustering of pigment on the surface of the tumor. The tumor may show a slightly more hyperemic and orange-red color if the overlying pigment epithelium and glial tissue have not hypertrophied to any degree. The overlying retina may show considerable signs of scarring and glial proliferation or may be atrophied, particularly on the dome of the enlarging tumor. The retina may be dependently detached secondarily and show some transudate, white residual edema, and particularly some cystoid changes.

Ancillary diagnostic examinations. The most useful ancillary diagnostic examination is fluorescein angiography, which may show an immediate filling of the choroidal tumor in the choroidal flush phase of the angiogram. The tumor then proceeds to fluoresce remarkably because of the large vascular channels, lacunas, and concentrations of fluorescein. Some of the fluorescein may stain the scar tissue surrounding the large vascular channels, and the fluorescence may persist into the late venous phase. However, most of the blood-fluorescein mixture appears to be washed from the hemangioma more rapidly than it is from a malignant melanoma.

A blanching of the choroidal hemangioma can be seen when pressure is exerted on the globe either digitally or by suction ophthalmodynamometry. The tumor may blanch markedly and may decrease in size as the pressure is elevated above the inflow pressure. This feature is most characteristic of a choroidal hemangioma.

Ultrasonography may also show the tumor to be more loculated and vascular in nature than a more solidly characterized tumor, such as a malignant melanoma or metastatic carcinoma.

The ^{32}P radioisotope test can be helpful in differentiating this tumor from other growths, although it does occasionally show a concentration of the isotope in the hemangioma, as is usually demonstrated with malignant melanomas.

Visual field examination may occasionally show sector defects caused by cystic degeneration of the overlying retina.

Bone-free roentgenographic examination of the eye rotated in various positions may reveal the presence of calcium and bone. Intracranial calcifications can be seen with the meningeal hemangiomas of the Sturge-Weber syndrome.

Indications for photocoagulation. A choroidal hemangioma less than 3 to 4 DD in diameter and located at least 1 DD away from the optic nerve can be considered for photocoagulation if it can be well visualized in its entirety.

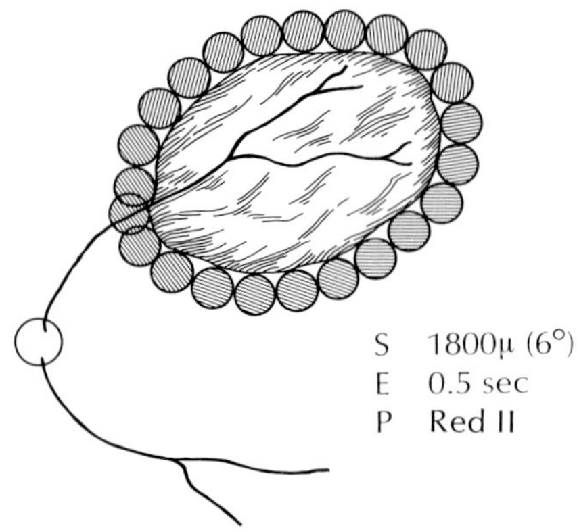

Fig. 8-17. Placement of punctate, linear, contiguous 6° (1,800μ) xenon-arc coagulations around the periphery of the choroidal hemangioma to obliterate the choroidal blood supply coming into the tumor (Stage 1).

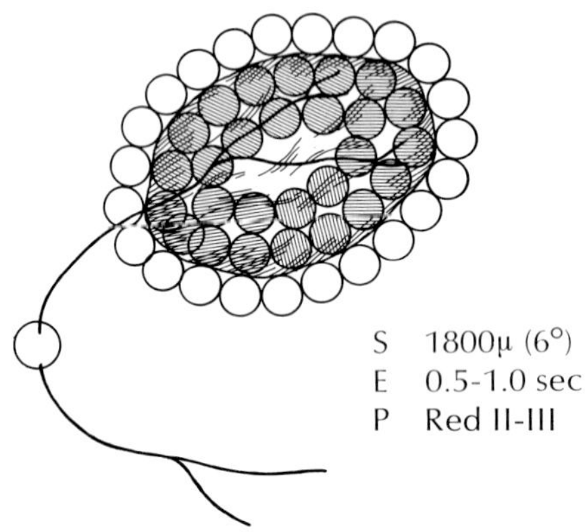

Fig. 8-18. Application of xenon-arc photocoagulations within the previous ring of treatment, as shown in Fig. 8-17, with longer exposures and slightly higher energy (Stage 2). The choroidal hemangioma tissue should shrivel immediately on application of the photocoagulation energy. An interval of 3 to 4 weeks should elapse between each of the 3 stages of treatment.

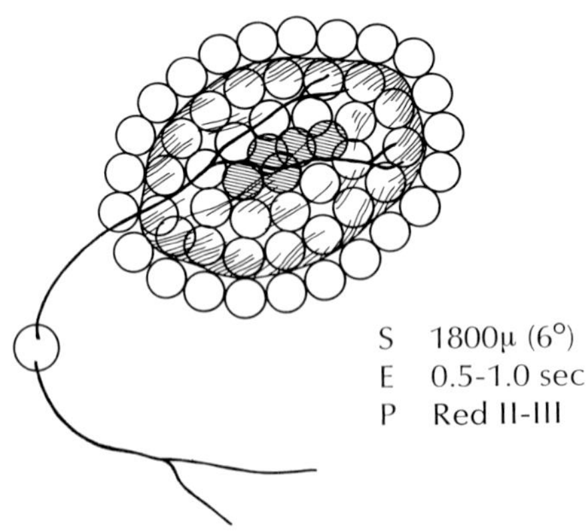

Fig. 8-19. Treatment of the central region of the choroidal hemangioma with Grade 4 xenon-arc photocoagulations of intensities similar to those noted previously. The entire tumor should be covered with a coagulum at this treatment session (Stage 3), and treatment should be repeated at monthly intervals until the vascular neoplasm has been destroyed.

Any choroidal hemangioma with the previous specifications can be treated if the elevation into the vitreous does not exceed 2 mm and the surface glial tissue does not prevent the photocoagulation beam from penetrating the tumor mass.

Photocoagulation approach. The patient must be informed that the photocoagulation procedure is being employed in an attempt to save the eye rather than the vision, although hopefully both can be saved.

A retrobulbar injection to obtain anesthesia and akinesia is required during the first few treatments with the xenon-arc instrument. Later, no anesthetic other than proparacaine administered topically may be necessary, since the sensory nerves in the treated outer layers of the eye will have been destroyed. Argon laser photocoagulation usually requires a retrobulbar and a topical anesthetic. A contact lens to neutralize the corneal power is also necessary with the latter instrument.

The xenon-arc instrument is the preferred photocoagulation source with which to treat a choroidal hemangioma, because the infrared component of the beam has a greater penetration through the highly vascular tumor than that of other photocoagulation emissions. Argon laser photocoagulation usually causes a coagulum on the surface of the blood-filled tumor and does not have the advantageous penetration of xenon-arc photocoagulation into the depths of the vascular mass.

Photocoagulation should be directed to the periphery of the tumor in a manner similar to that employed with malignant melanomas. In these cases however, there usually is less pigmentation, and it is important to use powers sufficient to destroy the vascular tissue and the surrounding choroidal feeder vessels to the tumor.

After half of the perimeter of the tumor has been coagulated with intense **6°** coagulations of **Red II** intensity for approximately **0.5 sec,** the treated region is allowed to heal and scar for approximately 4 to 6 weeks. The remaining half of the perimeter is then photocoagulated, and the reparative process is allowed to continue for approximately 1 month (Fig. 8-17).

The central regions of the tumor are later coagulated directly with high intensities (**Red II to III, 6°** coagulations for **0.5 to 1.0 sec**) repeatedly, until the tumor is considered to be arrested or obliterated (Figs. 8-18 and 8-19).

The tumor is evaluated at 3-month intervals for any sign of recurrence or regrowth (Fig. 8-20).

Complications. The most common complication is hemorrhage caused by excessive coagulation of the wall of a vessel under moderately high blood pressure. In these cases the wall herniates and eventually ruptures through the weakened coagulated zone, causing a large and sometimes disastrous vitreous or retinal hemorrhage. The point of proposed photocoagulation should be examined carefully before treatment to determine whether a large naked vessel without glial reinforcement is involved in that particular area. Rather than attacking them directly, photocoagulation should be employed around these more obvious large, weak-walled vessels.

As with any other photocoagulation procedure where very large amounts of energy are required for proper treatment of the tumor mass, vitreous contraction, retinal detachment, and excessive scarring can occur.

Macular striae, excessive glial proliferation, cystic formation, and pigmentary degeneration of the central retina have been observed as late occurrences that are possibly associated with the previous photocoagulation treatment.

Follow-up. The patient should be seen at approximately 1-month intervals and should be given cycloplegic and steroid drops during this interval. This medication should be

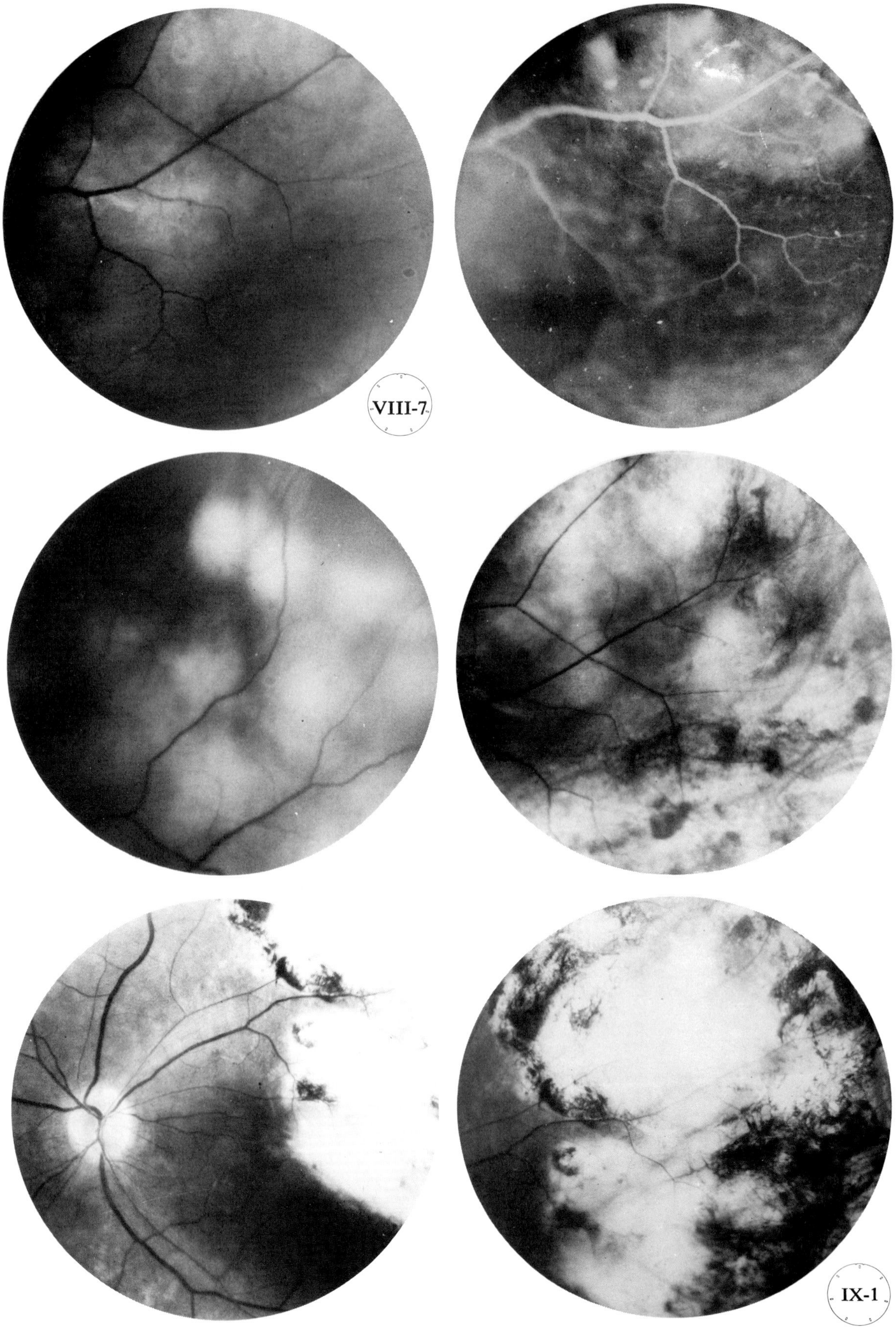

Fig. 8-20. For legend see opposite page.

continued throughout the course of treatment, which may last for 1 year. Further coagulation should be attempted, if healing has progressed satisfactorily, at 4- to 6-week intervals; the tumor tissue should be rephotocoagulated in an attempt to destroy all existing channels.

When the tumor has been destroyed by photocoagulation, the obliterated site must be evaluated carefully at 3-month intervals for the regrowth of neovascular tissue.

Fig. 8-20. A, A choroidal hemangioma was discovered in a 36-year-old man who complained of blurred vision of 5 months' duration in his left eye. The superotemporal mass was found to fluoresce during fluorescein angiography and to blanch when the globe was compressed. Ultrasonography also supported this diagnosis. **B,** Fluorescein angiogram showing marked concentration and retention of the dye in lacunas throughout the tumor mass. **C,** Xenon-arc photocoagulation directed to the outer rim of the choroidal hemangioma and later to the central choroidal mass. **D,** Xenon-arc photocoagulation causing coagulation and obliteration of the vascular channels in the central region of the hemangioma. Note that the peripheral aspects of the choroidal hemangioma have already been destroyed by previous photocoagulation. **E,** Posterior polar region, showing destruction of a large area of the superotemporal quadrant formerly occupied by the choroidal hemangioma. The foveal area was not damaged by the photocoagulation, and the vision was retained at 20/80, the level before photocoagulation. **F,** Wide-angle view of the entire area of photocoagulation treatment, showing complete obliteration of the choroidal hemangioma.

SECTION TWO

Macular diseases

Chapter 9

Classification

It is essential that macular disease syndromes be classified morphologically and etiologically before photocoagulation of macular diseases is discussed. This classification of macular diseases can be based on the pathologic findings as visualized during ophthalmologic examination; these findings are correlated with the histopathologic examination specimens submitted to the laboratory. Macular diseases can also be considered in terms of their cause, and this consideration is important when photocoagulation therapy is involved. A morphologic classification of macular diseases consists of the following categories.

- I. Macular interrretinal defects
  - A. Macular serous abnormalities
    - 1. Detachment of the pigment epithelium*
      - a. Degenerative*
      - b. Neovascular*
    - 2. Detachment of the sensory retina (degenerative)*
      - a. Central serous choroidopathy*
      - b. Idiopathic*
  - B. Macular hemorrhagic abnormalities
    - 1. Detachment of the pigment epithelium*
      - a. Degenerative*
      - b. Neovascular*
    - 2. Detachment of the sensory retina*
      - a. Degenerative*
      - b. Neovascular*
- II. Macular intraretinal abnormalities
  - A. Intracellular edema
    - 1. Retinal artery occlusion
      - a. Branch retinal artery
      - b. Central retinal artery
  - B. Extracellular edema
    - 1. Retinal vein occlusion*
      - a. Branch retinal vein*
      - b. Central retinal vein*

*Those particular diseases that can be considered for photocoagulation.

2. Diabetic maculopathy*
3. Hypertensive maculopathy
4. Irvine-Gass syndrome (aphakia)*
5. Vitreitis (peripheral uveitis)
6. Toxic maculopathy (epinephrine)

C. Microvascular abnormalities (telangiectasia*)

III. Miscellaneous macular diseases

A. Macular hole* or cyst
B. Preretinal fibrosis
C. Toxoplasmosis retinochoroiditis*
D. *Toxocara canis* or *T. cati* infestation*
E. Pigment epitheliopathy*
F. Angioid streaks*
G. Choroidal (subretinal) neovascularization*

An etiologic classification of macular diseases, as compiled by Maumenee, places the various macular diseases into seven general categories, depending on their suspected cause.

1. Degenerative
   a. Central serous choroidopathy (retinopathy)*
   b. Senile choroidal macular degeneration
   c. Retinal vascular disease (diabetes and hypertension)*
2. Inflammatory
   a. Histoplasmic choroiditis*
   b. Histoplasmiclike choroiditis*
   c. Toxoplasmosis retinochoroiditis*
   d. *T. canis* ocular infestation*
   e. Solar retinitis (foveomacular retinitis)
   f. Preretinal membrane contracture
   g. Acute multifocal posterior placoid pigment epitheliopathy (AMPPPE)
3. Metabolic
   a. Heredomacular degenerations (vitelliform, Stargardt's, flavimaculatus, and so on)
   b. Tapetoretinal degenerations (retinitis pigmentosa)
   c. Cerebromacular degeneration (Tay-Sachs and Niemann-Pick)
4. Neoplastic
   a. Nevus
   b. Malignant melanoma*
   c. Choroidal hemangioma*
   d. Metastatic
5. Traumatic
6. Toxic maculopathies (chloroquine retinopathy)
7. Congenital anomalies

I prefer to categorize the various macular problems according to their morphologic characteristics rather than their possible cause, since the latter may be open to debate. There is no doubt that knowledge of the underlying cause of the macular disease is important. The indications for, and the various parameters applicable to, photocoagulation and the particular photocoagulation approach for a disease process depends almost entirely on the morphologic derangement in the macular region. The photocoagulation procedure simply scars, seals, or obliterates a disease process before the lesion can directly or indirectly affect other, more widespread or vital, areas of the macular region. Basically, the presence of a breakdown of the anatomic barriers in the macular region or the proliferation of neovascular tissue is an indication for photocoagulation, provided the abnormality is at least ⅔ DD (1,000μ) from the central foveola (umbo). The following outline categorizes certain macular defects that may prove amenable to photocoagulation.

Macular defects amenable to photocoagulation

I. Anatomic barrier breakdown
  A. Bruch's membrane defect
    1. Angioid streaks
    2. Serous detachment of the pigment epithelium
  B. Pigment epithelial defect (serous detachment of the sensory retina, central serous choroidopathy)
  C. Retinal vessel breakdown
    1. Arteriole
      a. Diabetes
      b. Vasculitis
      c. Hypertension (?)
      d. Leber's retinopathy (miliary aneurysms)
      e. Coats' disease
      f. Occlusion
    2. Vein
      a. Occlusion
      b. Diabetes
      c. Eales' disease
  D. Retinal cellular breakdown
    1. Hypoxia
      a. Arterial occlusion (?)
    2. Structural
      a. Irvine-Gass syndrome (?)
      b. Preretinal membrane contracture
      c. Macular holes
II. Neovascular proliferation
  A. Retinal
  B. Choroidal

Chapter 10

Macular interretinal abnormalities

MACULAR SEROUS ABNORMALITIES

Detachment of the pigment epithelium

Degenerative

Clinical symptoms. A degenerative detachment of the pigment epithelium may cause no symptoms if it does not impinge on the foveal area. The most likely symptom is distorted vision caused by a tilting of the foveal area by the serous detachment. The occasional blurring of vision noted can be partially corrected by a hyperopic or astigmatic correction. Vague scotomas, as well as metamorphopsia, micropsia, and occasional photopsia, can also be observed by the patient.

Ophthalmoscopic appearance. A serous detachment of the pigment epithelium can occupy any area from an extremely small serous detachment to a large disc-shaped, blisterlike mound occupying the entire macular and paramacular region (Fig. 10-1). Most serous detachments are small, but intermediate ones the size of the optic disc can be seen frequently in the macular and perifoveal areas. These dome-shaped, blisterlike elevations appear to be firm, and there is little interruption of the overlying pigment epithelium or sensory retina in the immature stage. As the serous detachments mature, the pigment epithelium becomes more hypertrophied, clumped, and disorganized, and the overlying sensory retina may be atrophic or edematous. Glial changes or some vascular tortuosity in the retina can also be seen. In the late stages the entire pigment epithelium may be replaced by glial tissue proliferation, which creates a whitish appearance on the detachment dome and is usually surrounded by drusen or smaller serous detachments of the pigment epithelium. Hypertrophy of the pigment epithelium is usually a prominent component with more mature serous detachments of the pigment epithelium, and a typical "hot cross bun" appearance from proliferated pigment can be seen frequently.

Ancillary diagnostic examinations. Fluorescein angiography, particularly stereo fluorescein angiography, is of considerable importance because serous detachments of the pigment epithelium start to fill during the late choroidal flush phase and continue to concentrate dye throughout the arteriolovenular fluorescein transit. The fluorescence from the pooling of the fluorescein in the serous detachment beneath the pigment epithelium becomes extremely bright, and the margins are well defined, usually without leakage into the overlying subretinal space or into surrounding sub-pigment epithelial areas. In the area of pooling the pattern is homogeneous throughout the fluorescein transit. There is no

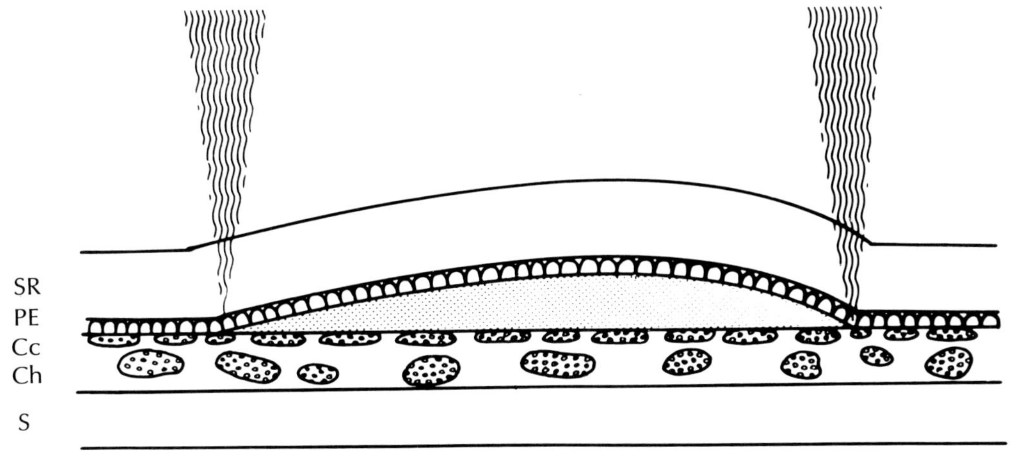

Fig. 10-1. Typical serous detachment of the pigment epithelium with elevation of the neuroepithelium and fluid between the pigment epithelium and Bruch's membrane. These lesions can degenerate, producing neovascularization extending into the serous cavity. Choroidal scarring and attenuation of the choriocapillaris can be observed.

mottling or fragmentation unless clumping and hypertrophy of the pigment layer are present. The pooling fluorescence persists strongly into the later venular phase.

Indirect fluorescein ophthalmoscopy should be performed on all patients immediately after fluorescein angiography, to detect more peripheral or unusually located leakage areas.

Stereo fundus color photography is valuable for following the progress of the slowly developing pigment epithelial defects, because these defects are most commonly seen in the very accessible posterior polar region, particularly in the macular and paramacular zones.

Visual field tests usually show vague relative scotomas on careful plotting in the region of the serous detachments. These results may be valuable for the long-term evaluation of these defects.

The beam from a direct ophthalmoscope can be directed to the margin of a serous detachment, and a large portion of the pigment epithelial detachment will glow from the scattered and reflected light within the detachment. Serous detachments of the sensory retina may glow slightly but without the intensity and sharp margin observed with the retinal pigment epithelial detachment.

Indications for photocoagulation. Immature macular serous detachments of the pigment epithelium less than 2 DD in width and with little pigment epithelial disruption and no defects of the overlying sensory retina can be evaluated carefully at 3-month intervals unless these detachments are located in the perifoveal region or subfoveal zone and are causing metamorphopsia or other visual symptoms. In these cases photocoagulation can be considered to alleviate the visual defects (Fig. 10-2).

Mature macular serous detachments of the pigment epithelium less than 1 DD in extent and with no changes in the overlying sensory retina should be watched closely by fluorescein angiography at 2- to 3-month intervals, because these lesions can undergo neovascular change. Mature serous detachments of the pigment epithelium in the macular region should be considered more seriously for photocoagulation if they occupy a perifoveal position and are not located in the papillomacular bundle. The increased

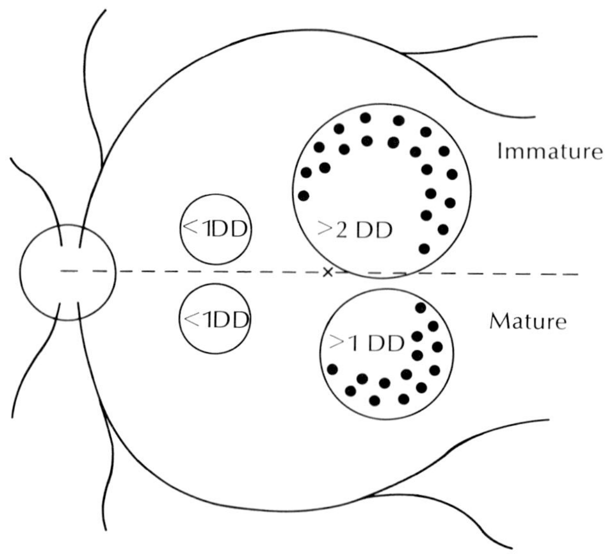

Fig. 10-2. Indications (black dots) for photocoagulation of immature (>2 DD) and mature (>1 DD) serous detachments of the pigment epithelium. Indications for photocoagulation depend on the proximity of the serous detachment to the umbo.

pigment clumping in the papillomacular region can lead to overlying nerve fiber defects if photocoagulation is attempted. However, photocoagulation is still indicated if underlying neovascular change is suspected.

All immature macular serous detachments of the pigment epithelium should be strongly considered for photocoagulation if their extent exceeds 2 DD. Mature serous detachments larger than 1 DD should also be photocoagulated. The possibility of neovascular change in serous detachments is greatly enhanced when pigment epithelial defects attain these, or larger, sizes.

Small subfoveal detachments of the pigment epithelium (<½ DD) cannot be treated because of their precarious location (Fig. 10-3). Any attempt at photocoagulation usually will injure the foveal region irreparably. Larger subfoveal serous detachments (>½ DD) can be treated along the temporal periphery of the detachment; hopefully, this procedure will cause the entire detachment to flatten.

Regardless of size or maturity, all macular serous detachments of the pigment epithelium with an overlying serous detachment of the sensory retina should be photocoagulated when recognized, provided that coagulations are not placed less than 1,000μ from the umbo. The occurrence of choroidal neovascularization is high in this condition and should be strongly suspected if overlying retinal edema, exudates, or hemorrhages exist around the serous detachment. Treatment for subfoveal serous detachments of the pigment epithelium with an overlying sensory retinal detachment should not be attempted because of the central location of these detachments.

If the macula of the fellow eye has been destroyed by a neovascularized or degenerated retinal pigment epithelial detachment, there is a stronger indication for treatment of the macular serous detachment. The defect should be watched closely by fluorescein angiography, and treatment should be instituted if there is any suggestion of neovascular proliferation or if there is definite evidence of enlargement, provided that the lesion is more than 1,000μ from the umbo. The prognosis is much poorer when there is evidence of neovascularization in the region of the detachment.

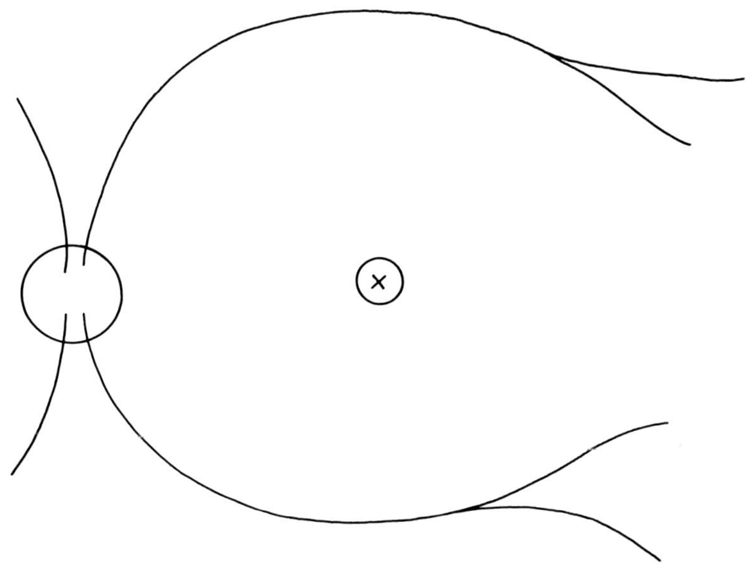

Fig. 10-3. A small (less than ½ DD) serous detachment of the pigment epithelium in the subfoveal location should not be treated because of its central location.

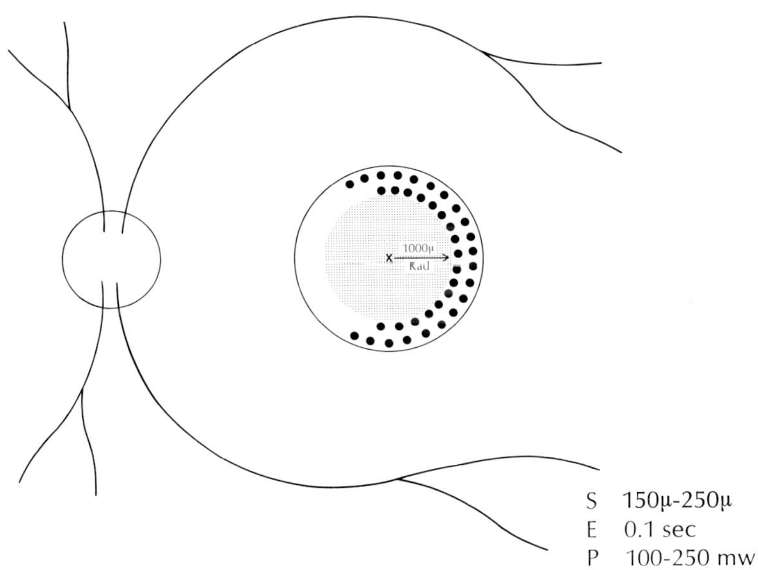

Fig. 10-4. Serous detachments of the pigment epithelium greater than 1 to 2 DD and located in the subfoveal area can be treated, depending on their maturity, with moderately intense 200μ coagulations in a temporal C pattern, provided that coagulations are not placed within 1,000μ of the umbo.

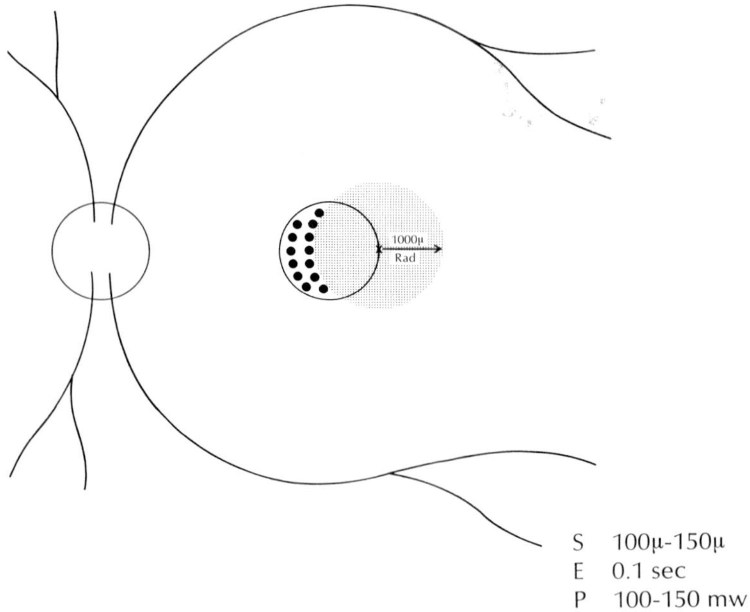

Fig. 10-5. Smaller serous detachments of the pigment epithelium located in the papillomacular bundle and impinging on the fovea can be treated, depending on their maturity, with a modified nasal C pattern at lower intensities, provided that coagulations are not placed within 1,000μ of the umbo.

Photocoagulation approach. Mature (>1 DD) and immature (>2 DD) serous detachments of the pigment epithelium located in the macular or paramacular region should be treated with **150μ to 250μ** coagulations in an interrupted speckled pattern. Coagulations should be created at least 200μ apart, with intensities ranging from **100 to 250 mw** at a **0.1-sec** exposure (Fig. 10-4). This dosage will vary, depending on the extent of overlying retinal edema and the prominence of the pigment epithelium. A soft-white, medium-intensity coagulation (Grade 3) should be produced. The entire dome of the serous detachment can be treated if the detachment lies in the paramacular or peripheral macular region. If the serous detachment occupies the macular zone impinging on the fovea, only the outer, more peripheral half of the serous detachment away from the fovea should be treated. Coagulations should not be attempted within 1,000μ of the umbo (⅔ DD). Coagulations can be made across the papillomacular bundle, provided that the coagulations are of slight (Grade 2) intensity (Figs. 10-5 to 10-7).

Fig. 10-6. A, A typical serous detachment of the pigment epithelium below the foveal area and other macular degenerative changes in a 49-year-old man who had complained of progressively decreasing vision in his left eye. **B,** Fluorescein angiogram during the early venular phase, demonstrating the concentration of the dye in the serous detachment of the pigment epithelium below the fovea. **C,** Multiple 150μ photocoagulations were applied to the pigment epithelial detachment. **D,** Healed serous detachment of the pigment epithelium 6 weeks after photocoagulation; vision has been retained at the 20/40 level. **E,** Fluorogram during the early venular phase, showing complete destruction of the serous detachment of the pigment epithelium and staining of the reparative glial tissue around the photocoagulation site.

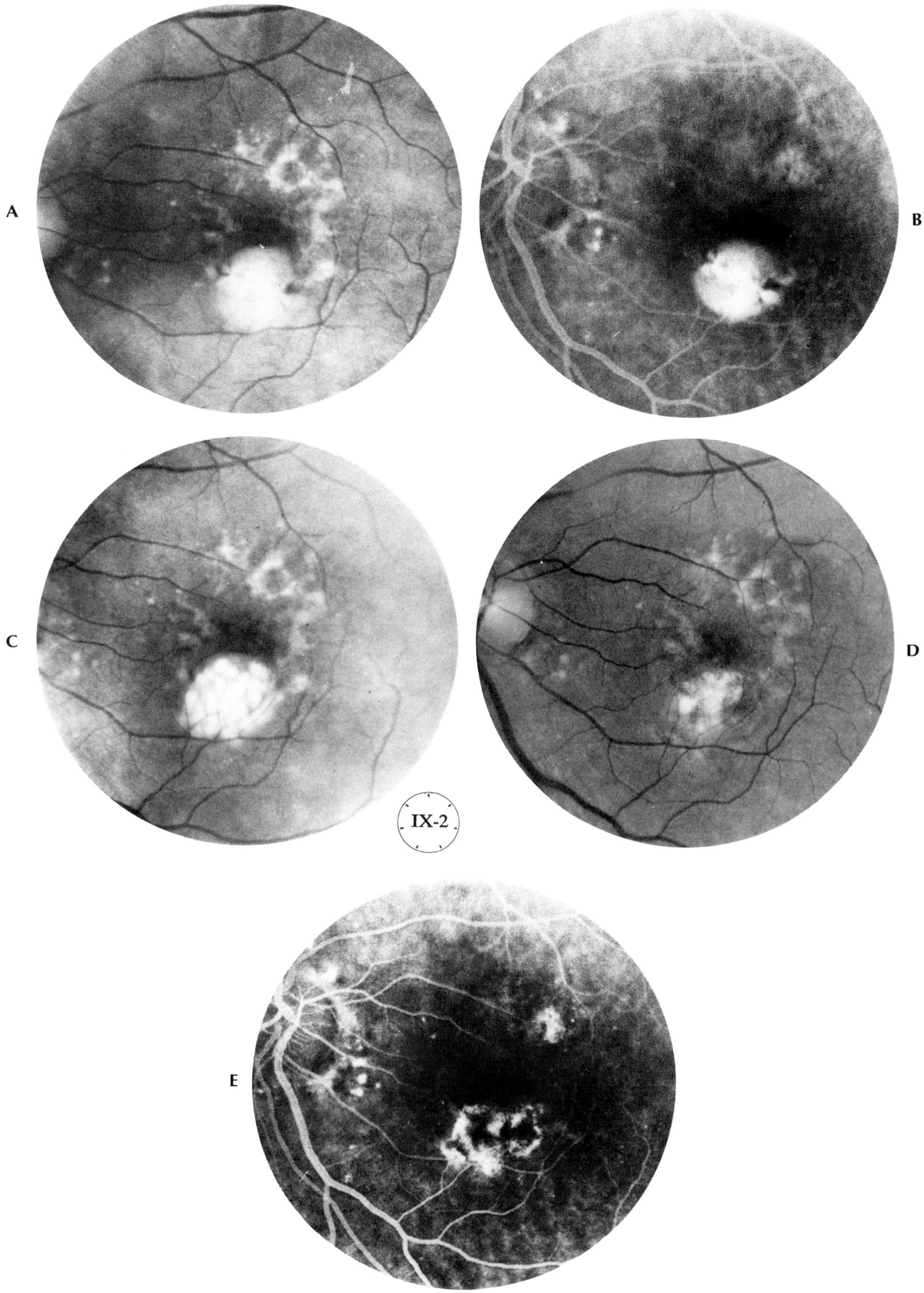

Fig. 10-6. For legend see opposite page.

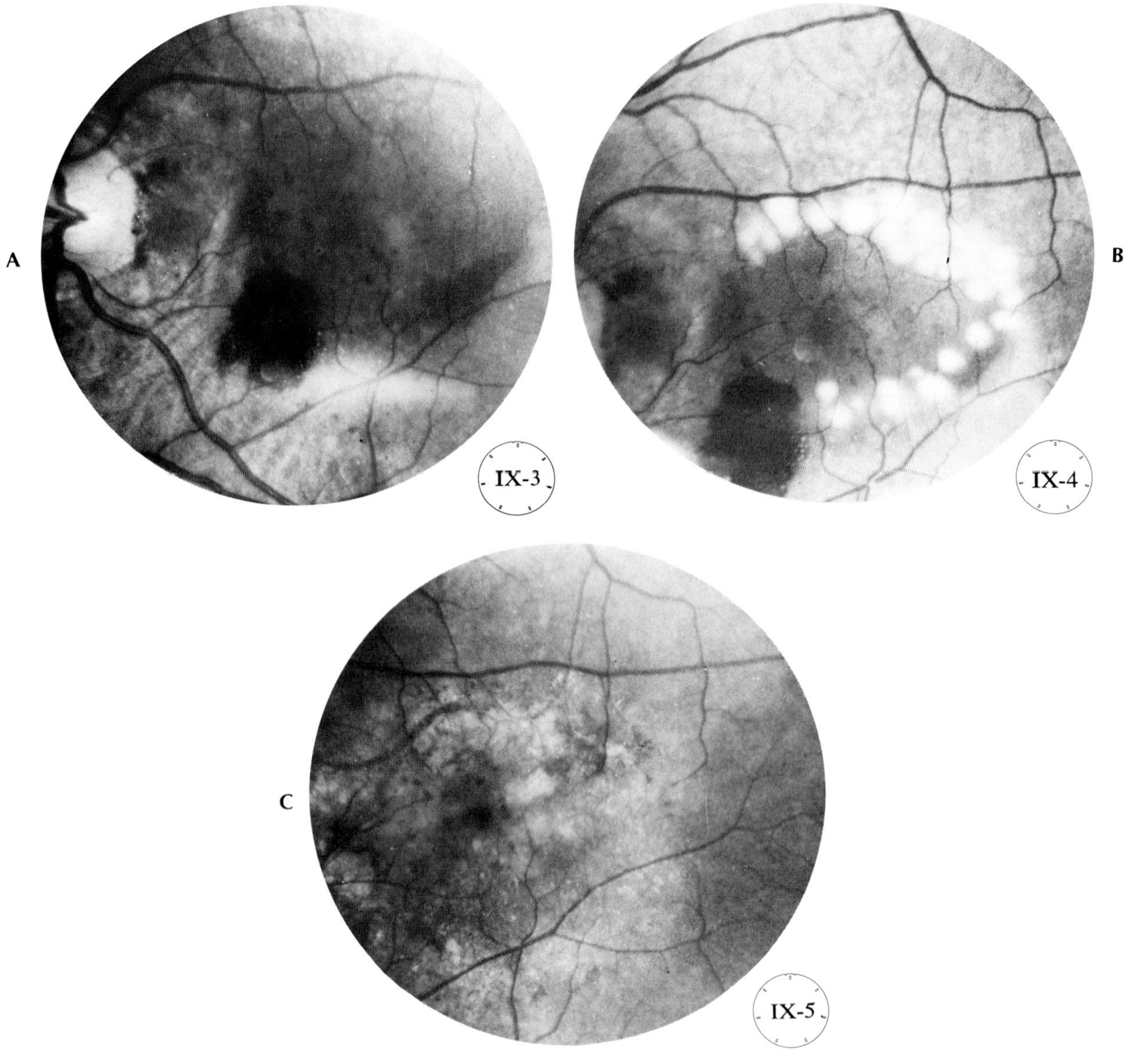

Fig. 10-7. A, A 2-DD serous detachment of the pigment epithelium with surface pigment speckling and a subretinal hemorrhage in a 48-year-old woman whose vision was 20/100. **B,** Pigment epithelial detachment immediately after photocoagulation with 200μ coagulations placed in a temporal C pattern approximately 1,000μ from the umbo. **C,** Serous detachment of the pigment epithelium 2 months after photocoagulation. The serous detachment is absent, and vision has been retained at 20/100.

Subfoveal serous detachments (>1 DD) causing visual symptoms can be treated by interrupted patterned coagulations, provided that the coagulations are of medium intensity (Grade 2) and do not approach closer than approximately ⅔ DD or 1,000μ to the umbo. In this manner the outer portions of the perifoveal serous detachment of the pigment epithelium will be treated with coagulations, and this treatment may be sufficient for collapsing the serous detachment without causing injury to the foveal and perifoveal receptor elements.

Extremely large serous detachments of the pigment epithelium commonly occupying areas greater than 3 to 4 DD and usually including the subfoveal region can be approached by coagulating the peripheral extent of the serous detachment during multiple photocoagulation sessions. Stronger (Grade 3) coagulation intensities may be required; typical settings are a **200μ** spot size, power levels of **200 to 400 mw,** and a **0.2-sec** exposure. Higher power densities are frequently necessary because of the retinal edema and some glial proliferation commonly present, as well as the atrophy of the pigment epithelial layer (Fig. 10-8). Starting peripherally and working centrally toward the foveal zone, coagulations are produced at the periphery of the serous detachment blister. The coagulations should be patterned, and they should not extend inward more than 3 coagulations during any treatment session. For extremely large serous detachments the coagulations should not come within 1,000μ to 1,500μ of the foveal region during the course of the treatment sessions. In many cases the coagulations will take the form of horseshoe patterns, with the open end encompassing the papillomacular bundle. During the subsequent photocoagulation sessions the horseshoe-type coagulations can be produced in smaller concentric patterns. It must be emphasized that the coagulations should not be extended too far centrally and that total collapse of the serous detachment may not be necessary to stabilize these large central serous detachments of the pigment epithelium (Fig. 10-9).

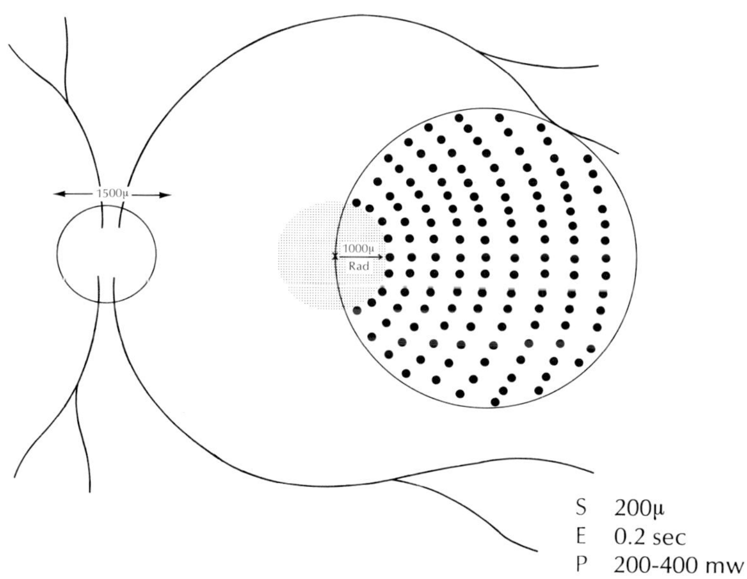

Fig. 10-8. Extremely large serous detachments (2 to 4 DD) of the pigment epithelium impinging on the subfoveal area should be treated with a modified temporal C technique, provided that coagulations are not placed within 1,000μ of the umbo. Coagulations should be placed at the periphery of the serous detachment initially and concentric coagulations produced more centrally during subsequent treatment sessions 1 to 2 months apart.

A 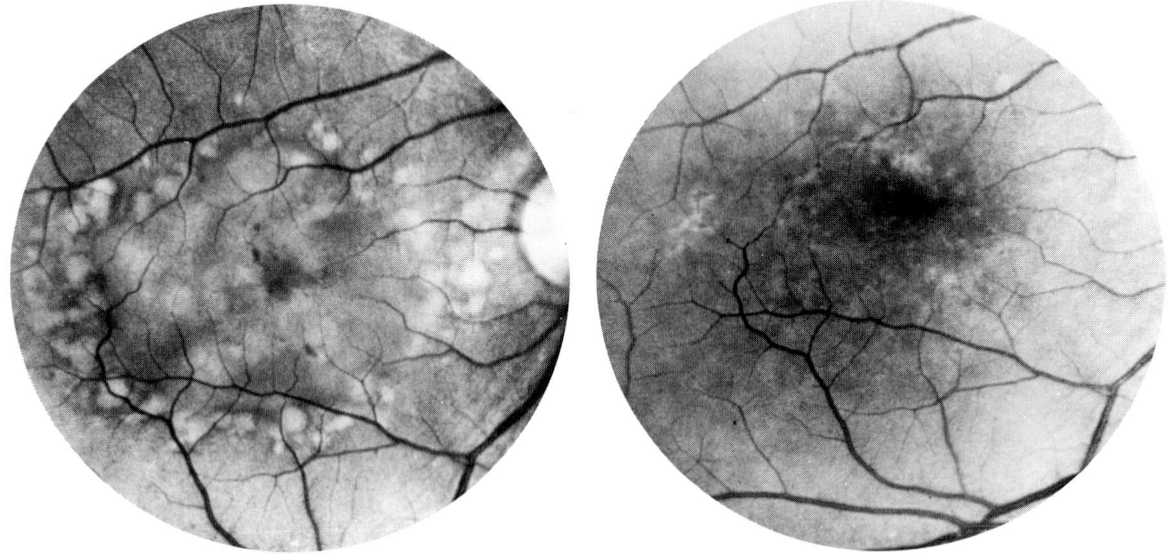 B

Fig. 10-9. A, An extremely large serous detachment of the pigment epithelium in a 67-year-old woman with a 20/100 visual acuity. **B,** Area of previous detachment 4 months after successful argon laser photocoagulation to the periphery of the detached area. Vision has been stabilized at 20/100 during a 2-year follow-up period.

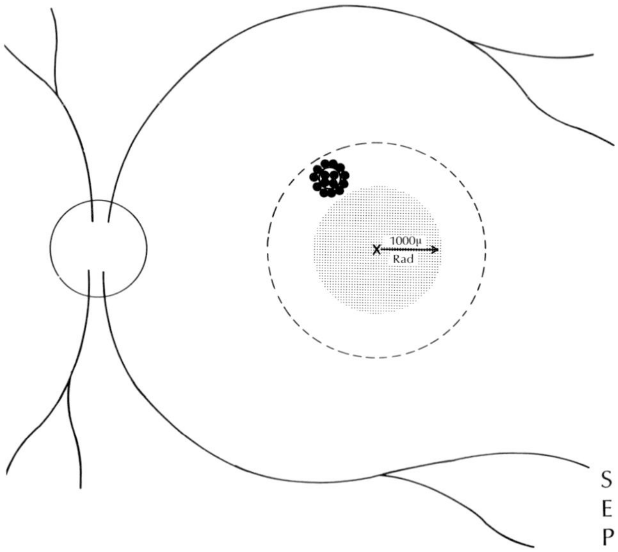

Fig. 10-10. Serous detachments of the pigment epithelium associated with serous detachments of the sensory retina (large dotted circle) should be treated completely with Grades 3 to 4 coagulations, provided that the serous detachment of the pigment epithelium is more than 1,000μ from the umbo.

Serous detachments of the pigment epithelium associated with serous detachments of the sensory retina should be treated with intense **150μ to 200μ** coagulations at power levels of **200 to 400 mw** and exposures of **0.2 sec** or longer (Fig. 10-10). Only the pigment epithelial detachment should be treated, and coagulations should not be placed within 1,000μ of the umbo (Fig. 10-11).

Intervals of 1 or 2 months are allowed between photocoagulation sessions to allow the peripheral detachment areas to collapse and seal down to the underlying Bruch's membrane. The eye can then be reassessed, and further photocoagulation treatments can be administered if the neuroepithelium is still highly detached.

Complications. The most common complication is the production of retinal striae that involve the foveal region, causing persistence of the distorted vision. This problem can be obviated by the use of low-intensity coagulations at a distance of at least 1,000μ (⅔ DD) from the foveal region (umbo).

With large serous detachments of the pigment epithelium (>2 DD) occupying a subfoveal position, coagulations closer than 1,000μ to 1,500μ to the foveal region sometimes appear to disrupt the nutrient supply to the receptor elements in the fovea, resulting in a concurrent decrease in visual acuity. The approach to the foveal region should not be closer than ⅔ DD.

Hemorrhage has occurred but is extremely rare unless underlying neovascularization has not been detected and is inadvertently photocoagulated.

Follow-up. After photocoagulation all patients with serous detachments of the pigment epithelium should be followed by serial color photography and ophthalmoscopic examination at intervals of 2 to 3 weeks.

Three to 6 weeks following treatment, a fluorescein angiogram should be taken to evaluate the effectiveness of the therapy. Fluorograms should be recorded within 1 week after photocoagulation if neovascularization was suspected originally.

Patients with successfully treated serous detachments of the pigment epithelium should be followed by fluorescein angiography at 3-month intervals to detect any

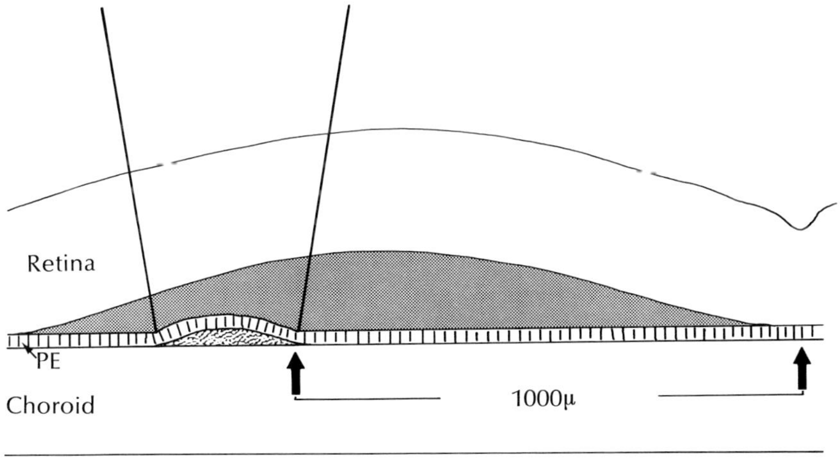

Fig. 10-11. Cross-sectional view of argon laser photocoagulation of a serous detachment of the pigment epithelium in the presence of a serous detachment of the sensory retina. In these cases only the pigment epithelial detachment should be photocoagulated; coagulations are not placed within 1,000μ of the umbo.

neovascular change or other deterioration. The patient should be given an Amsler grid chart to take home so that he can detect any early changes in his macular vision.

Neovascular

Neovascular degeneration of a serous detachment of the pigment epithelium must be treated with intense photocoagulation to effect obliteration of that area of the choroid and retina. Neovascularization is diagnosed by an unusual amount of exudates in the region of the serous detachment, as well as by edema of the overlying sensory retina. The blister fluid becomes more turbid, and a fluorescein angiogram may reveal the presence of a filamentous, vessellike area that stains and leaks profusely. If neovascularization is suspected, photocoagulation should be directed to the area and intense chalk white coagulations (Grade 4) produced. Coagulations can be produced in a central direction up to, but not within, a zone occupying a radius of 500μ from the umbo. Because of the disastrous nature of neovascular change in the macula, all attempts should be directed toward eradication of the neovascularization by 1 or more photocoagulation sessions.

Detachment of the sensory retina

Degenerative: central serous choroidopathy

Clinical symptoms. The most common symptoms of central serous choroidopathy include graying or blurring of the central vision, metamorphopsia, micropsia, and occasionally a defect in color perception. The severity of these symptoms may fluctuate from day to day or from hour to hour and may be associated with periods of stress.

Ophthalmoscopic appearance. The foveal region is almost always involved, as is indicated by the patient's blurred or distorted central vision, and one can usually detect a disciform elevation of the perifoveal, macular, or even paramacular sensory retina (Figs. 10-12 and 10-13). This elevation does not appear to be as firm as that noted with the serous detachments of the pigment epithelium, but there is no fluctuation or dependent shifting of the subretinal fluid with changes in the patient's position. The detachment of the sensory retina may be highly elevated and may show slight overlying edema of the sensory retina. Conversely, the serous detachment may be quite shallow and the edema of the sensory retina more pronounced. Underlying pigment epithelial or choroidal defects are not usually observed unless the patient has had similar occurrences in the past. The vision can usually be improved by increasing the hyperopic correction, and the difference in refractive measurement between the choroid and elevated retina can be obtained by retinoscopy of the eye with ordinary white light on the choroid and red-free light on the elevated retina.

Ancillary diagnostic examinations. A fluorescein angiogram will usually show the presence of a solitary focus, or occasionally multiple foci, of leakage through the pigment epithelium into the subretinal space. The leakage will start in the late arteriolar phase and become more pronounced during the arteriolovenular and venular phases of the retinal circulation. The leakage influx through the pigment epithelium may show a superiorly directed stream, caused by convection currents, from the pigment epithelial defect into the serous cavity. Eventually, the fluorescein concentration in the subretinal fluid may be sufficient to produce fluorescence in the detached area of the sensory retina. This serous accumulation beneath the sensory retina can be distinguished from a serous detachment of the pigment epithelium because the latter condition shows homogenous pooling in the detached area; this pooling starts during the late choroidal flush stage and grows in intensity throughout the fluorescein transit. With serous detachments of the pigment

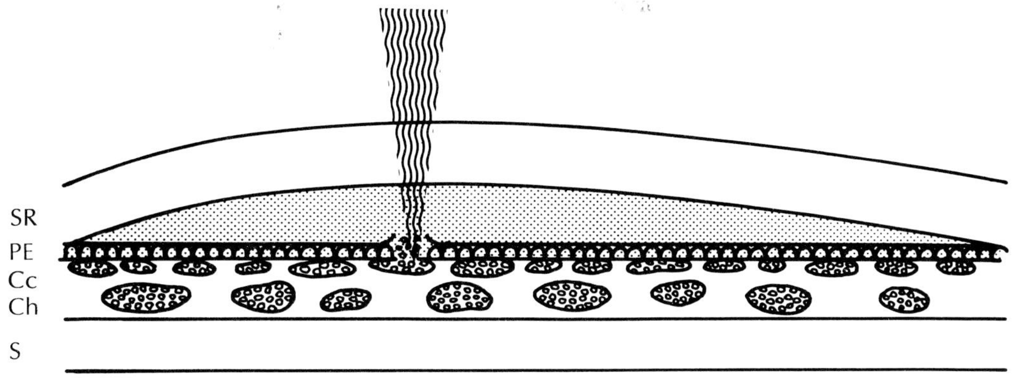

Fig. 10-12. Serous detachment of the sensory retina (central serous choroidopathy or central serous retinopathy), showing elevation of the sensory retina caused by breakdown and leakage of serous fluid (allowed by increased permeability of the pigment epithelial layer) from the choriocapillaris layer through Bruch's membrane into the subretinal space.

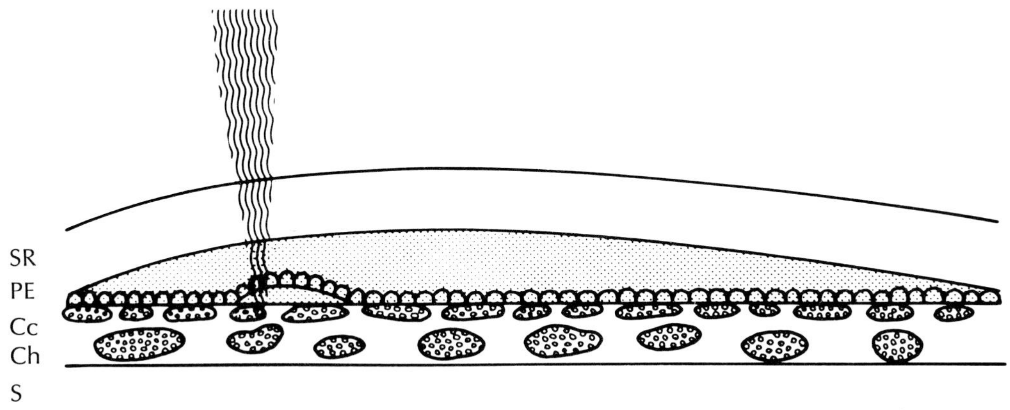

Fig. 10-13. Serous detachment of the sensory retina (central serous choroidopathy or central serous retinopathy) caused by leakage through the pigment epithelial layer from a small area of serous detachment of the pigment epithelium.

epithelium, the fluorescein pooling is intense and confined to a well-demarcated area, as opposed to the very light pooling in the ill-defined area of the serous detachment of the sensory retina. Stereo fluorescein angiography may provide further assistance in differentiating these and other conditions.

Indirect fluorescein ophthalmoscopy should be performed on all patients immediately after fluorescein angiography, to detect more peripheral or unusually located leakage areas.

Stereoscopic color photography can be of assistance in defining the extent of the serous detachment of the sensory retina (central serous choroidopathy) and may actually provide identification of the normally placed pigment epithelial layer behind the subretinal fluid.

A visual field examination may show a relative scotoma in the region of the sensory retinal detachment. This finding is significant in the evaluation of the progress of the disease.

Indications for photocoagulation. Photocoagulation can be attempted if the leakage area is greater than 1,000μ (⅔ DD) away from the umbo and the fluorescein leak is active, causing fluorescein to stream profusely into the subretinal fluid. Fluorescein leakage can be considered active, indicating a higher flow of serum through pigment epithelial–Bruch's membrane layers from the choriocapillaris, if it commences during the arteriolovenular phase and becomes much more prominent during the later phases. If the leakage zone is within 1,000μ of the central foveola (umbo), or if the leak is passive during the arteriolovenular or venular phases, photocoagulation should be withheld and the patient watched closely at 2- to 3-week intervals. In essence, when an area of active fluorescein leakage through the pigment epithelium is located outside a 1,000μ radius of the central foveola, the defect is usually treated as soon as it is recognized. Steroids are not usually helpful, although tranquilizers may be beneficial during the course of the disease.

If the leakage area is multifocal, all leaks outside a radius of 1,000μ from the umbo are treated, but more central leaks are not. Diffuse areas of leakage are investigated more thoroughly, and epithelial or choroidal neovascularization should be suspected. Under these conditions heavy steroid therapy given systemically can be tried for several weeks, and photocoagulation, if utilized, should be intense (Grade 4).

Photocoagulation approach. The leakage areas should be well enveloped with contiguous, mild coagulations of a mucoid character (Grade 2). Usually, spot sizes of **150μ** at power levels of **100 to 150 mw** and a **0.1-sec** exposure are required to seal the pigment epithelial leaks (Fig. 10-14). These settings may vary, depending on the amount of edema in the sensory retina, the distribution of pigment, disruptions in the pigment epithelial layer, and the amount of turbidity of the subretinal fluid. Coagulations should involve and overlap onto normal retina surrounding the leakage area for a short distance (Figs. 10-15 to 10-17).

If an active leakage point is located within the radius of 1,000μ from the central foveola, an auxiliary procedure can be used; it consists of producing mild coagulations in the dependent portion of the central serous choroidopathy bleb, provided that this region lies outside the 1,000μ radius. These small coagulations around the rim of the blister produce a disruption of the pigment epithelial–Bruch's membrane barrier and serve to function as an egress route for the subretinal fluid. This procedure usually will flatten the bleb in most regions other than the actual leakage zone and may improve the metamorphopsia and micropsia (Fig. 10-18).

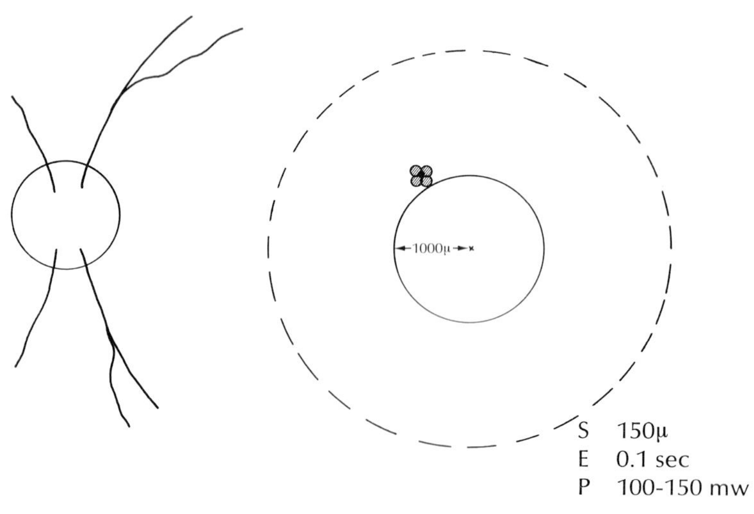

Fig. 10-14. Placement of contiguous, punctate Grade 2 coagulations in the region of the pigment epithelial leakage outside a radius of 1,000μ from the umbo.

A B

C D

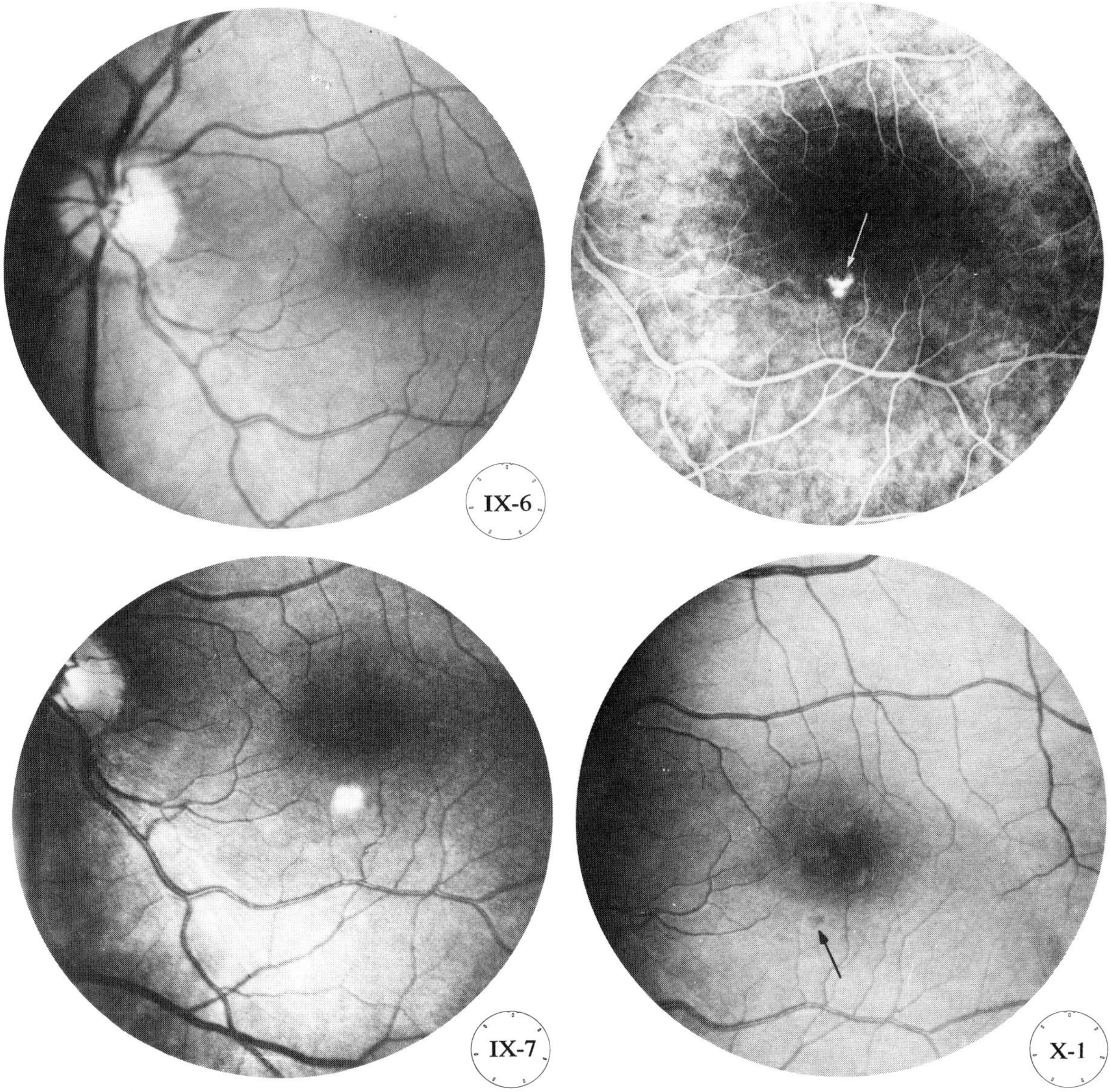

Fig. 10-15. A, A moderately elevated serous detachment of the sensory retina (central serous choroidopathy) in a 53-year-old man. Metamorphopsia and ophthalmoscopic evidence of the central serous choroidopathy condition had been present for 4 months, and there had been no improvement. The subretinal fluid was clear, subretinal precipitates were not present, and the leakage defects could not be determined ophthalmoscopically **B,** Fluorescein angiogram during the arteriolovenular capillary phase, showing the location of the pigment epithelial defect and a minute serous detachment of the pigment epithelium (arrow). The remainder of the choroidal and retinal vascular pattern was within normal limits. **C,** Four discrete, contiguous, punctate, Grade 2 coagulations were placed in the region of the fluorescein leakage so as to envelop the pigment epithelial defect and extend slightly into normal portions of the pigment layer. **D,** The area 14 days after photocoagulation, showing early pigment epithelial proliferation, scarring, and obliteration of the pigment epithelial defect (arrow). Most of the fluid beneath the serous detachment has disappeared, and vision has improved from $20/50^{-2}$ to $20/20^{-2}$ with correction.

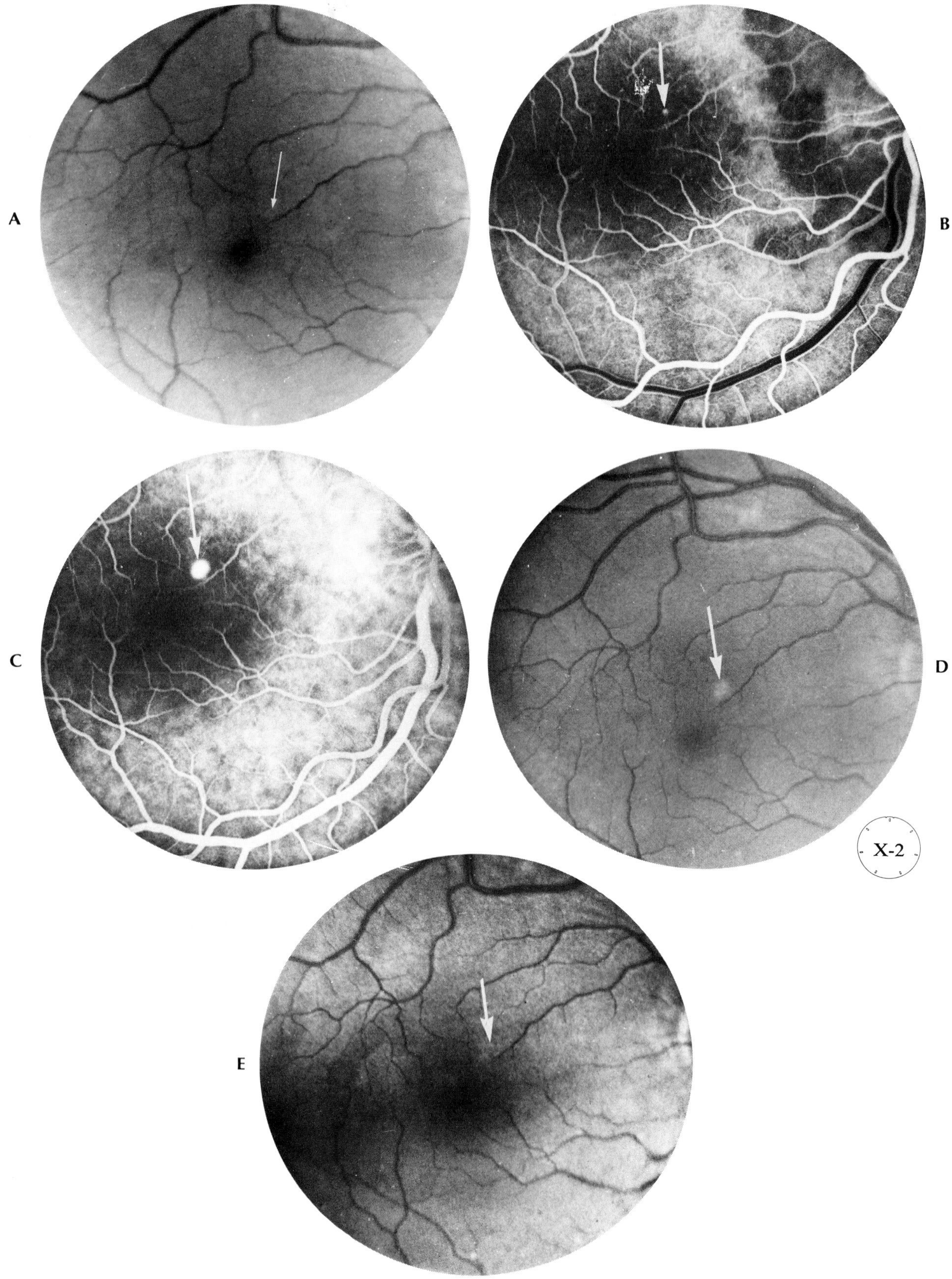

Fig. 10-16. For legend see opposite page.

Complications. Intense coagulations, particularly if the ruby laser is used, can produce small hemorrhages at the impact site. These hemorrhages are extremely rare; however, they are more common when short exposures, such as those delivered with ruby laser photocoagulation, are employed.

Treatment of an area of neovascularization or potential areas of neovascular change can stimulate the production of vessels from the choroid resulting in the eventual complete disruption of macular function. If a pigment epitheliitis or neovascular problem is suspected in the area of leakage, the patient must be evaluated closely, ophthalmoscopically and by fluorescein angiography, at 3- to 4-day intervals and treated with intense photocoagulation when neovascular proliferation has been documented. To afford better evaluation and therapy, the scattering produced by overlying sensory retina edema can be decreased, and the turbidity of the subretinal fluid can be lessened by the systemic administration of high doses of steroids (60 to 100 mg of prednisone daily under the direction of the patient's internist). If a problem other than the classic central serous choroidopathy is suspected initially, the patient must be evaluated extensively, and more intense photocoagulation must be considered from the onset.

Macular striae and hyperproliferation of the pigment epithelium in the region of the photocoagulation has been reported but is not common, particularly if mild mucoid coagulations (Grade 2) are produced at the leakage zone.

Follow-up. The patient should be investigated by fluorescein angiography approximately 4 weeks following photocoagulation to ensure that the leakage areas have been obliterated. The patient should be reevaluated thereafter at monthly intervals for several months. If neovascularization or epitheliitis was suspected originally, the patient should be examined 3 to 4 days following photocoagulation; fluorograms should be obtained at that time and at frequent intervals during the posttreatment period. The patient should be given an Amsler grid chart to take home so that he can detect any early changes in his macular vision. Fluorescein angiography at 6-month intervals may be indicated for some patients.

Idiopathic

If an inflammatory condition of the pigment epithelium or a neovascular change is suspected because of a more widespread leakage area, more intense staining, and other fluorescein characteristics, the patient should be investigated thoroughly and the possibility of giving steroids systemically or intense photocoagulation, or both, should be considered. Leakage may also occur around old choroidal or chorioretinal scars that may be located a considerable distance from the foveal region. Choroidal leakage areas producing

---

Fig. 10-16. A, A small punctate area of pigment epithelial atrophy at the 11 o'clock position (arrow) beneath a moderately elevated detached sensory retina in a 47-year-old man who had complained of blurred vision and distortion of 2 months' duration. **B,** Fluorescein angiogram during the late arteriolar phase, showing the early appearance of the fluorescein dye at the pigment epithelial defect (arrow). **C,** Fluorescein angiogram during the early venular phase, showing more extensive leakage of the fluorescein through the pigment epithelial defect into the subretinal space (arrow). **D,** Grade 2 contiguous coagulations were placed so that they covered the entire pigment epithelial defect and extended a slight distance onto normal pigment epithelium (arrow). **E,** Healed area 16 days after photocoagulation, showing a small chorioretinal pigmented scar (arrow) and complete disappearance of the subretinal fluid.

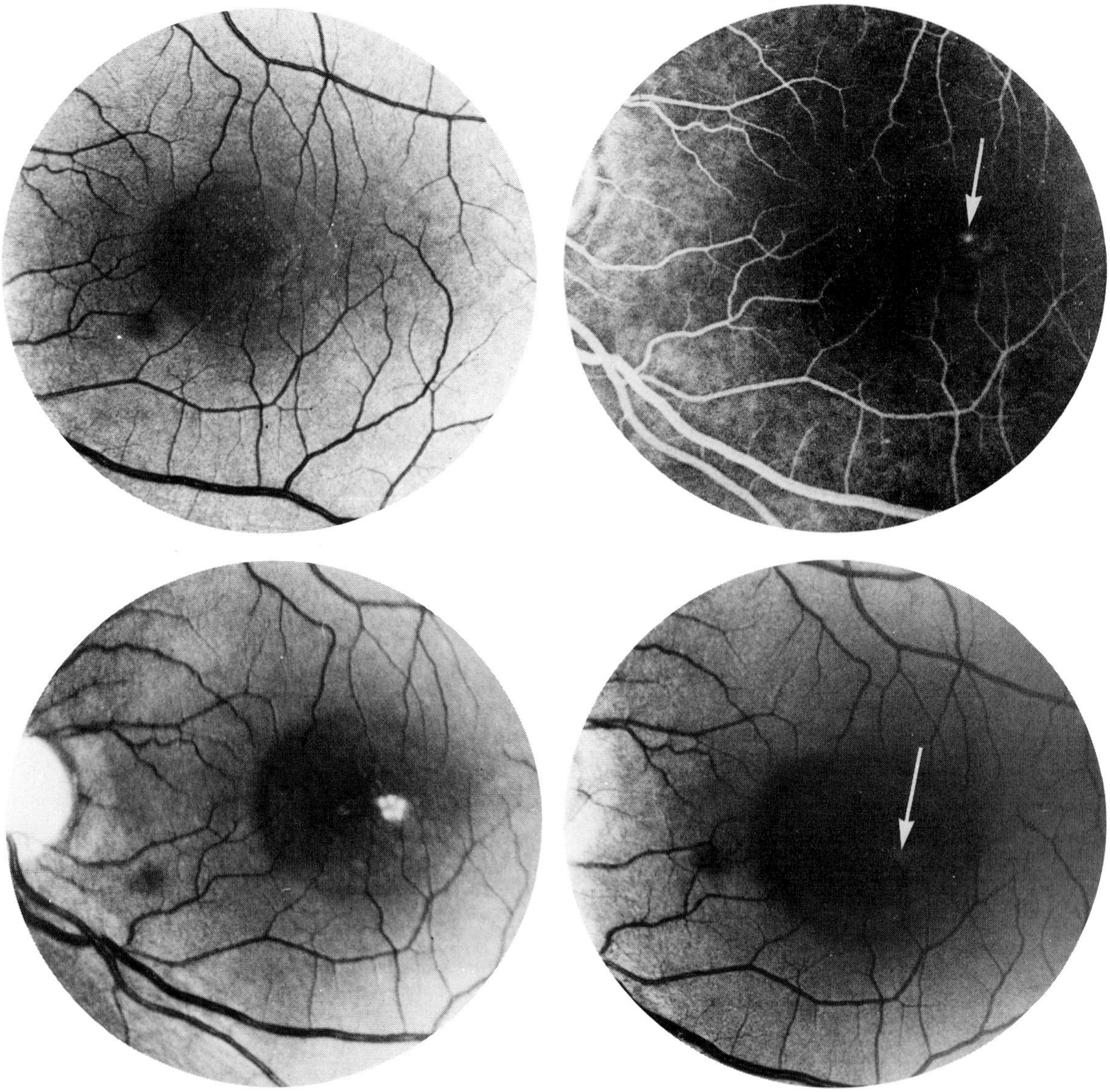

A B C D

Fig. 10-17. A, A 2-DD serous detachment of the sensory retina in a 51-year-old man who had a 3-week history of metamorphopsia and blurred vision in his left eye. **B,** Fluorescein angiogram during the arteriolovenular phase, showing a small perifoveal pigment epithelial leak (arrow), which increased during the later stages of the fluorescein transit. **C,** Five 40μ argon laser (before commercial lasers) photocoagulations were placed in the region of the pigment epithelial leak to seal that area. **D,** Macular region 6 weeks after argon laser photocoagulation, showing a small chorioretinal scar (arrow) and complete absorption of the serous detachment of the sensory retina. Vision has improved from $20/50^{-2}$ to $20/20^{-2}$.

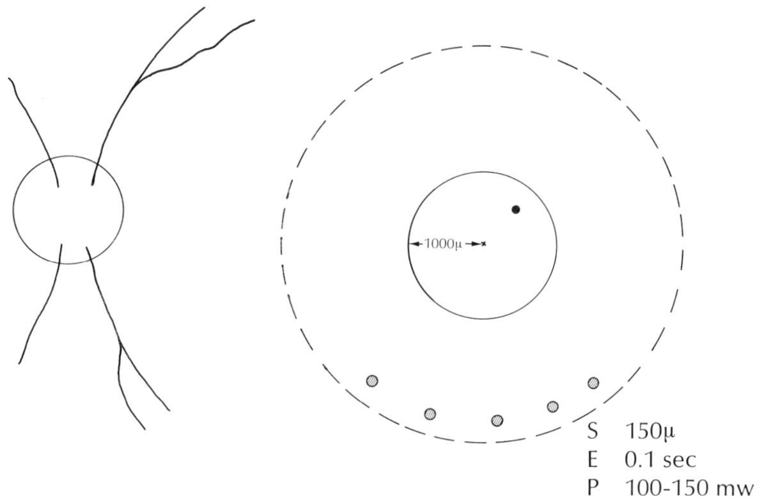

Fig. 10-18. Placement of interrupted, punctate Grade 2 coagulations at the peripheral inferior extent of the serous detachment of the sensory retina when active fluorescein leakage is within a radius of 1,000μ from the umbo.

serous elevations of the macular sensory retina have been observed outside the temporal vascular arcades and outside the ordinary field of view of the 30° fluorescein angiography camera. Therefore, all posterior polar areas should be investigated to determine the cause of the serous detachment of the sensory retina.

MACULAR HEMORRHAGIC ABNORMALITIES

Detachment of the pigment epithelium

Degenerative or neovascular

Clinical symptoms. Hemorrhagic detachment of the pigment epithelium can cause moderate to marked blurring of vision, distortion, micropsia, and occasionally photopsia or lightning flashes. If an overlying serous detachment of the sensory retina also is present, the distortion, blurring, and decrease of visual acuity may be more pronounced.

Ophthalmoscopic appearance. A hemorrhagic detachment of the pigment epithelium appears in its early stages as a grayish brown, elevated, circular disc-shaped mound, usually located in the perifoveal region or in the macular zone (Fig. 10-19). In later stages the rim of the mound becomes more highly pigmented, and the dome of the mound may become yellowish and gliotic. A typical signet ring appearance becomes apparent at this stage, and small vessels on the dome of the hemorrhagic detachment may be seen under higher magnification. In very late stages the entire hemorrhagic detachment may undergo organization and gliosis; whitening of the elevated region may be caused by gliosis and atrophy of the overlying retina (Fig. 10-20).

If a serous detachment of the sensory retina accompanies the hemorrhagic detachment of the pigment epithelium, the sensory retina is usually elevated concentrically over the hemorrhagic detachment of the pigment epithelium (Fig. 10-21). The intervening subretinal fluid may be turbid, and accumulations of proteinaceous material may form on the posterior aspect of the sensory retina. If neovascularization has occurred on the surface of the hemorrhagic detachment, the fluid will become extremely turbid, resulting in an increase in the posterior retinal precipitates, an increase in overlying retinal edema, and

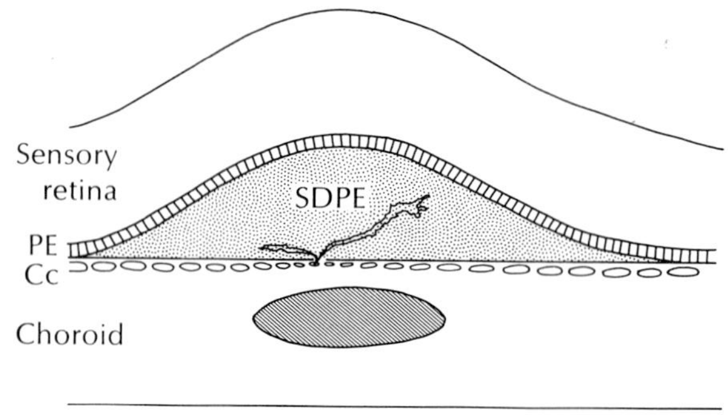

Fig. 10-19. Cross section of the choroid and retina, showing the possible early stage of the continuum leading from a serous detachment of the pigment epithelium *(SDPE)* to a hemorrhagic detachment of the entire neuroepithelium. Diagram shows a serous detachment of the pigment epithelium *(PE)* and early neovascularization extending from the choriocapillaris *(Cc)* through Bruch's membrane into the retinal pigment epithelial detachment.

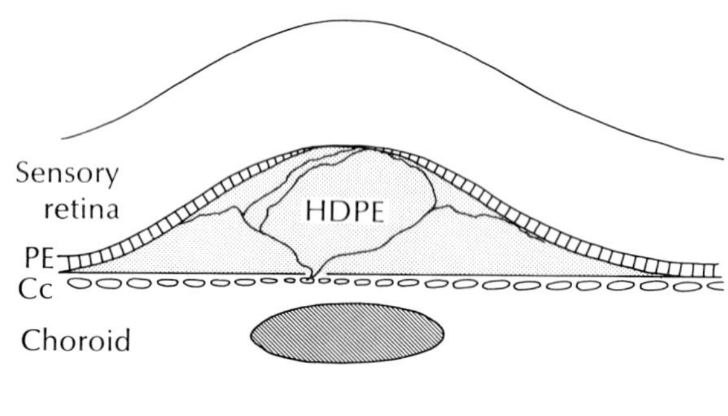

Fig. 10-20. Formation of a hemorrhagic detachment of the pigment epithelium *(HDPE)* probably caused by rupture of the subretinal neovascularization. Atrophy of the pigment epithelium *(PE)*, gliosis of the dome, and surface neovascularization are present during later stages.

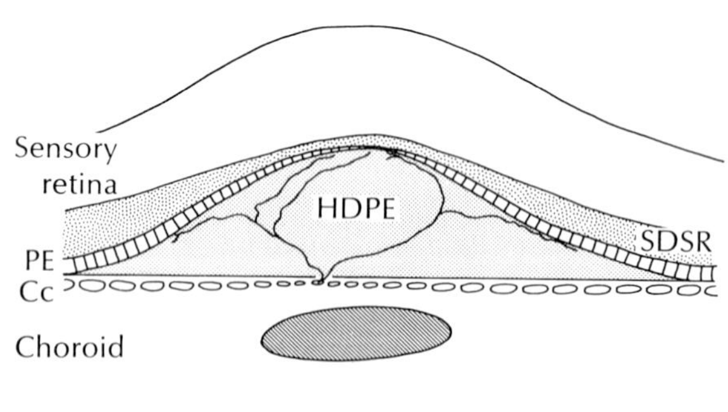

Fig. 10-21. A later stage of the continuum: Leakage from the neovascularization on the surface of the hemorrhagic detachment of the pigment epithelium *(HDPE)* into the subretinal space beneath the sensory retina, producing a serous detachment of the sensory retina *(SDSR)*.

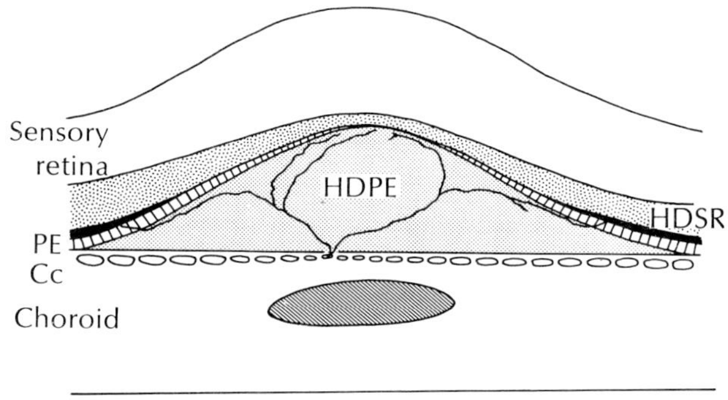

Fig. 10-22. Rupture of the neovascularization on the surface of the hemorrhagic detachment of the pigment epithelium *(HDPE)* into the subretinal space, producing a serosanguinous or hemorrhagic detachment of the sensory retina *(HDSR)*.

the precipitation of hard exudates surrounding the region of edematous sensory retina (Fig. 10-22).

Ancillary diagnostic examinations. A fluorescein angiogram will define the perimeter of a hemorrhagic detachment of the pigment epithelium with concentric zones of nonfilling and blockage, increased staining, and increased leakage during the arteriolovenular phase and later phases of the fluorogram. This rim of leakage surrounds the blood beneath the pigment epithelium at this early stage, but there may be no fluorescein leakage from the dome of the lesion. Indirect fluorescein ophthalmoscopy should be performed on all patients immediately after fluorescein angiography, to detect more peripheral or unusually located leakage areas.

As the hemorrhagic detachment of the pigment epithelium matures, wispy, threadlike neovascularization may be observed on the surface of the dome of the detachment during the early fluorescein transit. This neovascularization is followed by more intense, smudgy leakage during the later phases of the angiogram. If an overlying serous detachment of the sensory retina exists, this leakage can extend into it, causing the neovascular area to be grossly indistinct.

During the late stages, neovascularization may be extremely prominent, involve areas other than the hemorrhagic detachment, and be seen to coalesce and migrate along the pigment epithelium from the region of the original hemorrhagic detachment. The overlying serous detachment of the sensory retina will also accumulate fluorescein, which may be intermixed with a hemorrhage in the subretinal space.

Stereoscopic color photography of the lesion, usually with magnification, can be valuable for detecting a slight detachment of the overlying sensory retina, as well as for following the course and elevation of the hemorrhagic detachment of the pigment epithelium.

Tangent screen field testing will demonstrate areas of damage, presumably to the receptor elements or pigment epithelium in the region of the hemorrhagic detachment. This scotoma will be absolute and should be differentiated from a relative scotoma produced by the serous detachment of the overlying sensory retina.

Indications for photocoagulation. Any hemorrhagic detachment of the pigment epithelium should be strongly considered for photocoagulation if its border is located more than 1,500μ (1 DD) from the umbo (Fig. 10-23). Even in the early nonneovascular stages, photocoagulation is warranted because of the great propensity for these lesions to eventually develop neovascularization.

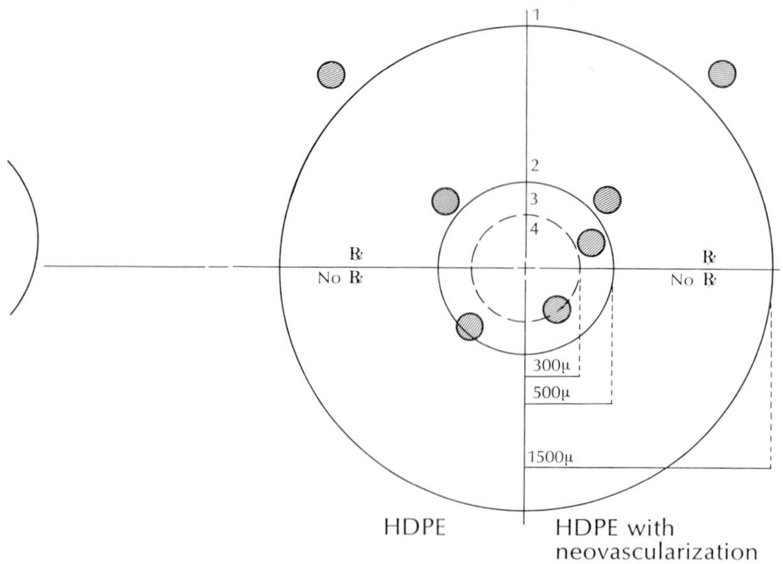

Fig. 10-23. Various zones (*1,* 1,500μ or more from the umbo; *2,* 500μ to 1,500μ from the umbo; *3,* 300μ to 500μ from the umbo; and *4,* less than 300μ from the umbo) determining which particular photocoagulation technique is used for a hemorrhagic detachment of the pigment epithelium *(HDPE).* Whether treatment is recommended (top half of circle) or not (bottom half) for simple hemorrhagic detachments of the pigment epithelium (left side) and those complicated by the presence of neovascularization (right side) is indicated.

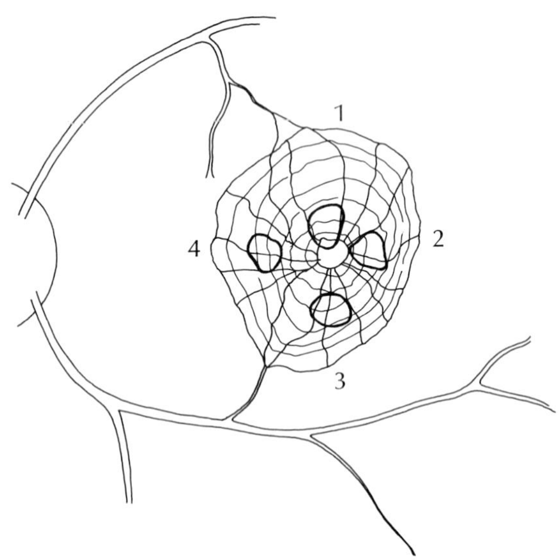

Fig. 10-24. A neovascularized hemorrhagic detachment of the pigment epithelium should not be treated if its border falls within the perifoveal capillary network, *1;* it should cautiously be considered for photocoagulation if its border impinges on the perifoveal capillary network, *2;* and it should be coagulated as soon as it is recognized if its border is more than 125μ (1 disc vein width) from the inner border of the perifoveal capillaries, *3* and *4.*

If the central border of the hemorrhagic detachment lies within a 500μ to 1,500μ radius of the umbo, photocoagulation is indicated as soon as the detachment is recognized.

A hemorrhagic detachment whose border is within 500μ of the umbo should be treated only if neovascularization is present, if treatment can be limited to an area outside a 300μ radius of the umbo, away from the perifoveal capillary network border, and if the neovascularization can be completely coagulated (Fig. 10-24).

A hemorrhagic detachment of the pigment epithelium with an overlying serous detachment of the sensory retina should be treated immediately, provided that the border of the hemorrhagic detachment is more than 500μ from the umbo.

A hemorrhagic detachment of the pigment epithelium with a serosanguinous detachment of the sensory retina should be treated only if the hemorrhagic detachment can be completely visualized without interference from overlying blood and if it lies more than 750μ from the umbo.

A pigment epithelial hemorrhagic detachment with a dense hemorrhagic detachment of the overlying sensory retina should not be considered for photocoagulation until the subretinal blood has been absorbed.

Photocoagulation approach. A retrobulbar injection of 2% lidocaine is required for adequate akinesia and anesthesia, because of the length of exposure and intensity of the coagulation. Topical use of an anesthetic and a plano contact lens of the suction or hand-held variety are also necessary.

A hemorrhagic detachment of the pigment epithelium whose border is located more than 1,500μ from the umbo should be treated with intense coagulations at any stage of development. Coagulations of **200μ to 300μ** diameter with exposures of **0.2 to 0.5 sec** at power ranges (**300 to 600 mw**) sufficient to produce a chalk white intense (Grade 4) coagulation are necessary for the eradication of the neovascularization on the surface and more deeply located areas of the detachment. These coagulations should extend beyond the border of the detachment, as noted by a fluorescein angiogram, and onto normal retinal tissue.

If the edge of the hemorrhagic detachment is located between 500μ and 1,500μ of the umbo, a row of **50μ** intense coagulation spots (at power levels of **150 to 200 mw** and an exposure of **0.05 sec**) should be placed in a contiguous manner along the central border of the hemorrhagic detachment to delimit the detachment from the foveal retina (Fig. 10-25). This row of coagulations may operate as a fire wall against the conduction of heat from the domo of the hemorrhagic detachment into the foveal region, but it also delineates the

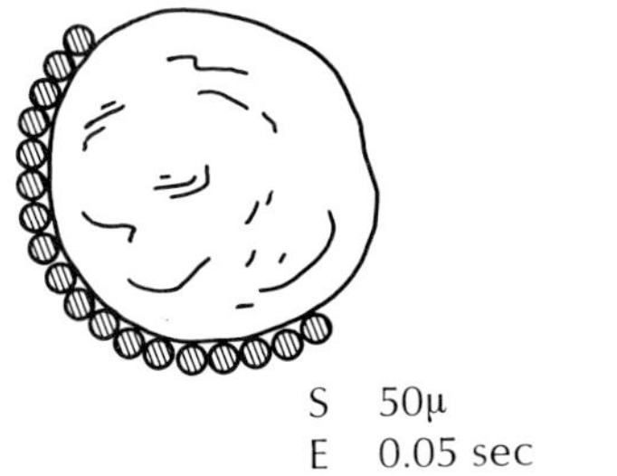

Fig. 10-25. Punctate, linear, contiguous 50μ coagulations at the junction of the hemorrhagic detachment of the pigment epithelium and the normal pigment epithelium in the region toward the fovea.

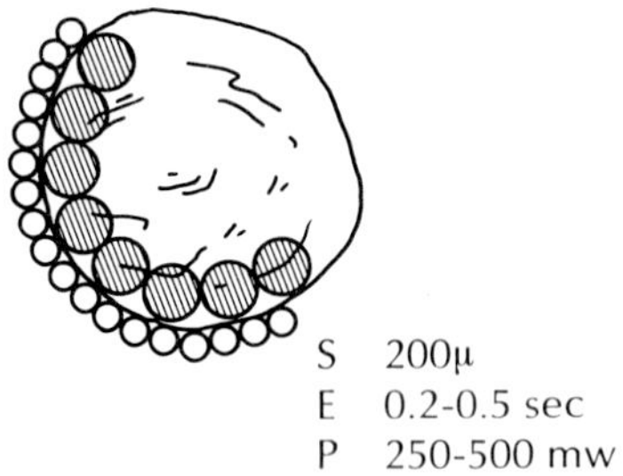

Fig. 10-26

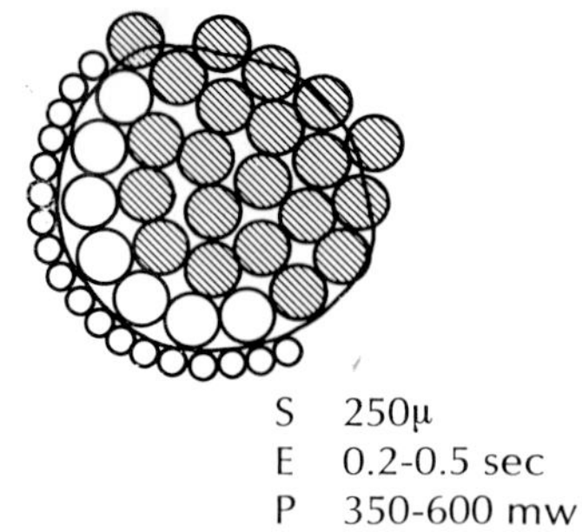

Fig. 10-27

Fig. 10-26. Punctate, linear, contiguous 200μ coagulations in the substance of the hemorrhagic detachment of the pigment epithelium in a concentric row more distal from the fovea than the previously placed coagulations.

Fig. 10-27. Application of punctate, barrage-type, overlapping 250μ coagulations to the entire area of the hemorrhagic detachment of the pigment epithelium and to a small rim of normal pigment epithelium.

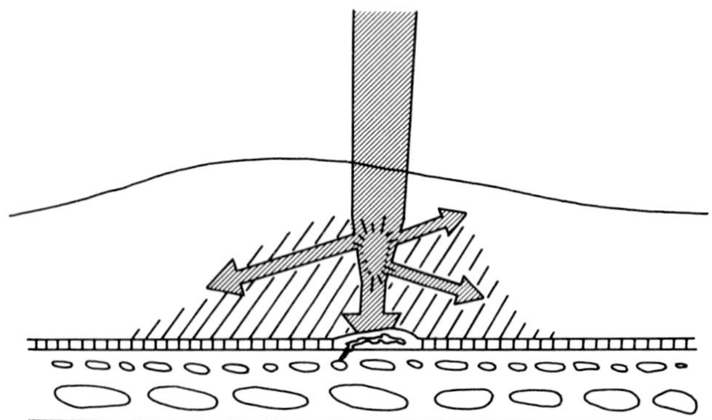

Fig. 10-28. Scatter and decreased effectiveness of the photocoagulation beam in the treatment of a pigment epithelial serous or hemorrhagic abnormality caused by overlying sensory retina edema.

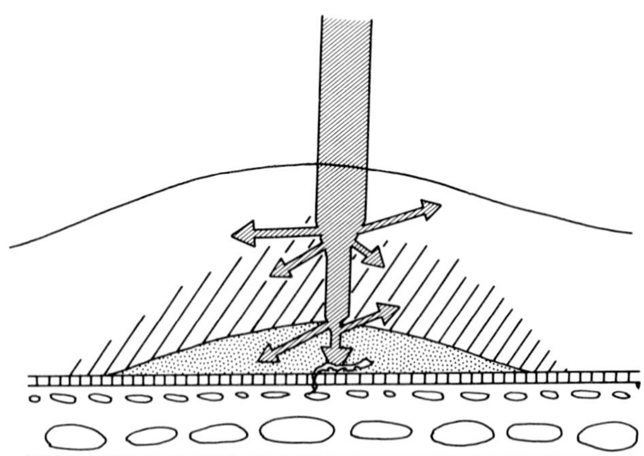

Fig. 10-29. Scatter and decreased effectiveness of the photocoagulation beam in the treatment of a pigment epithelial or subpigment epithelial serous or hemorrhagic abnormality caused by edema of the sensory retina and dispersion in the subsensory retinal detachment region.

detachment for later, more intense destructive photocoagulation purposes. When the 50μ diameter delimiting coagulations have been produced, coagulations of approximately **200μ to 250μ** diameter are then used at **0.2- to 0.5-sec** exposure intervals with intensities of **250 to 600 mw** to produce an intense chalk white coagulation (Grade 4) of the hemorrhagic detachment (Figs. 10-26 and 10-27).

If a hemorrhagic detachment of the pigment epithelium is located within a 500μ radius of the umbo and the neovascularization occupies and has originated from the outer portion of the hemorrhagic detachment, intense coagulations of the outer half of the dome can be created in a more heroic attempt to obliterate the neovascularization. Coagulations should not be placed within a 300μ radius of the umbo under any circumstances. This technique sometimes can restrict the neovascularization to a degree where smaller, more precise coagulations can be introduced at a later date. Photocoagulation of the outer extent of these hemorrhagic detachments of the pigment epithelium should be done with the techniques and settings discussed in the previous paragraph. The more centrally located coagulations are produced first; coagulations farther away from the fovea are produced secondly. If the central neovascularization cannot possibly be destroyed without damaging foveal vision, photocoagulation is contraindicated, and the lesion should not be treated.

If the overlying sensory retina is edematous (Fig. 10-28) or detached from the pigment epithelial surface by a serous or serosanguinous layer of fluid (Fig. 10-29), the turbidity of this fluid layer and the sensory retinal edema can be cleared to some extent by high doses of steroids given systemically (60 to 100 mg of prednisone daily). The clearing of this edema and turbidity allows one to visualize and coagulate the neovascularization more effectively with lower-power coagulations because of minimization of the adverse scattering of the laser beam. Higher power levels are usually required if the edema or turbidity remain, because of the dispersion of the laser beam before its impingement on the neovascular tissue and the hemorrhagic detachment of the pigment epithelium.

In these cases with overlying serous or serosanguinous detachments of the sensory retina, only the hemorrhagic detachment and areas of neovascularization should be

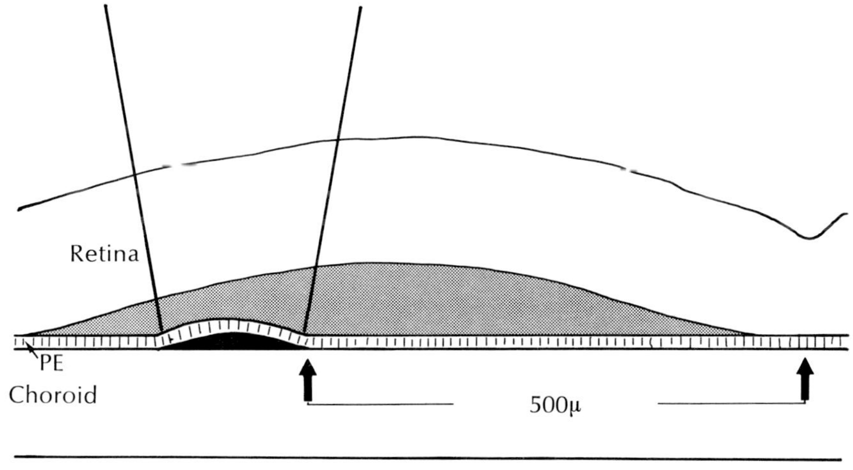

Fig. 10-30. Photocoagulation technique for a hemorrhagic detachment of the pigment epithelium *(PE)* and an overlying serous detachment of the sensory retina. The border of the lesion should be more than 500μ from the umbo, and photocoagulation should be directed to the detachment of the pigment epithelium only. Photocoagulation should not be applied closer than 750μ to the umbo if the sensory retinal detachment is serosanguinous.

treated. The entire hemorrhagic detachment should be covered with coagulations; but with overlying serous detachments treatment should not be attempted closer than 500μ of the umbo, and with overlying serosanguinous detachments of the sensory retina treatment should not be attempted closer than 750μ of the umbo (Fig. 10-30). Power settings will depend on the amount of subretinal fluid present. Usually, it is advisable to start treatment with **100μ** diameter spot sizes at an exposure of **0.1 sec** and a **200-mw** power intensity. The power can then be increased in 50-mw steps to **400 mw** to obtain a dirty white (Grade 3) or chalk white (Grade 4) coagulation. Occasionally, these power settings prove inadequate, and the exposure interval must be increased to **0.2 sec.** In these instances the power level should be reduced to **200 mw** initially and then increased as before to obtain the desired coagulation intensity (Figs. 10-31 to 10-34).

Complications. The most common complication is hemorrhage at the time of coagulation or during the immediate postoperative period. This hemorrhage can be caused by undertreatment or overtreatment or by the inadvertent increase in venous pressure in the head and eye vessels created by the patient during the Valsalva maneuver or during other bodily movements. The patient must be cautioned not to bend over suddenly or strain at stool and to avoid coughing or lifting heavy objects. To decrease the chance of rupture and

A

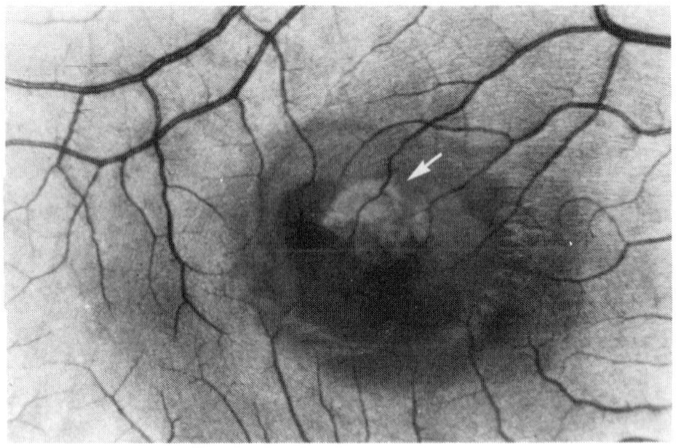

X-3

Fig. 10-31. A, A neovascularized hemorrhagic detachment of the pigment epithelium superior to the fovea (arrow) and small extravasations of blood beneath the sensory retina in a 14-year-old girl with a 3-week history of vision blurred to 20/70. **B,** Fluorogram during the choroidal flush phase, showing fluorescence of neovascularization on the surface of the hemorrhagic detachment of the pigment epithelium (long arrow). Note the cilioretinal artery (short arrow). **C,** Fluorogram during the arteriolar phase demonstrating early leakage from the area of neovascularization on the surface of the hemorrhagic detachment of the pigment epithelium. **D,** Barrier of 50μ coagulations along the border of the hemorrhagic detachment of the pigment epithelium, adjacent to the fovea. **E,** Photocoagulations of 200μ were applied to the body of the hemorrhagic detachment of the pigment epithelium, adjacent to the previously formed coagulation barrier. **F,** Treated hemorrhagic detachment of the pigment epithelium 2 months after photocoagulation, showing complete destruction of the lesion and minimal gliosis and hypertrophy of the pigment epithelium. The fovea remains intact, and the vision has improved to 20/25. **G,** Overall view of the macular and papillary region, illustrating the lack of peripapillary atrophy, hyperpigmentation, and peripheral atrophic chorioretinal spots, which would not be suggestive of the histoplasmosis syndrome.

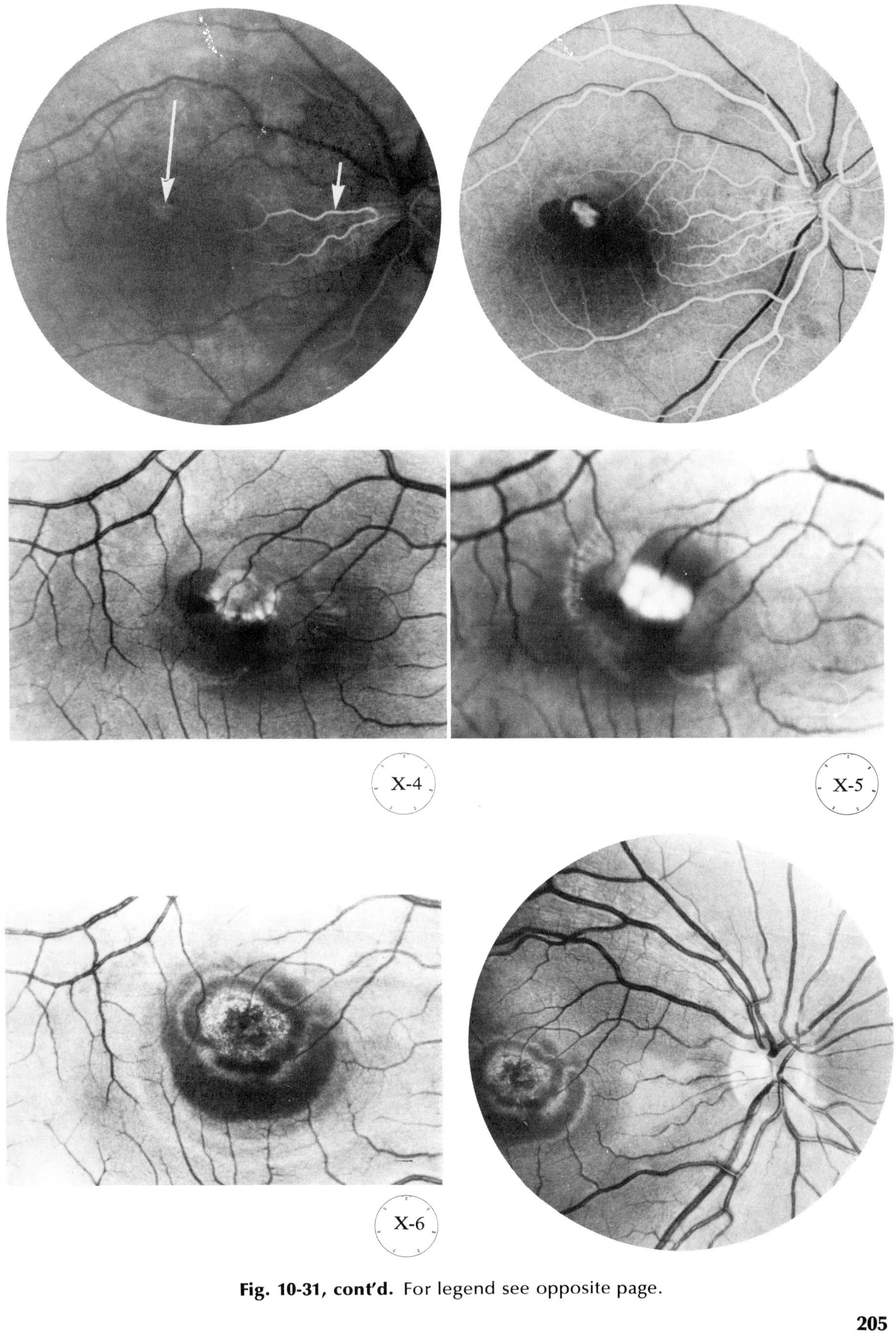

Fig. 10-31, cont'd. For legend see opposite page.

to avoid stimulating the regrowth of a partially coagulated vessel, photocoagulation must encompass the entire area of abnormality and possible neovascularization.

Atrophy of the receptor elements in the foveal zone and striae of the macular region have been observed to result from the intense photocoagulations that are necessary to control and eradicate nearby neovascularization. The problem of macular striae is not important, considering the possible consequences of allowing the neovascular process to run its course without photocoagulation. Damage to the receptor elements of the foveal region can be minimized by not treating areas of neovascularization within 500μ of the umbo if there is a considerable serous accumulation beneath the sensory retina extending from the area of treatment to the subfoveal region. In cases with serosanguinous subretinal fluid, photocoagulation should be limited to regions 750μ or more from the umbo to lessen the chances of heat conduction through the proteinaceous fluid to the fovea.

If the neovascularization is not obliterated entirely, the neovascular response may be stimulated and the lesion made considerably worse. Neovascularization can grow dramatically within several weeks and encompass a much larger area. Therefore, the initial photocoagulation attempt should produce coagulations that will eradicate the neovascularization at that session. Careful fluorescein angiography 2 weeks after photocoagulation will demonstrate any areas of patent or proliferative neovascularization. Rephotocoagulation of these residual neovascular zones should be done immediately.

Follow-up. The patient should be seen at biweekly intervals during the postoperative period, and a fluorescein angiogram should be taken at each of these visits. If neovascularization can be demonstrated, photocoagulation sbould be attempted at that time. Several months later a fluorescein angiogram may show leakage or staining points in the area of scar tissue; these points can be watched closely without photocoagulation intervention. The patient should be given an Amsler grid chart to take home so that he can detect any early changes in his macular vision. However, at the least suggestion of neovascularization, photocoagulation therapy should be introduced. The patient should then be evaluated by fluorescein angiography at 6-month intervals during the next several years.

Detachment of the sensory retina

Degenerative or neovascular

Clinical symptoms. Hemorrhagic detachment of the sensory retina or serosanguinous detachment of the sensory retina can occur from rupture of a hemorrhagic detachment of the pigment epithelium or from a spontaneous break or degeneration of the pigment

---

Fig. 10-32. A, A typical signet ring hemorrhagic detachment of the pigment epithelium in a 51-year-old man with a 3-week history of blurred vision of $20/80^{-2}$. The hyperpigmented signet ring (arrow) surrounds the gliotic dome of the hemorrhagic detachment of the pigment epithelium. **B,** Fluorogram during the early arteriolar venular phase, demonstrating the early leakage from the neovascularization on the surface of the hemorrhagic detachment. **C,** Fluorogram during the early venular phase, illustrating the more profuse leakage from the neovascularized hemorrhagic detachment of the pigment epithelium. **D,** Dense Grade 4 coagulum after the barrier and barrage photocoagulation techniques have been applied to the hemorrhagic detachment of the pigment epithelium. **E,** Treated hemorrhagic detachment of the pigment epithelium 7 weeks after photocoagulation, showing hyperproliferation of the pigment epithelium and a small surrounding rim of chorioretinal atrophy (arrow). Vision has improved to 20/30.

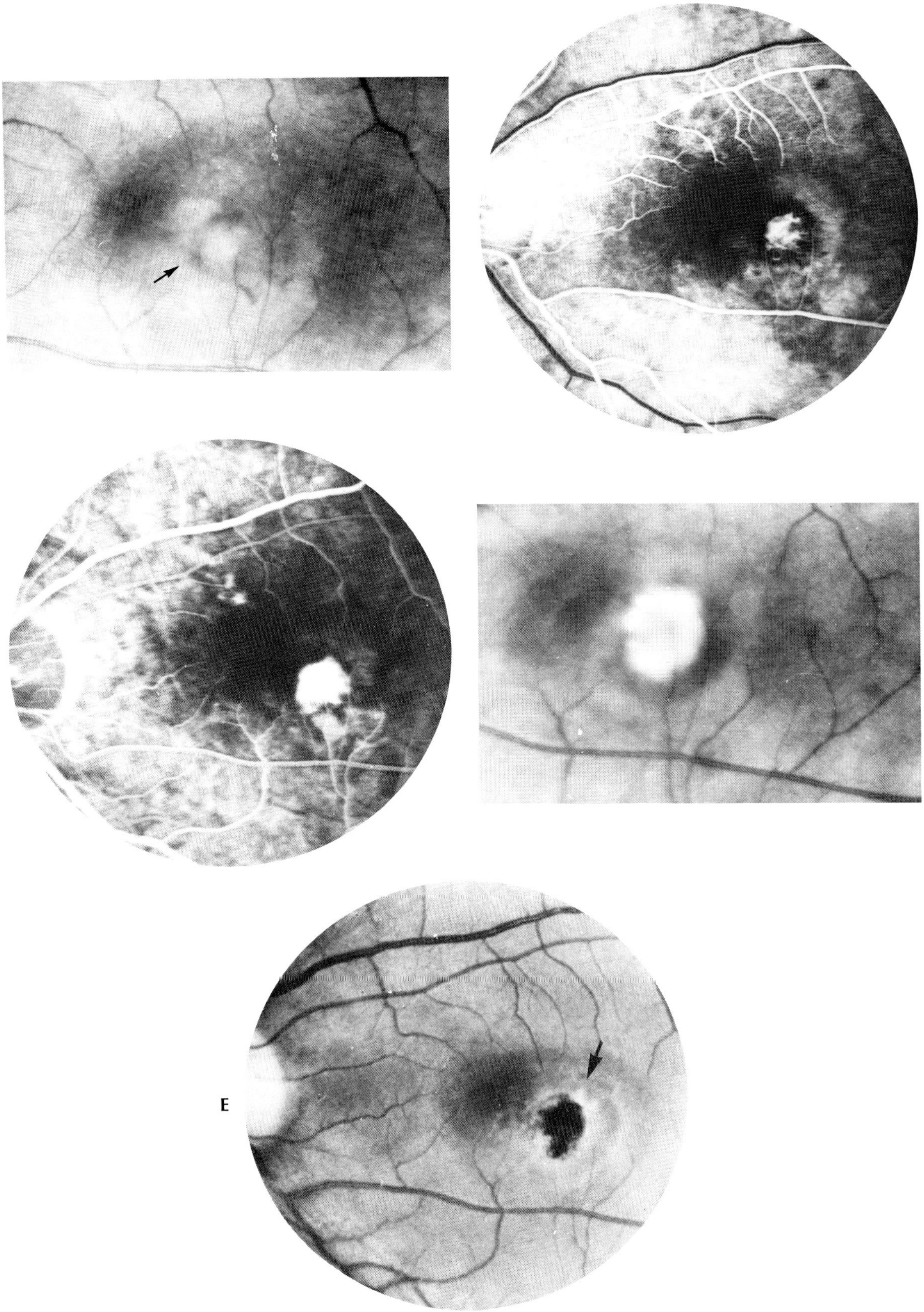

Fig. 10-32. For legend see opposite page.

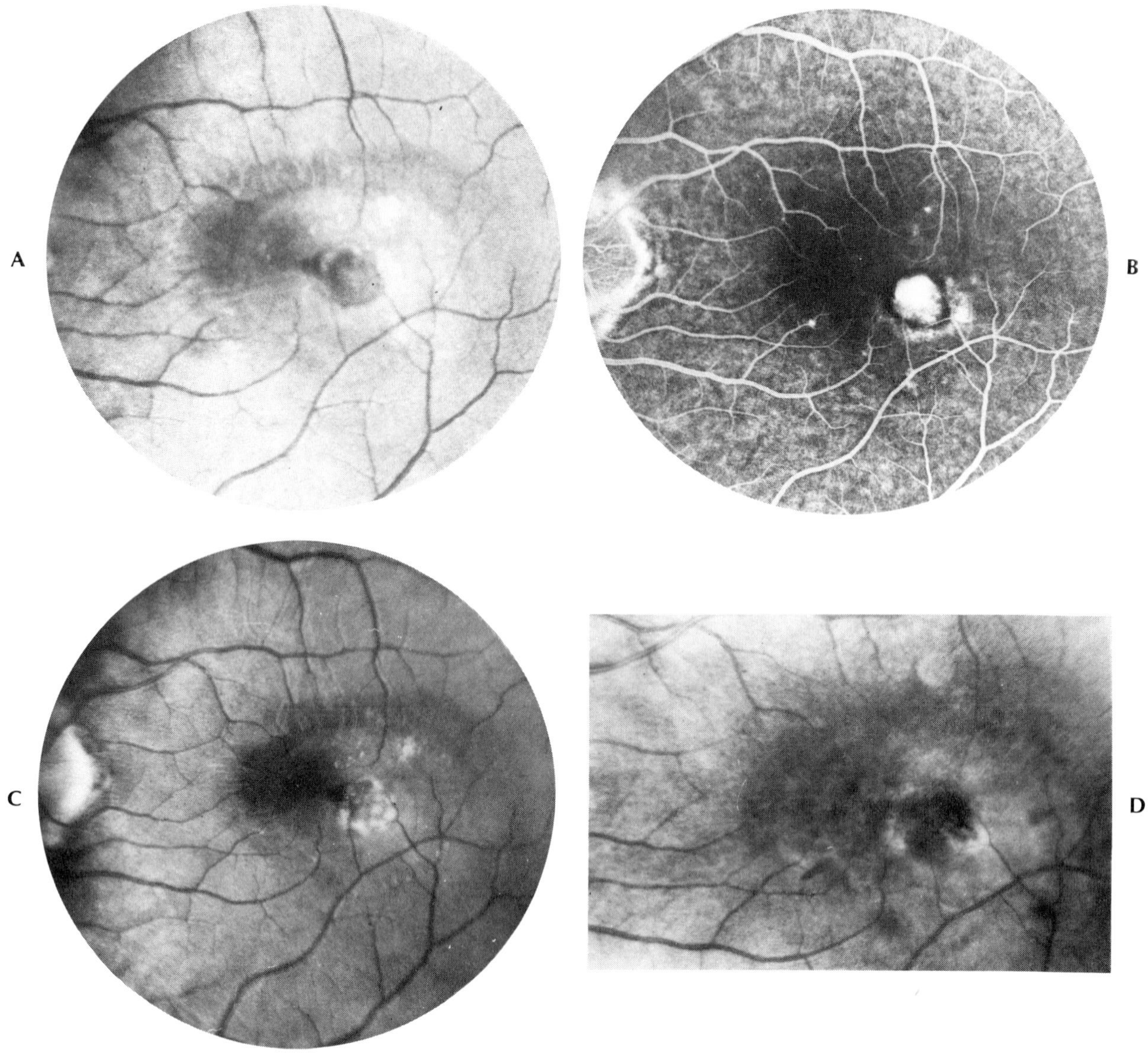

Fig. 10-33. A, A hemorrhagic detachment of the pigment epithelium and a small overlying serous detachment of the sensory retina in a 27-year-old man who had complained of metamorphopsia. His vision had decreased to 20/100, and he had definite macular field defects. **B,** Fluorogram during the arteriolovenular phase, demonstrating extensive leakage in the region of the neovascularized hemorrhagic detachment of the pigment epithelium. **C,** Variable-sized photocoagulations from 50μ to 200μ diameter were applied to the entire region of the hemorrhagic detachment of the pigment epithelium and to a small surrounding rim of normal chorioretinal tissue. **D,** Healed hemorrhagic detachment of the pigment epithelium and serous detachment of the sensory retina 9 weeks after photocoagulation therapy. Vision has improved to 20/40, and the serous detachment of the sensory retina has disappeared.

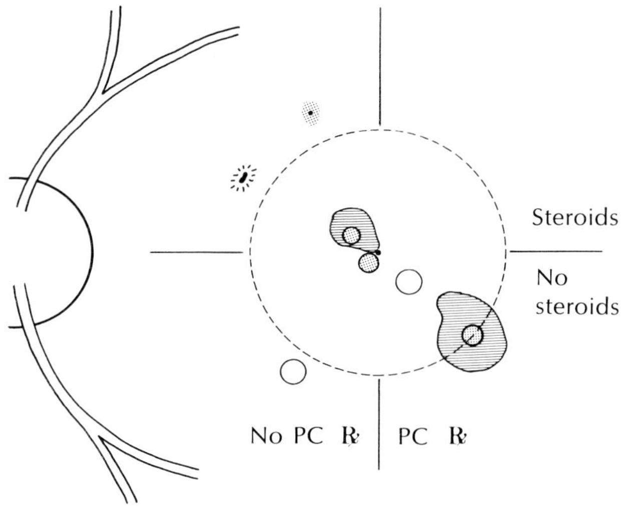

Fig. 10-34. Histoplasmosislike macular syndrome, showing the possible use of systemic steroids for yellow nodules (10 o'clock position), for orange plaques (11 o'clock position) and, for hemorrhagic detachments of the pigment epithelium when overlying sensory retinal detachments are too close to the fovea for photocoagulation *(PC)*. Serous detachments of the pigment epithelium (open circles) and solitary hemorrhagic detachments with or without overlying sensory retinal detachments are treated according to their appearance and distance from the umbo.

epithelial–Bruch's membrane region. This break or degeneration may be in the zone of old choroidal or pigment epithelial scarring and may cause marked blurring and distortion of the central vision if it affects the macular region. Patients may also notice flashing lights and photopsia.

Ophthalmoscopic appearance. The retina appears elevated in the zone of detachment, and red blood is present beneath the sensory retina. This blood may be lying dependently in a boat-shaped fashion at the lower portion of the bleb, or it may be irregularly positioned about the excursion of the sensory retinal detachment. The retinal vessels can be seen coursing over the blood-filled detached area, and there may be a moderate amount of edema, gliosis, or atrophy of the overlying sensory retina.

Ancillary diagnostic examinations. Fluorescein angiography may be of no help once the hemorrhage has occurred beneath the sensory retina, since the leakage area may be covered by the large accumulation of blood. Fluorescein angiography is of value, however, in the stages before the hemorrhagic detachment occurs, when the defect in the pigment epithelial–Bruch's membrane region may be detected as an area of hyperfluorescence or leakage. After the area has undergone organization and resolution of the hemorrhage, a fluorogram may be useful in detecting any further changes, such as the proliferation of neovascular tissue.

Stereo or regular color fundus photography is extremely helpful in detecting the areas of maximal hemorrhagic, gliotic, or absorption activity during the course of the disease. Photocoagulation can be more accurately directed in many cases if these observations have been documented.

Indications for photocoagulation. Hemorrhagic detachments of the sensory retina should not be photocoagulated, because the large amount of blood can act as a nidus for the conversion of light energy to heat energy and can interrupt the overlying nerve fiber elements.

If large accumulations of blood are present beneath the sensory retina but the source of the hemorrhage can be located away from the mass of blood, photocoagulation can be considered.

In the early stages, when severe leakage or small amounts of blood are discovered at the pigment epithelial–Bruch's membrane region, photocoagulation can be directed to the area of leakage in order to cauterize and seal that particular region.

Photocoagulation approach. The coagulations should be intense (**300-mw** power at a **0.5-sec** exposure) and occupy a diameter of at least **150μ to 200μ**. The coagulations should encompass the area of leakage and extend into an area of normal choroid, if possible. In the late stages, after absorption, the coagulations should simply be employed to delimit and obliterate areas of possible leakage or neovascularization.

Complications. The complications of hemorrhage, macular striae, receptor damage in the fovea, and activation of the neovascularization have all been discussed previously.

Follow-up. The patient should be seen at 1- to 3-month intervals following photocoagulation of the defect. In this way the occurrence of any new neovascularization or new areas of leakage or hyperstaining can be seen by fluorescein angiography. Once the lesion is stabilized, the intervals between follow-up evaluations with fluorescein angiography may be lengthened to 6 months.

Chapter 11

Macular intraretinal abnormalities

INTRACELLULAR EDEMA

Branch retinal artery occlusion

Clinical symptoms. Clinical symptoms of a branch retinal artery occlusion are usually sudden loss or disturbance of vision, distortion, metamorphopsia, micropsia, and photopsia or flashing. The loss of vision usually affects only one segment of the visual field but is dense.

Ophthalmoscopic appearance. The usual ophthalmoscopic view of a branch artery occlusion may show a sluggish blood flow and a boxcar appearance of the small segments of erythrocytes in the veins and arteries. An embolism or the site of occlusion can occasionally be located, and the distribution of the artery may show early swelling of the inner layers of the retina and hazy edema in these regions. The macular region appears edematous and distorted.

Ancillary diagnostic examinations. A fluorescein angiogram will show that very little fluid, if any, is entering the arterial occlusion area and can usually determine the site of occlusion. The degree of leakage beyond this point can be noted with certainty. Fluorescein angiography is most effective in the later stages of a branch artery occlusion if neovascularization has occurred. In these cases the areas of neovascularization leak fluorescein profusely, and any areas of abnormal intraretinal shunting or tortuosity of the vessels can be documented easily.

Stereo color photography of the fundus can also be useful for determining the long-term course of the disease after the initial occlusion.

Indications for photocoagulation. There are no indications for photocoagulation during the early course of arterial occlusion. However, several months to years later the presence of a neovascular response that is proliferating and possibly bleeding into the vitreous body should be documented closely and carefully by fluorescein angiography, and the areas of tuft formation should be treated by intense photocoagulation.

Photocoagulation approach. Photocoagulation should be directed only to those areas or tufts of neovascularization in the late stages, several months or years after the initial occlusion (Fig. 11-1). Photocoagulation should only attempt to obliterate those areas of leakage or hemorrhage; it should not attempt to interrupt the intraretinal shunting mechanisms or the other compensatory vascular devices that have been created to relieve the arteriovascular occlusion. Coagulation diameters should always be larger than the neovascularization (usually **200μ**), and the coagulations should be approximately **0.2 to 0.5**

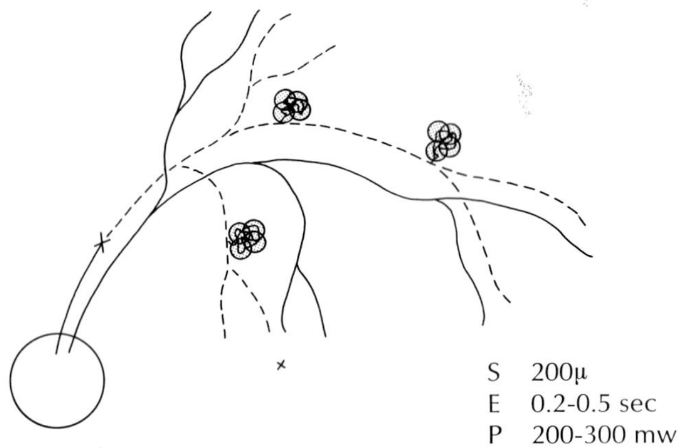

Fig. 11-1. Placement of contiguous or overlapping argon laser coagulations in the area of neovascularization or vascular leakage. Coagulations of 200μ at Grade 3 intensity are usually necessary for obliteration of the neovascularization or leaking vessels.

sec in duration, having power levels sufficient (usually **200 to 300 mw**) to cause a moderately intense coagulatory effect (Grade 3) (Fig. 11-2).

Complications. Occasionally, hemorrhage will result from treatment of the neovascularization, but I have not found this to be a great problem. Coagulations should be moderately intense (Grade 3) but not chalk white (Grade 4), and they should encompass the entire area of neovascularization so that no area of neovascularization is damaged rather than obliterated.

Follow-up. Patients should be followed at weekly intervals during the first 2 months after photocoagulation and then at 2- to 4-month intervals following stabilization of the process. Fluorescein angiograms should be taken at 2- to 3-month intervals for the first year following photocoagulation and then at 6-month intervals thereafter.

Central retinal artery occlusion

Clinical symptoms. A clinical symptom of central retinal artery occlusion is an immediate and sometimes dense loss of vision, which may fluctuate during the early stages.

Fig. 11-2. A, Increased hemorrhagic activity in a 59-year-old hypertensive man who was found to have had a superotemporal branch artery and vein occlusion 2 years previously. One episode of bleeding into the vitreous has occurred. **B,** More distal portions of the superotemporal region, showing numerous tufts of retinal neovascularization and large and well-entrenched intraretinal and interhemispherical shunts (arrow) between the superotemporal and inferotemporal vascular system. **C,** Fluorogram during the arteriolovenular phase, showing marked intraretinal shunting, fluorescein leakage (arrow), and tufts of neovascularization. **D,** Fluorescein angiography transit approximately 12 sec later, showing more marked leakage into the macular and paramacular region from the zone of the occluded arteriole and venule. **E,** Wide-angle view of the complete barrage-type Grade 3 coagulations applied in a contiguous manner to the zone of intraretinal vascular leakage and neovascularization. **F,** The area 2 months after argon laser photocoagulation, showing obliteration of the neovascular channels and leaking intraretinal vessels. Vision has been retained at the prephotocoagulation level of 20/40, and the hemorrhagic activity has been eradicated.

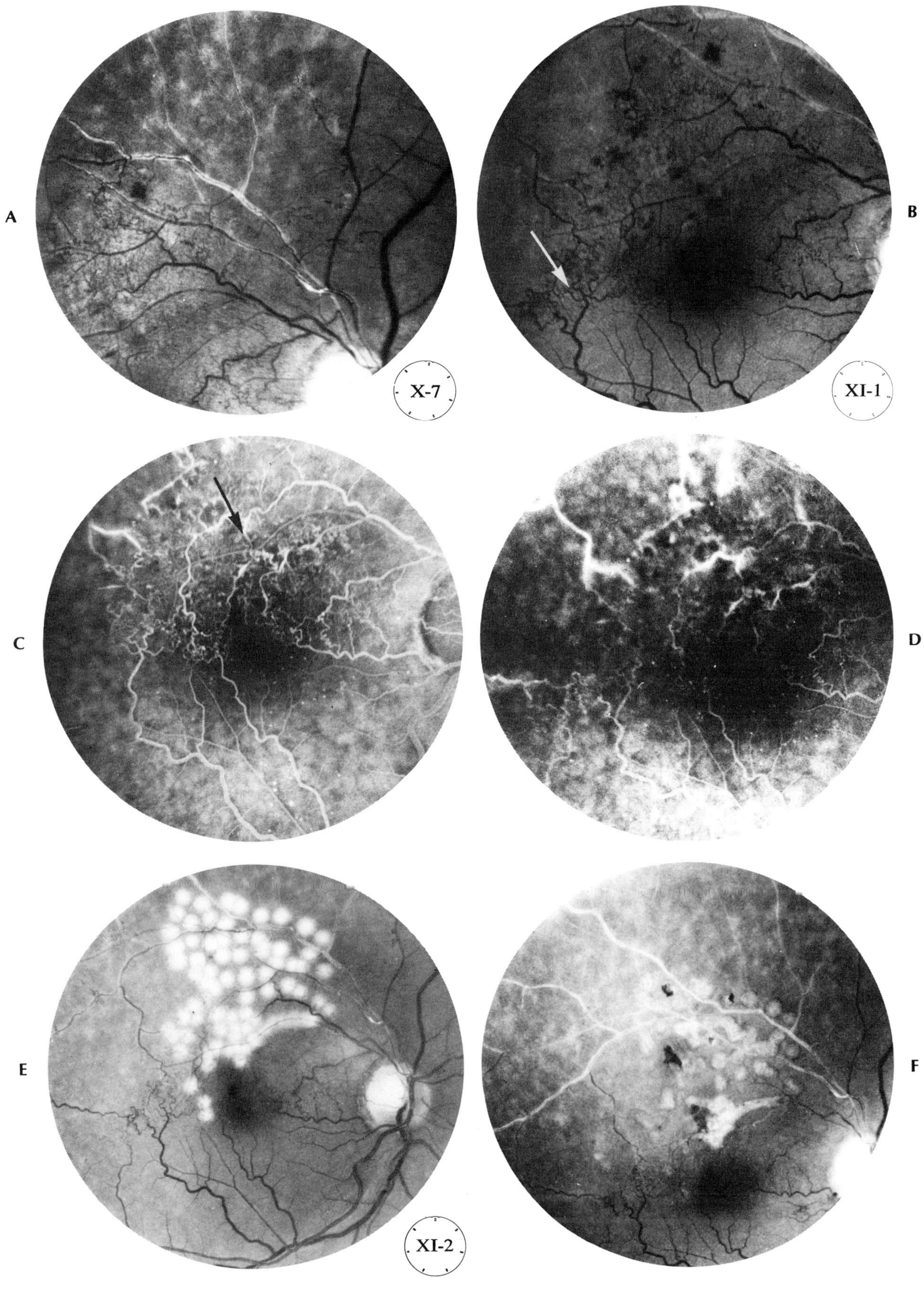

Fig. 11-2. For legend see opposite page.

Ophthalmoscopic appearance. The ophthalmoscopic appearance of a central retinal artery occlusion usually shows the various phenomena described in the section on Branch Retinal Artery Occlusion (p. 211) in all of the vessels extending from the optic disc. The foveal region appears much more red than the surrounding areas of retinal edema because of unimpaired visualization of the underlying choroidal blood supply. The retinal edema may increase with the passage of time from the moment of occlusion. Stagnation and attenuation of the vessels in the retina are most pronounced during the early stages.

Ancillary diagnostic examinations. A fluorescein angiogram will show an absence or paucity of blood flow into the retinal vessels and indicate the amount of blood flow into the retinal region.

Indications for photocoagulation. There are no indications for photocoagulation during the stage of acute onset.

If repair of the retina is accomplished later and a neovascular response, although unusual, is seen, particularly off the optic disc region, then the retinal ablation type of procedure can be considered 3 months to a year after the initial appearance of the neovascularization.

Photocoagulation approach. The photocoagulation approach to a central retinal artery occlusion with reestablishment of blood flow and possible neovascularization of the papillovitreal or retinovitreal variety is the retinal ablation procedure. Coagulations are performed from the paramacular region outward to the equatorial zone, as described under the section on the retinal ablation (PRP) technique for papillovitreal neovascularization of diabetic origin (p. 147). In this way the relative hypoxia is decreased, and the neovascularization appears to be decreased in a majority of cases.

Complications. The complications of photocoagulation are minimal, although occasional hemorrhages from an individual coagulation can be seen. These hemorrhages resolve quickly over a period of several weeks, and there have been no sequelae from this problem.

Follow-up. Follow-up examinations should be performed at 2- to 3-week intervals following photocoagulation during the initial course of treatment. The frequency of examinations can then be decreased, and fluorescein angiography can be performed at approximately 3-month intervals to follow the recovery of the fundus after photocoagulation therapy.

EXTRACELLULAR EDEMA

Branch retinal vein occlusion

Clinical symptoms. A branch retinal vein occlusion may have no clinical symptoms in a patient who is completely unaware of his problem and is simply found to have this condition during routine observation. More likely, the patient will complain of blurred vision, metamorphopsia, and micropsia. Some individuals complain of a decrease in light sensitivity or of wiggly lines in their central reading area. Many patients have hypertension or have been under considerable emotional stress. Occasionally, marked visual loss may be observed because of an intravitreal hemorrhage from the occluded area.

Ophthalmoscopic appearance. The obstruction of one of the branch veins in the eye can take any form. More commonly, the vein is obstructed within 1 to 2 DD of the optic disc, usually at the crossing of an arteriole. The entire distribution of the vein can be markedly edematous, and there can be many areas of deep and superficial retinal hemorrhages, microcystic changes in the macular region, and foveal macrocysts. The condition may be much more limited, and only a small terminal branch vein may be occluded. The same problems of edema, hemorrhagic activity, and microcystic changes can occur, however, and the results may be equally devastating. Branch retinal vein occlusions in the superonasal and inferonasal retina are not as common as in the temporal regions, but they do occur.

Ancillary diagnostic examinations. The most useful ancillary diagnostic examination is fluorescein angiography, which can show any of the characteristic defects from early retinal edema in the area of occlusion to marked microcystic changes and dye accumulation. As the process worsens, large segments of the blocked venous distribution become ischemic, the infarcted retina becomes more edematous, and deterioration ensues. To determine the healing capability of the eye and the possible indications for photocoagulation, fluorescein angiograms should be taken at approximately 2- to 3-month intervals during the evaluation of a branch retinal vein occlusion.

Stereo color photographs of the occluded venous area should be taken at 3- to 4-week intervals and reviewed to determine if there is any change in the elevation or extent of the retinal abnormalities.

Central visual fields should be tested at 3- to 4-week periods, and the results should be charted for red and green test objects as well as for white ones. The results of the field and Amsler grid testing should be compared at these intervals to determine if there is any extension of the blockage.

Contact lens biomicroscopy is very valuable for documenting the extent of edema, hemorrhagic activity, and particularly the coalescence of microcysts into macrocysts in the foveal and perifoveal regions.

Indications for photocoagulation. Most branch retinal vein occlusions are not treated for a period of 3 months following the commencement or recognition of their clinical symptoms. However, photocoagulation may be introduced before this time or at any interval after this time if the visual field is found to be deteriorating, if the microcystic disease is worsening and macrocysts are forming from the coalescence of the microcysts, if the visual acuity is decreasing, and if the edema and hemorrhagic activity are increasing. Furthermore, any degeneration reflected by increased infarct formation or marked pooling of the fluorescein during fluorescein angiography is also indicative of the marked deterioration that signals the decompensation of the eye during its natural reparative process. If the compensatory activity of the eye is failing, as noted previously, photocoagulation should be strongly considered.

Photocoagulation approach. The photocoagulation approach can be considered in three steps.

The arteriolar constriction or "crimping" technique. The rationale of this technique is to decrease the amount of arteriolar pressure being brought to bear on the occluded portion of retinal tissue. The technique is employed by placing coagulations at approximately ½-DD intervals along the arterioles in the region of venous blockage from the optic disc to a point perpendicular to the foveal region. In this manner the coagulations, which must be at least 50% larger than the vessel itself, are placed with sufficient intensity to cause the arterioles to go into spasm. The usual exposure is **0.2 sec**, and the usual coagulation diameter is approximately **200μ to 250μ** (Figs. 11-3 and 11-4). When the most proximal point along the arteriole feeding the area of the retinal branch vein occlusion has been thrown into spasm, the next coagulation is placed approximately ½ DD more distally on the same arteriole or any arterioles feeding the venous occlusion area. The power input should be decreased following the first arteriolar spasm, because the blood no longer flows as rapidly and less energy is needed for subsequent photocoagulation of the more distal

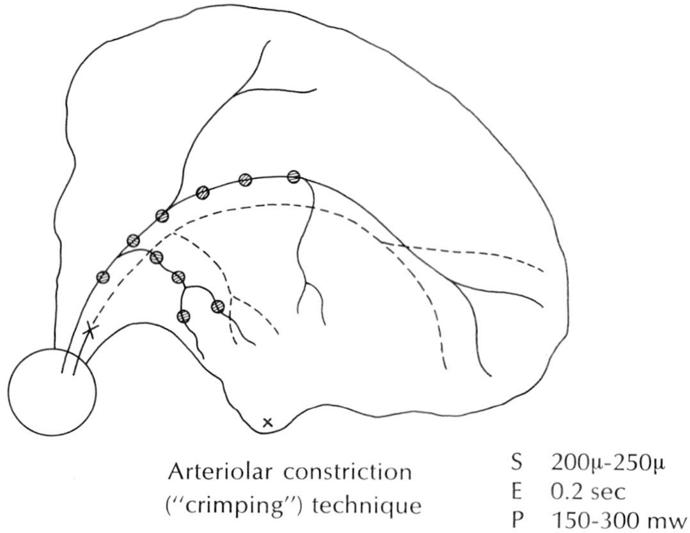

Fig. 11-3. Arteriolar constriction or "crimping" photocoagulation technique illustrating 200μ to 250μ coagulations placed ½ DD apart along the arteriole in the occluded zone distally to a point that would be perpendicular with the maculopapillar axis at the fovea.

arterioles. Within 2 to 3 min the arteriolar spasm will diminish and the arterioles will reopen; they can then be rephotocoagulated in an effort to damage the perivascular tissue sufficiently to cause eventual scarring and crimping of the arteriole at the point of coagulation. After the healing has been completed, this constriction causes a 10% to 15% decrease in the pressure along the arteriolar system by hemobarometry and appears to effectively reduce the load on the venous-obstructed system, allowing more adequate compensation by the retinal tissue. The vision may improve, and the edema and microcystic changes in this obstructed area may also decrease, as noted by subsequent fluorescein angiographic studies. If a beneficial effect is not accomplished and the fluorescein angiographic and perimetric evaluations remain unchanged, arteriolar crimping can be repeated with a similar follow-up and evaluation 1 to 2 months later.

The barrier technique. If the arteriolar crimping technique is unsatisfactory, even when repeated, the barrier technique can next be employed to decrease the pressure head on the macular and paramacular zone. In this way it is hoped that the microcystic disease and the marked edema and hemorrhagic activity will also decrease because of the restriction of the arteriolar flow into this area. The actual barrier technique consists of producing several rows of interrupted coagulations in an arcuate fashion approximately 1 to 1½ DD from the fovea in the region of the obstruction. These coagulations can be **200μ to 300μ** in diameter and are usually employed with intensities of **200 to 300 mw** at an exposure of **0.2 sec** (Figs. 11-5 and 11-6). The coagulations need not be chalk white but simply an off-white coagulation of moderate intensity (Grade 3). This technique usually decreases the amount of microcystic changes in the macular region and leads to some resolution of the edema and hemorrhagic activity.

The barrage technique. The barrage technique is used when the condition of the macular region is worsening because of the high arteriolar pressure and lack of venous return in the obstructed area. With this technique, coagulations of approximately **200μ to 500μ** in diameter are used at exposures of **0.2 to 0.5 sec** with sufficient intensity (usually **250 to 500 mw**) to cause an off-white discoloration (Grade 3) at the coagulation site (Figs.

A

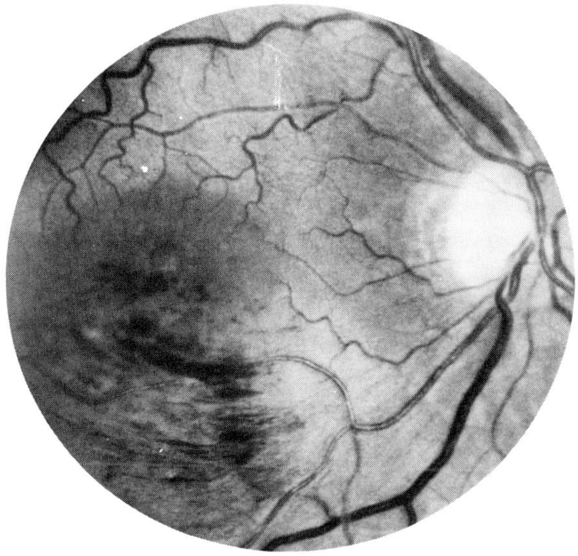

B

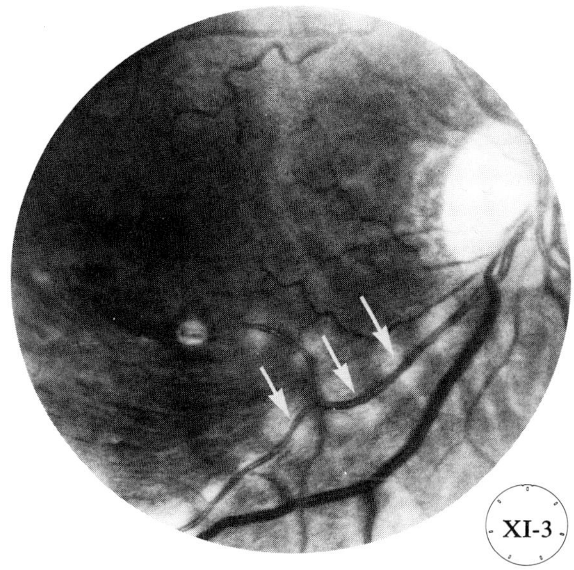

C

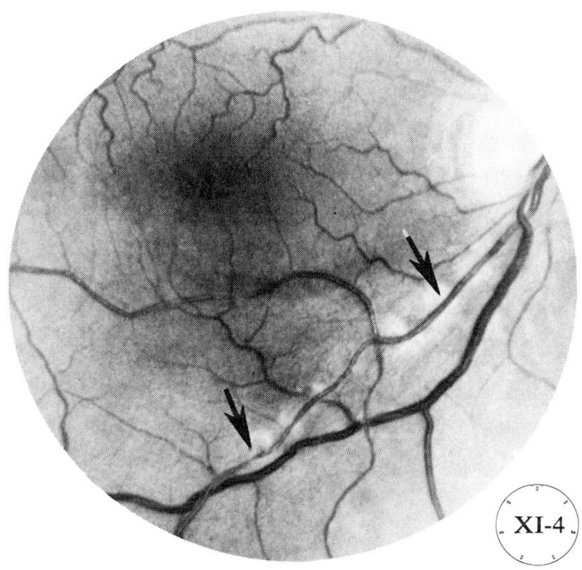

Fig. 11-4. A, An increase in microcystic, edematous, and hemorrhagic activity in a 59-year-old woman who had complained of blurred vision of 3 months' duration that was becoming progressively worse. There was also a loss of visual field, visual acuity, and increased leakage as demonstrated by fluorescein angiography. **B,** Multiple punctate, interrupted coagulations were applied to all arterioles in the occluded area at ½-DD intervals to a point perpendicular to the maculopapillar axis at the fovea. These coagulations were sufficient to cause a noticeable constriction and spasm of the arteriole at the impact site (arrows). **C,** Posterior polar region 11 weeks after arteriolar constriction by argon laser photocoagulation, showing a marked decrease in the edematous and hemorrhagic activity. Vision has improved from 20/80 to 20/25. Note the residual constriction of the arterioles at the previous photocoagulation site (arrows).

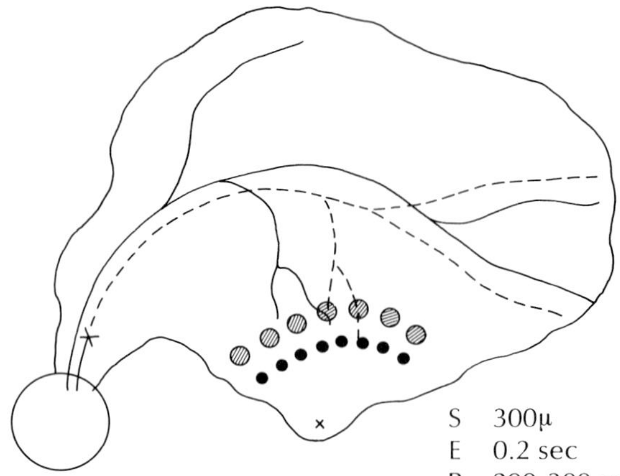

Fig. 11-5. Barrier argon laser photocoagulation technique for more severe branch vein occlusions or for those vein occlusions that do not respond to repeated arteriolar constriction photocoagulation therapy. Smaller coagulations are placed no closer than 1 DD to the fovea (lower parameters), and larger coagulations are produced more peripherally (upper parameters).

11-7 and 11-8). These coagulations are placed approximately 500μ apart throughout the distribution of the obstruction, somewhat in the manner of a retinal ablation. The coagulations do not come within 1½ to 2 DD of the fovea, and the coagulations can be produced with any of the photocoagulation devices. One can consider the use of the ruby laser as an initial photocoagulation source when using the barrage type of technique because of the high transmission through the nerve fiber layer, which may contain blood and other elements that are obstructing and and absorbent to the photocoagulation beam of the xenon-arc or argon laser instruments.

Complications. The complications noted with branch retinal vein occlusion are similar to those encountered with central retinal vein occlusion (p. 226).

Follow-up. The patient is advised to administer cycloplegic and steroid drops to the treated eye 3 times a day for 10 to 14 days after photocoagulation and to refrain from any strenuous activities or initiation of the Valsalva maneuver. The treated area is evaluated 2 weeks after treatment for any evidence of increased edema, cyst formation, vitreous traction, or hemorrhagic activity.

Fig. 11-6. A, A small macular branch vein occlusion from the inferotemporal arcade in a 36-year-old woman who had progressively blurred vision over a period of 4 months. Marked edema and exudate formation and extensive microcystic changes can be seen. **B,** Fluorescein angiogram showing dilated venules and leakage into the zone of the branch vein occlusion. **C,** Magnified view of the macular branch vein occlusion, showing the large area of exudate and edema formation (arrow). **D,** Venous occlusion area immediately after punctate, interrupted Grades 2 to 3 argon laser photocoagulations were applied approximately 1,000μ from the fovea in a concentric manner through the occluded zone (arrow). **E,** Healed photocoagulated area 6 weeks after barrier argon laser photocoagulation, showing decreased edema and hemorrhage and a slight reduction of exudates.

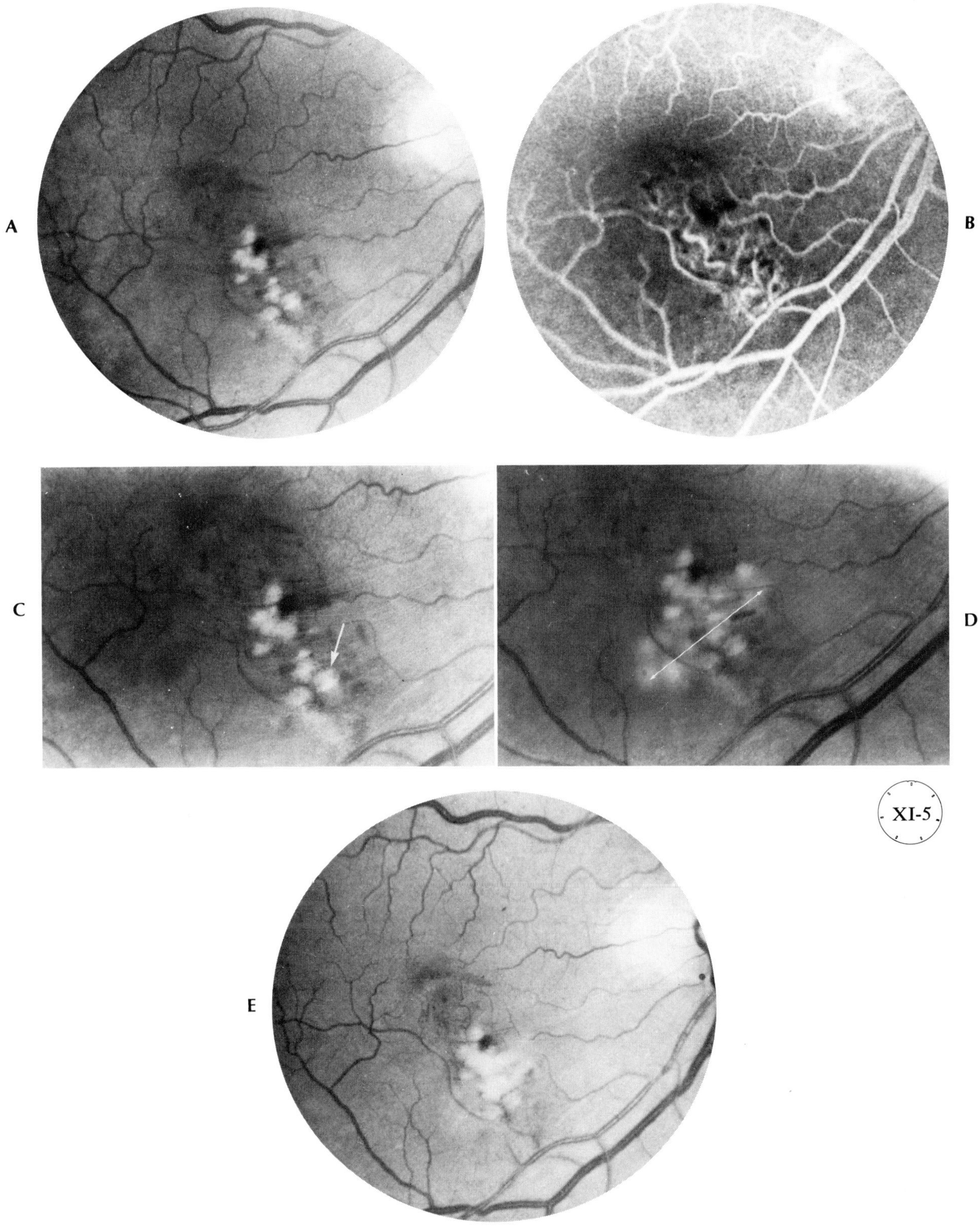

Fig. 11-6. For legend see opposite page.

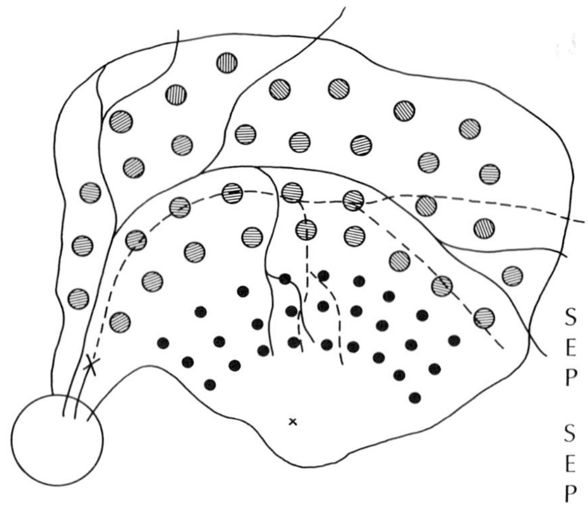

Fig. 11-7. Barrage argon laser photocoagulation technique for markedly severe branch vein occlusion or for those branch vein occlusions that do not respond to the arteriolar constriction or the barrier approach. Smaller coagulations are placed in the areas more proximal to the macula, and larger coagulations are placed in the more distal occluded zones. These coagulations are placed in all areas of the retina affected by the branch vein occlusion.

With any of these particular techniques, the patient must be followed very closely by indirect ophthalmoscopy, contact lens biomicroscopy, visual field examination, and fluorescein angiography. The fluorescein angiogram shows the pathophysiologic changes most accurately, and one should rely on this test frequently. Above all, photocoagulation intervention should be considered at any time when the integrity of the macular region appears to be greatly threatened.

Tufts of neovascularization may occur during the late reparative stage of a venous occlusion after intervals of several months to several years. These tufts of neovascularization must be watched closely ophthalmoscopically and by fluorescein angiography to determine whether any growth of the neovascular buds is taking place. Occasionally,

---

Fig. 11-8. A, A moderately severe occlusion of the superotemporal branch vein in a 68-year-old woman who had complained of marked loss of vision centrally and in the lower field of her left eye. Her condition was evaluated closely for approximately 4 months, and the hemorrhagic and edematous activity increased. There was a concurrent visual loss to 20/400 in that eye. **B,** Fluorescein angiogram demonstrating marked intraretinal shunting, leakage, infarcted areas (arrow), and total disruption of the outflow vasculature. **C,** Punctate, interrupted 250μ argon laser coagulations were placed in a barrage fashion approximately 1 DD from the foveal region peripherally over the extent of the branch vein occlusion. **D,** More peripheral view of the barrage argon laser photocoagulations to the area of the branch vein occlusion. Obvious hemorrhages and large tortuous vessels are avoided during photocoagulation. **E,** Posterior polar region 8 weeks after argon laser photocoagulation, showing a considerable decrease in hemorrhagic and edematous activity and in microcystic changes in the macular region. During this time vision improved to 20/50. **F,** Magnified view of the photocoagulated area 14 weeks after the argon laser photocoagulation barrage to the occluded zone, showing a moderate decrease in the residual hemorrhages and edema. Vision has improved to 20/40.

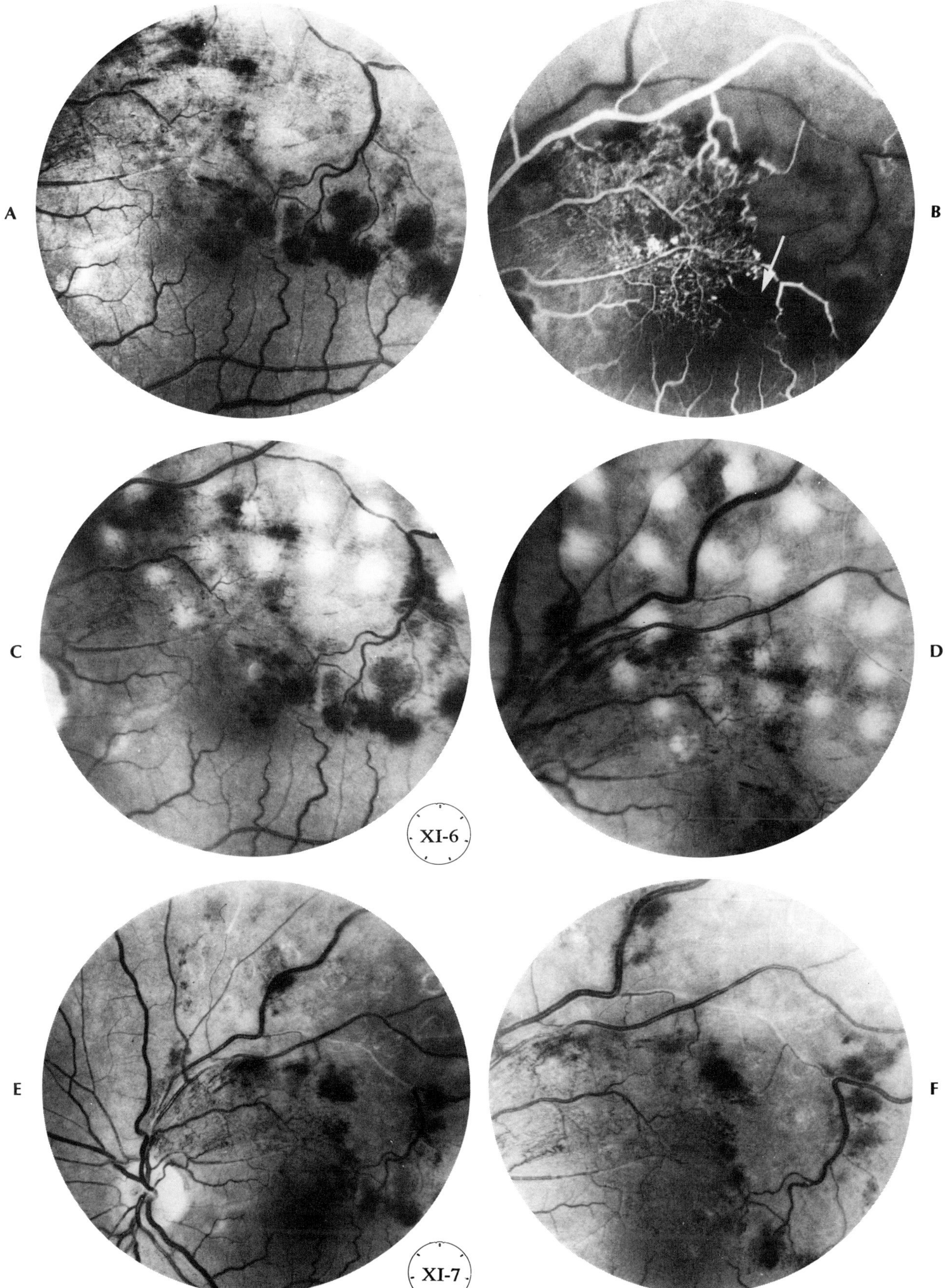

Fig. 11-8. For legend see opposite page.

hemorrhages into the vitreous occur from these neovascular sites, and these sites must then be photocoagulated directly. It is advisable to photocoagulate only the zones of neovascularization and not the areas of intraretinal dilated vessels or other shunting systems that have developed as a compensation response to the venous occlusion. Therefore, in the late reparative phase of branch venous obstruction, photocoagulation should be directed solely to the neovascularization, without interrupting the other vascular channels that have developed.

Central retinal vein occlusion

Clinical symptoms. The clinical symptoms of a central retinal vein occlusion usually include marked blurring and distortion of vision and considerable metamorphopsia. The visual sensitivity for light may be decreased, and the vision itself may be diminished to hand movements or less.

Ophthalmoscopic appearance. Because of the occlusion of the central retinal vein, the entire retina is usually markedly edematous and there are large areas of deep hemorrhages and especially of superficial hemorrhages. The hemorrhaging may be extended to the entire retina posterior to the equator, although the edema usually is much more marked in the posterior polar regions. The optic disc may be edematous and show a large amount of hemorrhagic activity. The central macular zone commonly encompasses a large cystic area, and multiple microcystic changes occur in the perifoveal and more peripheral macular regions. Attenuation of some of the arterioles can be seen because of previous arteriolosclerotic changes. The veins are markedly dilated and tortuous and may be beaded or sausagelike in configuration.

Ancillary diagnostic examinations. A fluorescein angiogram will demonstrate greatly reduced retinal vascular flow, the presence of marked blockage of the retinal vein in the region of the optic nerve, a breakdown of all the vascular elements, and fluorescein leakage into the retina throughout the posterior pole. A great accumulation of the fluorescein dye in the macular region is usually observed, particularly in the microcystic zones. The optic disc shows fluorescein leakage that can be quite extensive.

Fig. 11-9. A, A central retinal vein occlusion in a 48-year-old hypertensive man who had complained of a sudden loss of vision in his right eye 4 months previously. The visual acuity was 20/200, and there was extensive macular edema and hemorrhagic activity. During the subsequent 4 months, his vision declined to counting fingers, and the microcystic and edematous changes in the macular area increased. **B,** Fluorescein angiogram taken during initial examination, showing marked blockage of the venous system and leakage from the optic disc and other areas of the retinal vasculature. Considerable retinal and macular edema could be observed. **C,** Argon laser 300μ coagulations were placed in the perimacular area and outward to the equatorial region with a typical panretinal photocoagulation technique. The photocoagulation spared the macular area but came close to the nasal border of the optic disc. Coagulations were Grades 2 to 4 in intensity and were spaced approximately ½ to 1 DD apart (wide-angle view). **D,** Fluorescein angiogram during the arteriolovenular phase, 3 months after argon laser photocoagulation, showing a marked decrease in the macular edema and vascular leakage. **E,** Fluorescein angiogram during the late venular phase, showing some residual collection of fluid in the perifoveal retinal regions. **F,** Posterior polar region 3 months after argon laser photocoagulation, showing a marked decrease in the edematous and hemorrhagic activity. Vision has improved from a prephotocoagulation level of counting fingers to 20/50 (wide-angle view).

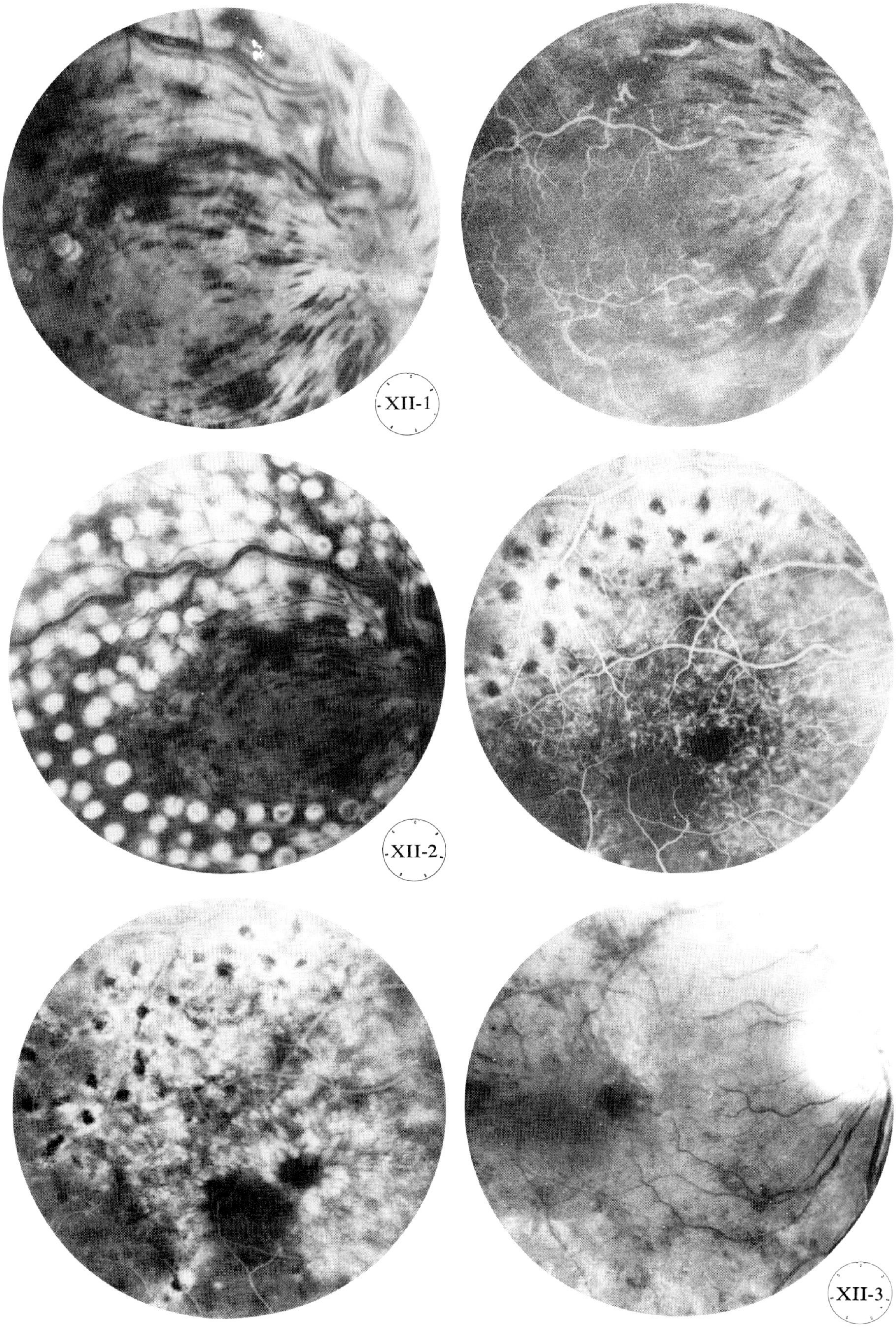

A B C D E F

Fig. 11-9. For legend see opposite page.

Stereo color photography of the posterior polar region is helpful in the continued evaluation of the process after the onset of the occlusion.

Regular visual field examinations may be useful for following the reparative course if the visual acuity is adequate for performance of the test.

Indications for photocoagulation. The most plausible indication for photocoagulation of a retina damaged by a central retinal vein occlusion is the presence of increasing edema, increasing microcystic changes, and increasing deterioration of macular function and visual perception. As the fluorescein picture worsens and there are increases in the areas of infarction and in the amount of edema and microcystic filling and proliferation, the possibility of photocoagulation intervention should be considered. To allow natural improvement and stabilization of the condition, if possible, it is advisable to delay therapy for a period of at least 3 months after occlusion. If the edema, hemorrhagic activity, and microcystic changes are decreasing, photocoagulation should be deferred.

The rationale for photocoagulation of a central retinal vein occlusion is to destroy retinal tissue, thereby decreasing the relative hypoxia of the retinal tissue affected. In addition, photocoagulation may increase the interchange between the choroid and the retina, thereby allowing an egress route for the retinal edema to escape into the choroid. It is also conceivable that the small amount of vascular flow that may be present in certain of these central retinal vein occlusions can then be utilized by the remaining functioning retina in a more efficient and effective manner after the photocoagulation procedure. It is expected that photocoagulation intervention will decrease the edematous and microcystic changes in the macular region that eventually lead to irreparable deterioration of the fovea if not treated.

Photocoagulation approach. Either the ruby laser, argon laser, or xenon-arc photocoagulation system can be used to produce a photocoagulation barrage in the manner described under instructions for retinal ablation (p. 147). Ruby laser photocoagulation seems to be preferable in those cases with extensive hemorrhagic activity, particularly when many hemorrhages exist in the superficial retinal layers. In these cases the ruby laser tends to penetrate to the pigment epithelial surface, resulting in less absorption by the superficially located blood than occurs with argon laser or xenon-arc photocoagulation. The ruby laser also seems to have less chance of interrupting the nerve fiber layer components during the photocoagulation process than the other two photocoagulation instruments because of the lack of coagulation in a region closely adjacent to the nerve fiber layer.

Fig. 11-10. A, Posterior polar region immediately after arteriolar constriction in a 57-year-old hypertensive man who had: a central retinal vein occlusion; marked hemorrhages, edema, and microcystic formation in the macular region; and a decrease in vision from 20/20 to 20/400. The eye was evaluated during a 3-month period, and some worsening of his vision and ophthalmoscopic appearance was noted. The arteriolar constriction crimping technique was then employed to all arterioles leading from the optic disc region to more fully compensate for the vascular abnormality. **B,** Inferotemporal arcade region following arteriolar constriction photocoagulation. Note marked hemorrhages and edema. **C,** Superotemporal vascular arcade region immediately following arteriolar constriction photocoagulation. **D,** Posterior fundus region 3 months after arteriolar constriction argon laser photocoagulation, showing complete clearing of the hemorrhages and edema and clearing of most of the microcystic changes. **E,** Macular and inferotemporal fundus region 3 months following photocoagulation, showing resolution of most of the hemorrhagic and edematous activity. Vision has improved from 20/400 to 20/50.

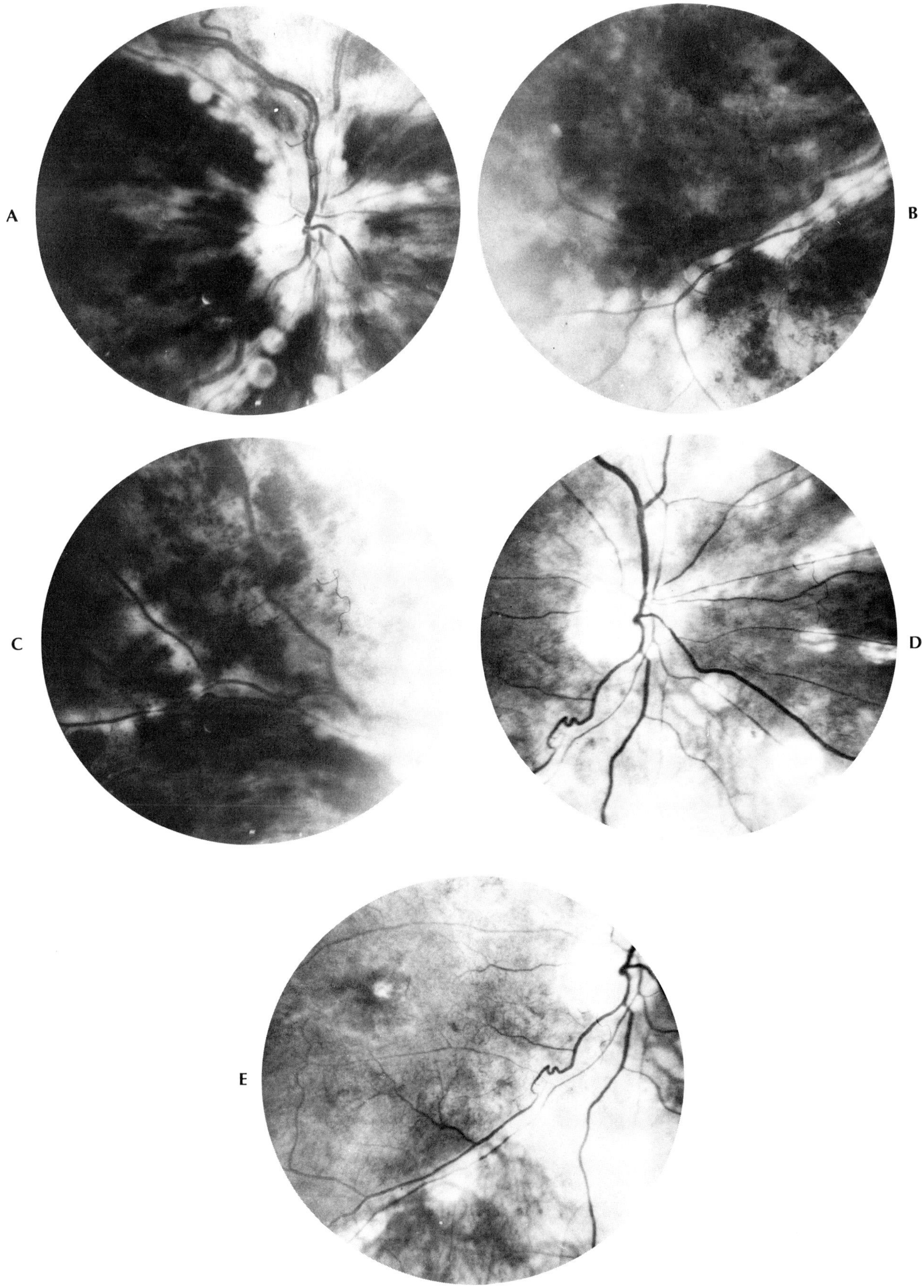

Fig. 11-10. For legend see opposite page.

Five-degree ruby laser impacts sufficient to produce a blanching of the pigment epithelial layer (Grade 1) or a small intraretinal bubble (Grade 2) should be employed with the barrage or panretinal photocoagulation technique. Usually, several sessions will be required for adequate treatment.

Argon laser photocoagulation can be used with **300μ to 500μ** diameter coagulations at a **0.2-sec** exposure and power levels of **300 to 500 mw**. With argon laser or xenon-arc photocoagulation an attempt must be made to avoid areas of hemorrhage because of the possible damage to the inner retinal layers that could result. To create an effective coagulation, edematous zones will require higher power inputs or longer exposures. Usually, a mild mucoid to off-white coagulation (Grades 2 to 3) in the deep retinal layers is adequate to produce a satisfactory result. The photocoagulation treatments should be divided into 3 sessions at least 1 week apart to minimize the irritation effect of the numerous coagulations (Fig. 11-9).

Once the retinal ablation has been performed, the patient should be seen again in approximately 3 weeks, and further photocoagulation should be considered 2 to 3 months later if there are any areas that have not been sufficiently treated or that show an inadequate response to photocoagulation.

The arteriolar constriction or crimping technique can be employed initially, as described in the section on Branch Retinal Vein Occlusion (p. 215). The resulting reduction of arteriolar pressure in the retina can be beneficial and provide adequate compensation and recovery of the occluded area. Additional arteriolar constriction photocoagulations can be performed 2 to 3 months later to produce a further effect, if necessary (Fig. 11-10).

Complications. The complications of treatment of a central retinal vein occlusion include hemorrhage into the retina or into the vitreous because of the inadvertent rupture or coagulation of a highly engorged or enlarged retinal vein or artery. Great care must be taken to coagulate around the markedly dilated vessels, particularly with ruby laser, which produces a "fast" explosive coagulation.

Marked glial response to the photocoagulation can sometimes be noted; there may be formation of striae along with retraction of the entire coagulated area along the plane of the retina toward the central portion of the vitreous. This response is most difficult to obviate during the photocoagulation procedure, unless one recognizes the attachment of the posterior hyaloid to an area of proposed treatment and subsequently reduces the intensity of the photocoagulation in that particular region. To minimize this complication, photocoagulations should not be placed within a 1½ to 2 DD radius of the fovea.

Retinal detachment has been noted in a localized portion of the posterior pole in rare instances and conceivably could be attributed to photocoagulation in an area with a very strong vitreoretinal adhesion. Areas of vitreoretinal adhesion must be avoided scrupulously.

Follow-up. The patient must be seen at 3-week intervals and be followed very closely by indirect ophthalmoscopy, contact lens biomicroscopy, and fluorescein angiography. The fluorogram ideally will show a decrease in the calibre of the vessels and the edema in the posterior pole. The amount of microcystic changes should be evaluated most closely during visits, and photocoagulation should be repeated if the microcystic changes have not improved or if they are worsening. Usually, photocoagulation sessions should be spaced at least 2 months apart to allow the eye to acclimate to the photocoagulation process and to its own hemodynamic condition.

Irvine-Gass syndrome

Clinical symptoms. The symptom of the Irving-Gass syndrome is gradual and painless loss of vision and moderate distortion. This symptom usually appears weeks to months following intraocular surgery, particularly cataract extraction.

Ophthalmoscopic appearance. Microcystic formation in the perifoveal and macular region can be diagnosed by direct ophthalmoscopy and by binocular biomicroscopy with the contact lens. Foveal cystic changes are usually observed when a large macrocyst is present. Edema of the macular retina and some disruption and disorganization of the pigment epithelium are common, and the internal limiting membrane is roughened and irregular. There may or may not be a posterior vitreous detachment associated with this syndrome.

Ancillary diagnostic examinations. Fluorescein angiography will show pooling of the fluorescein in the foveal microcysts during the late venular stages. Leakage into the extracellular space can also be seen in the macular and paramacular regions, and there is usually a relative lack of fluorescein concentration in the foveal zone. The fluorescein pooling and leakage intensifies for 10 to 20 min following fluorescein injection.

Stereo color fundus photography will also show the existence of edema and elevation of the macular region caused by the microcystic formation.

Indications for photocoagulation. The presence of microcystic disease for a period of longer than 1 year without improvement of vision along with evidence that the microcysts are coalescing to form macrocysts, resulting in a decrease in vision, are indications for cautious photocoagulation of the macular region. This therapy is being evaluated experimentally at this time and must be undertaken judiciously.

A large amount of preretinal fibrosis, the presence of an obvious macular vitreoretinal membrane under traction, and gross deterioration of the macula are considered contraindications for photocoagulation intervention.

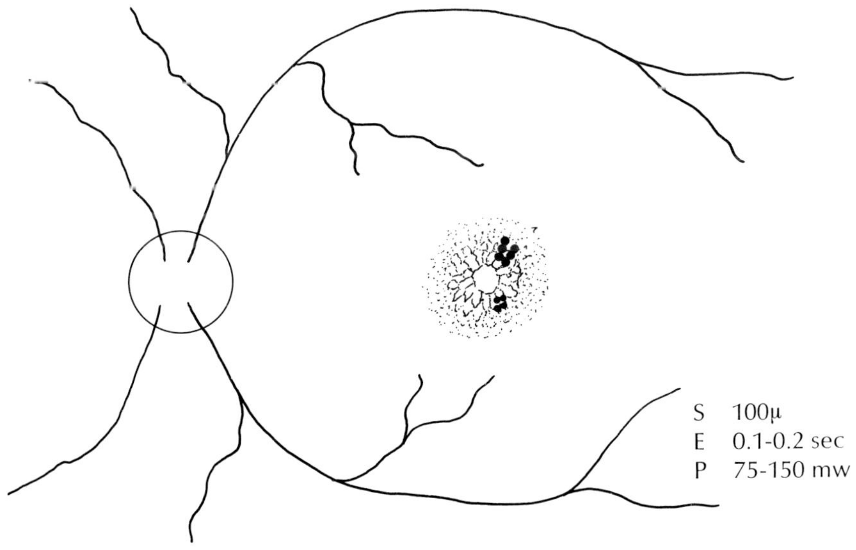

Fig. 11-11. Placement of argon laser coagulations in the region of most prominent intraretinal leakage at least ½ DD from the umbo. The use of argon laser photocoagulation for this disease is highly experimental at this time.

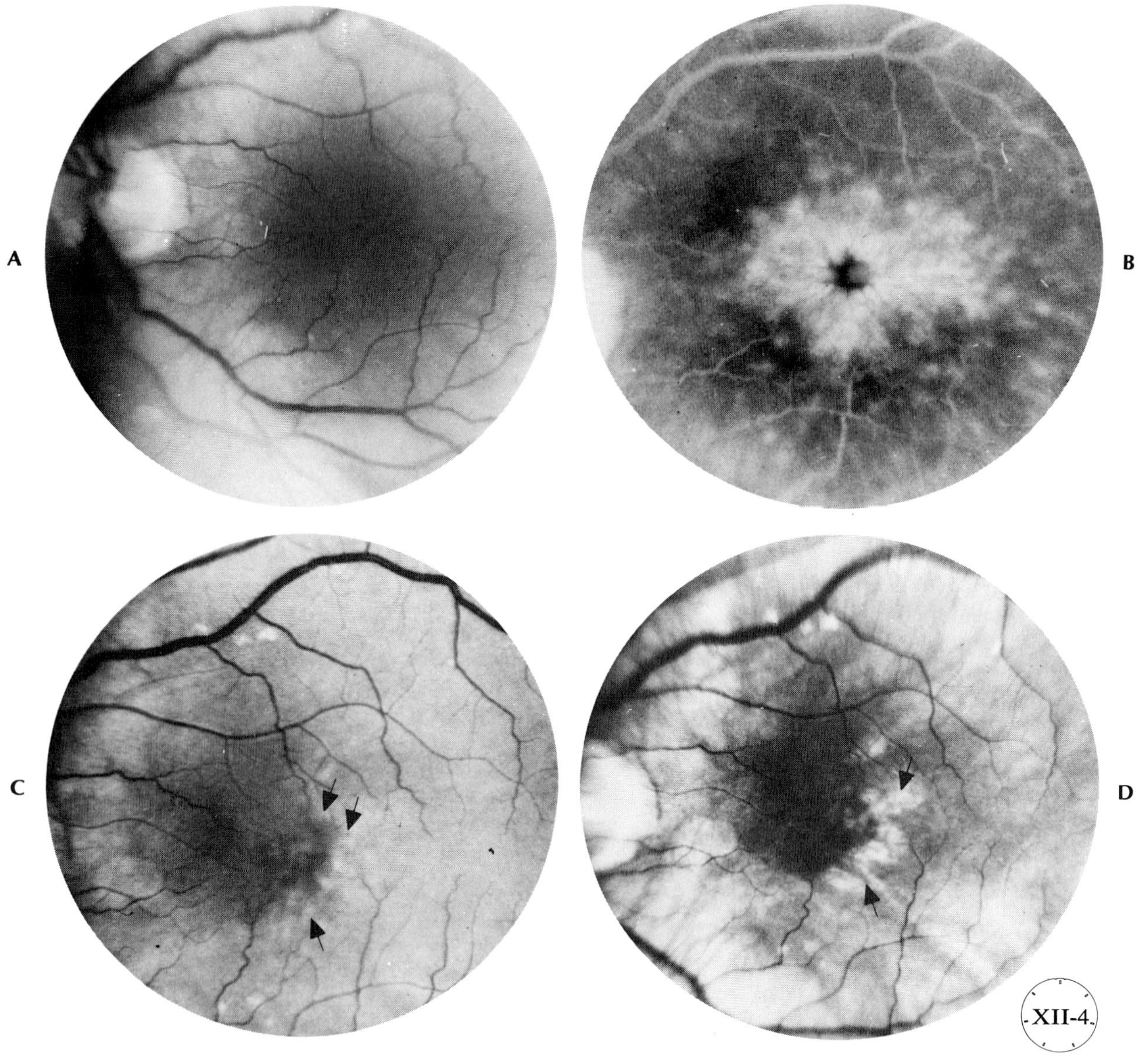

Fig. 11-12. A, Extensive microcystic edema in the macular region consistent with the Irvine-Gass syndrome of 1 year's duration in a 65-year-old woman who had undergone cataract surgery 2 years previously. Her vision had progressively become worse, from 20/200 to counting-fingers vision, over this period of time, and photocoagulation therapy was attempted on an experimental basis. **B,** Fluorescein angiogram showing marked microcystic accumulation of fluorescein dye in the macular region. **C,** Grade 2, 100μ punctate coagulations were applied to a limited area of prominent macular leakage (arrows). **D,** Macular zone 3 months later, showing scarring at the regions of previous argon laser photocoagulation (arrows) and reduction of the microcystic edema. Vision has improved to $20/60^{-2}$.

Photocoagulation approach. Photocoagulation is directed to a quadrant or segment of the macular region to test the response of the macula to the process of photocoagulation. Impacts of **100μ** at **0.1 to 0.2 sec** and at power levels sufficient to cause a very slight mucoid reaction (Grade 2) should be produced in the selected quadrant (Fig. 11-11). Usually, the quadrant with the greatest degree of microcystic change or fluorescein pooling is treated. Coagulations should be interrupted and placed in a closely approximated barrage fashion in an area at least 750μ (½ DD) from the umbo. The photocoagulation effect should be seen at the time of the treatment, and during the postoperative period the patient should be watched for a decrease in the amount of microcystic change and macular edema (Fig. 11-12).

If the microcystic changes and edema in the macular area are decreased after photocoagulation, it is then conceivable that additional photocoagulation could be performed in other segments or quadrants of the macular zone. All photocoagulations should be produced in the region of most advanced microcystic change, outside a radius of 750μ of the umbo.

Complications. Foveal and macular striae, as well as hypertrophy of the pigment epithelium and excessive glial production in the region of the treatment, can occur following photocoagulation. To obviate this problem, photocoagulation intensity should be minimal.

An increase in macular edema following photocoagulation has been observed, but the cause is not known. For this reason photocoagulations generally should not be directed to more than 20% to 25% of the macular region during a treatment session.

Follow-up. Patients should be followed at 4- to 6-week intervals so that the response to photocoagulation can be judged. Approximately 3 months following photocoagulation, a fluorescein angiogram should be taken and compared with the prephotocoagulation fluorograms. If the microcystic disease and the fluorescein pooling have decreased and the vision has improved, further photocoagulation can be considered.

Vitreitis

Clinical symptoms. The patient with vitreitis experiences a gradual blurring of vision and numerous floaters and other debris throughout the visual field. A dense graying of the central vision, distortion, and micropsia can be noted as the condition worsens. Conjunctival hyperemia can also be observed.

Ophthalmoscopic appearance. Some cells and flare can be noted in the anterior chamber in conjunction with a marked vitreous response with numerous white cells throughout the cortex of the vitreous body. Inflammation of the anterior retina and pars plana can be noted, particularly in the inferior portions. The macula, when seen clearly, can be edematous; there can be multiple microcystic changes and central macrocystic formation.

Ancillary diagnostic examinations. A fluorescein angiogram will show a dense pooling in the macular and paramacular regions, clustering and pooling of the fluorescein in the microcystic areas, and leakage into the surrounding macular retina.

Indications for photocoagulation. Photocoagulation has not been indicated for this particular disease.

Follow-up. Follow-up examinations should include fluorescein angiography and stereo color fundus photography as the vitreous clears so that microcystic changes in the macula can be documented. Conceivably, photocoagulation can be employed in the very late stages if the microcystic component persists.

Chapter 12

Miscellaneous macular diseases

MACULAR HOLES AND CYSTS

Clinical symptoms. The patient with macular holes usually complains of severe distortion and painless loss of vision over a period of several weeks. The vision is usually reduced to 20/200 or less once a macular hole has been formed. Patients with macular cysts usually have better visual acuity unless the cystic formation has been chronic.

Ophthalmoscopic appearance. A definite elevation of the macula and occasionally the paramacular area can be seen rising to an area of a central foveal cyst that may eventually break down to form a macular hole. The diagnosis of a cyst is made if stereo biomicroscopy with a precorneal or contact lens reveals the inner wall of the cyst to be intact. Once the hole has formed, the underlying pigment epithelium or choroid may be well seen; there is clumping of the pigment epithelium, and the remaining outer retina is irregular. The edges of the macular hole may be partially rolled outward, and there may be a slight retinal detachment surrounding the penetrating macular hole.

Ancillary diagnostic examinations. Fluorescein angiography will show the appearance of fluorescein within the macular cyst if a cyst is present. A fluorogram of lamellar macular hole may show very little change from a normal fluorogram, whereas that of a penetrating macular hole will demonstrate the choroidal flush phase prominently.

Stereo color photography will show the macular hole or cyst prominently and is extremely valuable for continued evaluation of the condition.

A visual field examination will indicate a very dense absolute scotoma if a macular hole is present; it will show a relative scotoma if a macular cyst is present.

Indications for photocoagulation. Photocoagulation should not be used for treatment of a macular cyst.

If the edges of a penetrating macular hole are progressively rolling outward to a greater degree or if the retinal detachment surrounding a penetrating macular hole is beginning to spread peripherally, photocoagulation to seal off the hole and prevent a more extensive retinal separation can be considered.

Photocoagulation treatment should not be considered for a lamellar macular hole, but the disorder should be watched closely.

Photocoagulation approach. Interrupted coagulations of **100μ** diameter are produced with a **0.1-sec** exposure and sufficient intensities (usually **150 to 250 mw**) to cause a very mild mucoid coagulation (Grade 2) at the outer extent of the retinal detachment where the

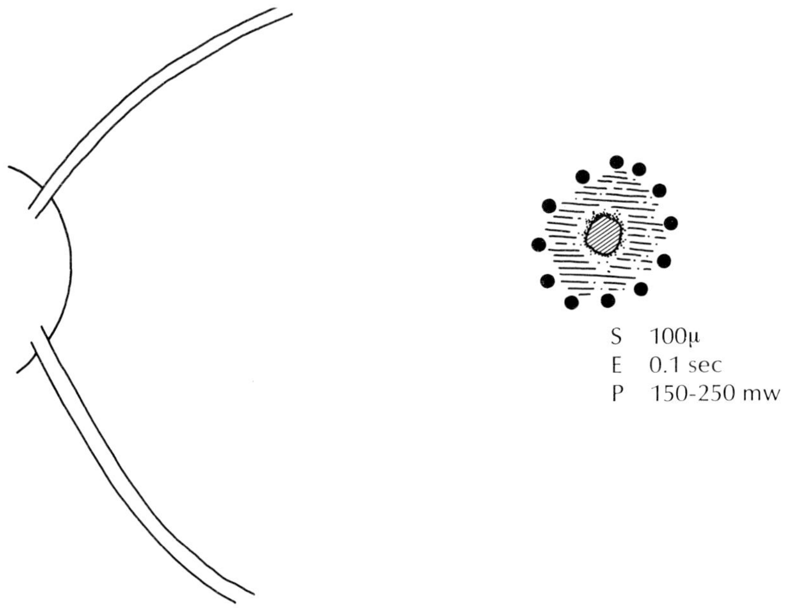

Fig. 12-1. Proper placement of 100μ coagulations away from the border of the macular hole and in an area of attachment of the sensory retina to the pigment epithelial layer.

sensory retina is still adherent to the underlying pigment epithelium (Fig. 12-1). The purpose of these coagulations is to prevent the occurrence of a full-sized retinal detachment by surrounding and sealing the macular hole and by blocking the extent of the subretinal fluid expansion. Individual photocoagulations should not be created closer than 300μ of each other and should be placed around the macular region in a linear fashion (Fig. 12-2).

Complications. If the coagulations are too intense, the process of rolling of the edges of the macular hole can be aggravated, the surrounding retinal detachment can be worsened, and treatment will be ineffective. Hemorrhage and gliosis are not unusually encountered, but macular striae can conceivably form if the coagulations are too intense.

Follow-up. Following photocoagulation, patients should be watched at 3-week intervals for any increase in the traction or size of the macular hole. Once stabilization has been accomplished, the patient can usually be followed by fundus photography and fluorescein angiography at 3- to 6-month intervals.

PRERETINAL FIBROSIS

Clinical symptoms. The patient with preretinal fibrosis usually experiences a very gradual decrease in visual acuity, increasing metamorphopsia, and an awareness of decreased light sensitivity in the central visual field. The onset of symptoms may be more sudden if the preretinal fibrosis is secondary to macular microangiopathy.

Ophthalmoscopic appearance. Moderate to marked wrinkling of the internal limiting membrane and patchy edema of the macular and paramacular regions are most commonly observed with this condition. The retinal vessels appear to be tortuous and kinked, and some intraretinal shunting vessels and dilated retinal capillaries can be seen in the macular zone. Early gliosis of the inner portions of the macular or paramacular area can be observed by slit lamp biomicroscopy.

Ancillary diagnostic examinations. Fluorescein angiography may show areas of patchy leakage from the retinal vessels and accumulation of the dye in the macular area. This pooling of dye will be more apparent in the late venular stages.

Stereo fundus photography with magnification will show the gross irregularity of the internal limiting membrane and the underlying retinal edema in the macular and paramacular regions.

Campimetry may indicate relative scotomas in the areas of greatest disruption and gliotic activity. These scotomas may be regional and limited to small portions of the macular area.

Indications for photocoagulation. Preretinal fibrosis must not be treated indiscriminately, although treatment to localized or segmental patches of gross edema of the retina in the macular or paramacular area may be beneficial. Photocoagulation must be performed discretely and must not be done in an area of extensive preretinal gliosis.

Photocoagulation should be performed only if leakage is extensive, as shown by fluorescein angiography, and if the vision has decreased markedly to the 20/80 or 20/100 level.

Progression of the visual field defect or rapidly decreasing visual acuity is an indication for the consideration of photocoagulation therapy.

Photocoagulation therapy for this disease is still being evaluated on an experimental basis. Photocoagulation should be considered cautiously and only for severe cases with marked leakage and edema.

Photocoagulation approach. Coagulations of **100μ** at a **0.1-sec** exposure are produced in an interrupted, noncoalescent patterned barrage to the area of maximum leakage (Fig. 12-3). This leakage area can be determined from the fluorescein angiogram, and the coagulations can be accurately placed with the aid of photographic enlargements. The area of photocoagulation must not exceed more than 10% to 15% of a sector of the macula at any one photocoagulation session. The macula must be allowed to heal from the photocoagulation, and the area is then reevaluated ophthalmoscopically and by fluorescein angiography approximately 2 to 3 months after the photocoagulation intervention. Further photocoagulation can be considered if leakage persists in large amounts, but no more than 10% to 15% of the macular sector should be treated during any individual future photocoagulation session (Fig. 12-4).

Complications. The gliotic response can be worsened by excessive photocoagulation, but this problem can be obviated by limiting the amount of photocoagulation to 10% to 15% of the macular sector at any one session.

Fig. 12-2. A, Right macular region of a 51-year-old woman who had noticed a loss of vision that had progressed over a 2-month period to a counting-fingers visual acuity. Her condition was evaluated closely, and the puckering, rolling of the edges of the hole, and tenting of the macular region were observed to have increased over a 3-month interval. **B,** Fluorescein angiogram of the right macular area, showing a faint transmitted fluorescence through the damaged pigment epithelium in the region of the macular hole. **C,** Grade 2 punctate, linear, interrupted 100μ coagulations were placed around the macular region in an area of attached retina. **D,** Right macular region 9 weeks after photocoagulation showing a faint pigmentation and disruption of the pigment epithelium in the area of the coagulations. There has been no further advancement of the macular disease. **E,** Magnified view of the right macular region, showing the macular hole, surrounding microcystic disease, and faint areas of pigment hypertrophy secondary to argon laser photocoagulation.

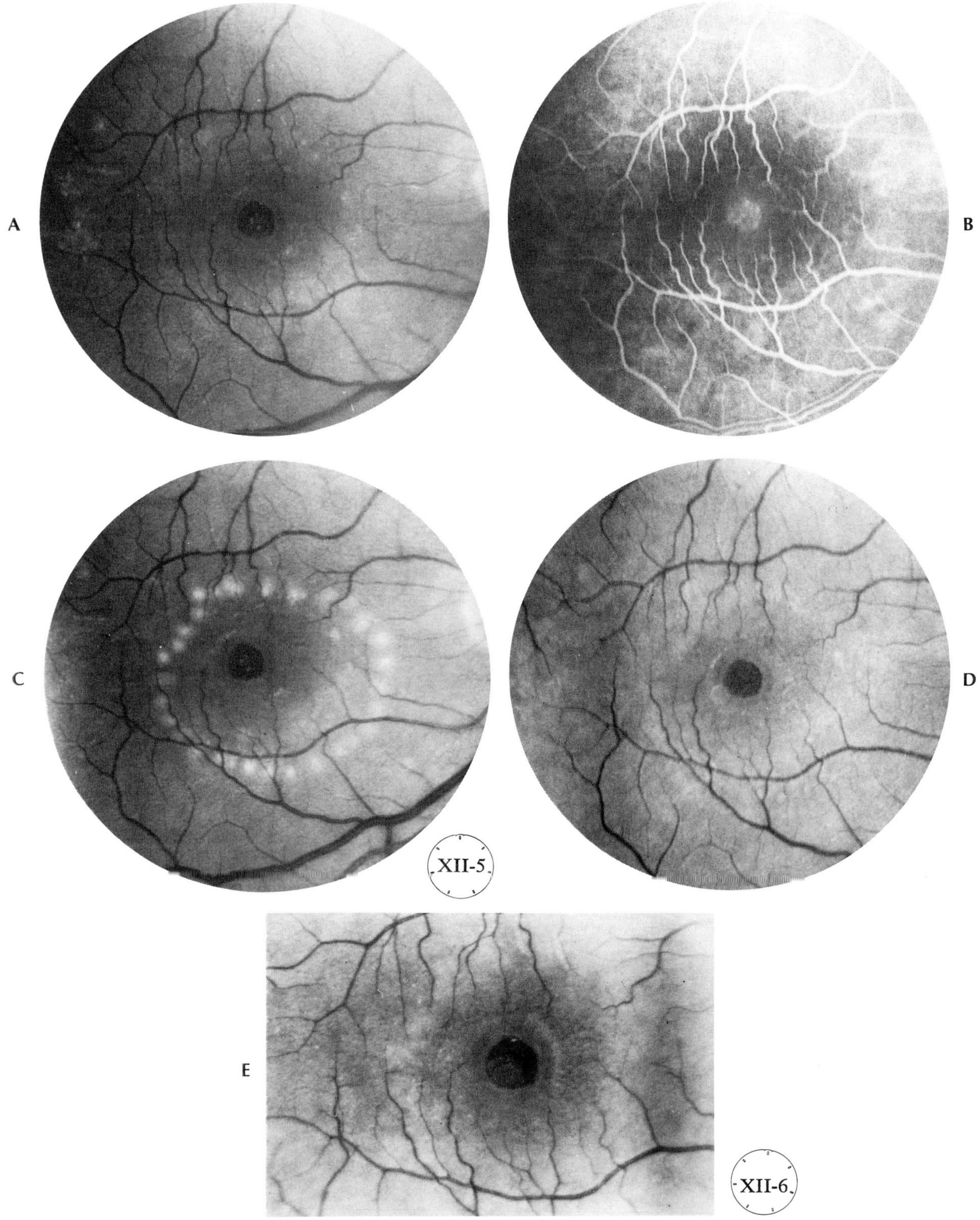

Fig. 12-2. For legend see opposite page.

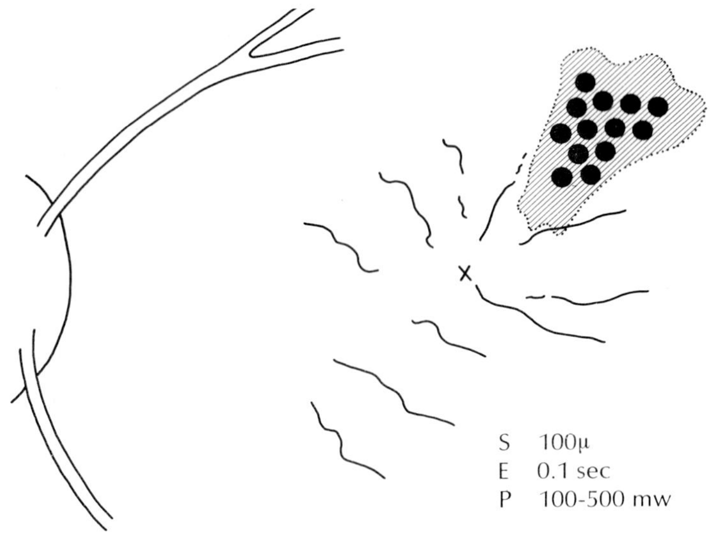

Fig. 12-3. Placement of 100μ punctate, interrupted, barrage coagulations in the region of maximal fluorescein leakage at least 1,000μ from the umbo. No more than 10% to 15% of the macular area should be treated at a single photocoagulation session.

Macular striae can be formed but are not significant if the leakage component can be diminished by photocoagulation.

The macular area can be involved by hemorrhage if the power input is excessive or if the scar tissue resulting from photocoagulation results in the tearing of a small macular vessel.

Follow-up. Following photocoagulation the healing response of patients should be evaluated at monthly intervals. Further photocoagulation should be considered only if marked benefit has been observed following the initial treatment and if large leakage areas persist.

TOXOPLASMIC RETINOCHOROIDITIS

Clinical symptoms. During the acute phase of toxoplasmic retinochoroiditis the vision may be markedly blurred and distorted because of many vitreous opacities and floaters. During the healed phase the patient may experience floaters and scotomas but no other subjective problems.

Ophthalmoscopic appearance. The acute lesion will show a moderately dense, white area of edematous retina and choroid, usually in the paramacular or posterior polar region. A large number of whitish vitreous opacities usually lie over the lesion or may involve the entire vitreous body. The inactive phase of the disease may show marked, well-delineated, punched-out areas of the atrophied or destroyed retina and choroid, complete disruption of these layers, and heavy pigmentation around the lesions. A few choroidal vessels may line the bottom of the inactive lesion, which may be 1 to 4 DD in extent, but usually there is a total destruction of the choroid and retina. Numerous vitreous floaters can persist during the inactive phase and be seen subjectively.

Ancillary diagnostic examinations. Stereo fundus photography is helpful in following the course of the disease process during the inactive phases.

Fluorescein angiography will demonstrate areas of pronounced retinal vascular leakage in the area of inflammatory activity. A combination of leakage and pooling of the dye that

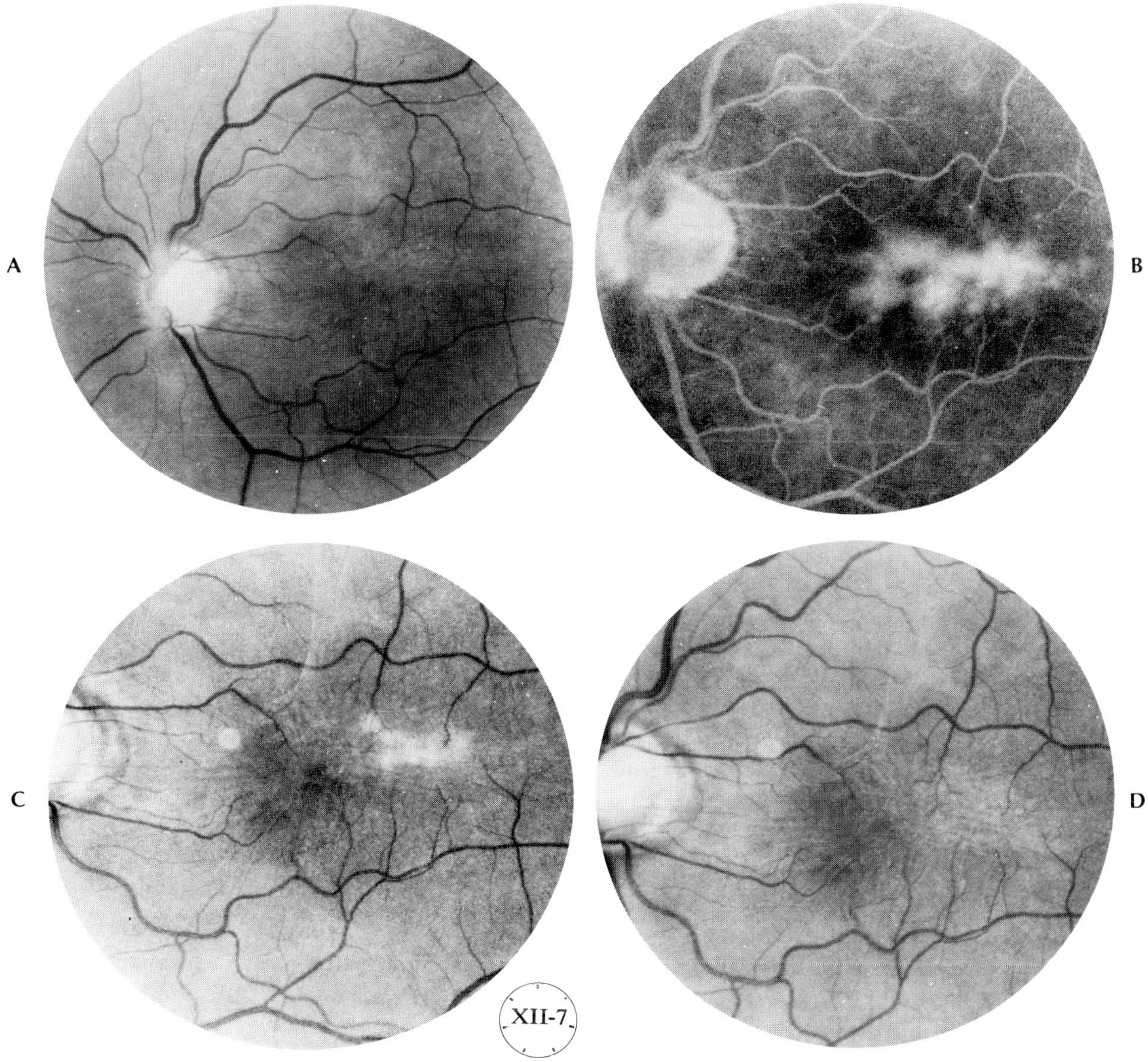

Fig. 12-4. A, Macular region of a 57-year-old woman who had complained of a gradually increasing visual loss and distortion. Marked wrinkling and thickening of the internal limiting membrane and macular retinal edema were observed. **B,** Fluorescein angiogram showing areas of marked leakage from the macular retinal vessels. **C,** Mucoid, Grade 2 100μ coagulations were placed in the area of maximal leakage temporal to the fovea in an interrupted barrage manner. **D,** Macular region 10 weeks after photocoagulation with cauterization of the temporal area of fluorescein leakage. Vision has improved from 20/100 to 20/50.

starts in the arteriolar phase and concentrates during the venular phase can be observed. This ill-defined, smudgy area of retinal leakage will correspond to the zone of activity as seen ophthalmoscopically.

Tangent screen visual field examinations can be most helpful in demonstrating involvement of a region of the macula or posterior pole by the inflammatory process. Amsler grid charts should be given to the patient so that he can detect any changes in macular function and report them to the ophthalmologist as soon as he recognizes them.

Indications for photocoagulation. Based on the rationale that the *Toxoplasma* cysts or antigenic tissue in the periphery of the toxoplasmic lesion can reactivate at any time, photocoagulation should be directed to these borders to destroy this tissue or these cysts and thereby prevent any reactivation and extension of the inflammatory process. This procedure is done most effectively during the inactive phase of the toxoplasmic infection, although it has been attempted during the active phase. Lesions in the periphery of the eye are usually not photocoagulated, and photocoagulation is limited to those posterior polar lesions that could threaten the macular region during reactivation.

Choroidal or retinal neovascularization at the borders of the toxoplasmosis scar should be photocoagulated as soon as it is recognized, provided that the neovascularization is located more than 1,000μ from the umbo. Neovascular change is not common, but one should be alert to its occurrence, since the results can be devastating.

Photocoagulation approach. The pigmented rim of the toxoplasmosis scar and portions of the surrounding normal retina are photocoagulated with **200μ to 500μ** spot sizes at a **0.2-sec** exposure and intensities of approximately **150 to 450 mw** (Fig. 12-5). These moderately intense coagulations are produced around the area of former destruction, and the entire toxoplasmic area is walled off or surrounded. Coagulations should be contiguous with one another, and all areas around the scar should be well coagulated. Smaller coagulations can be made in those areas closer to the fovea if the scar impinges on the macular region (Figs. 12-6 to 12-8).

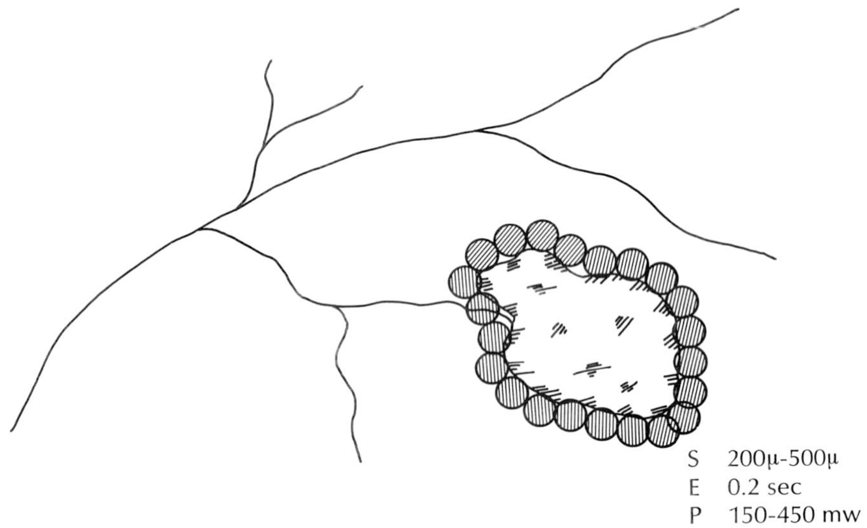

Fig. 12-5. Placement of 200μ to 500μ punctate, linear, contiguous coagulations around the border of an inactive toxoplasmosis scar. The coagulations should involve a large rim of surrounding healthy retina.

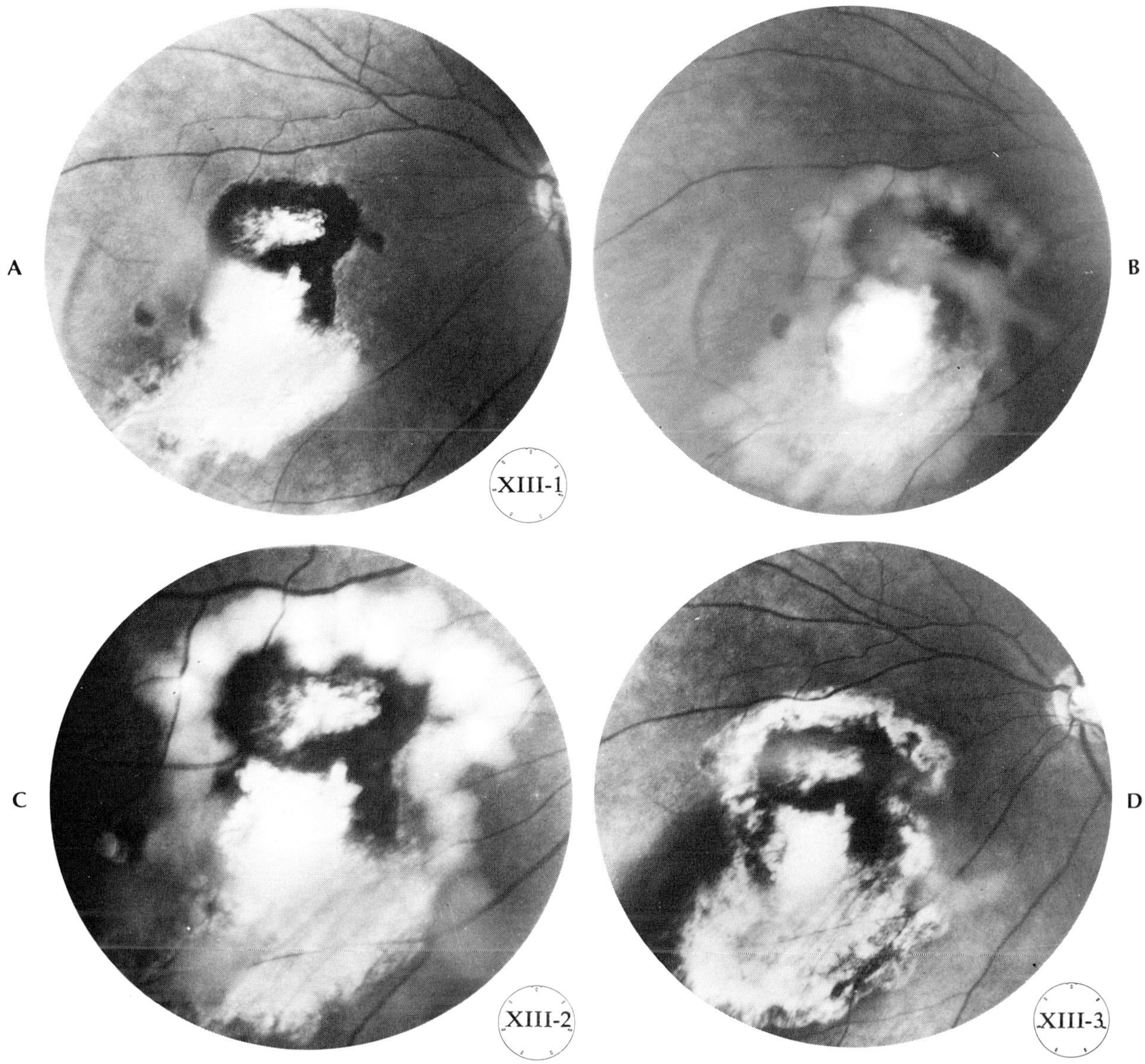

Fig. 12-6. A, Forty-five degree wide-angle Nikon photograph of the nasal fundus of a 33-year-old woman who had been experiencing frequent episodes of blurred vision caused by severe vitreous clouding. Her ophthalmoscopic lesion was diagnosed as toxoplasmic retinochoroiditis after a blood titer and skin test were strongly positive for toxoplasmosis. **B,** Wide-angle view after photocoagulation with 500μ contiguous coagulations around the border of the inactive toxoplasmosis scar. **C,** Toxoplasmosis scar immediately following photocoagulation to the border. **D,** Wide-angle view of treated toxoplasmosis lesion 7 weeks after photocoagulation, showing scarring, disruption, and gliosis of the border of the previously diseased area.

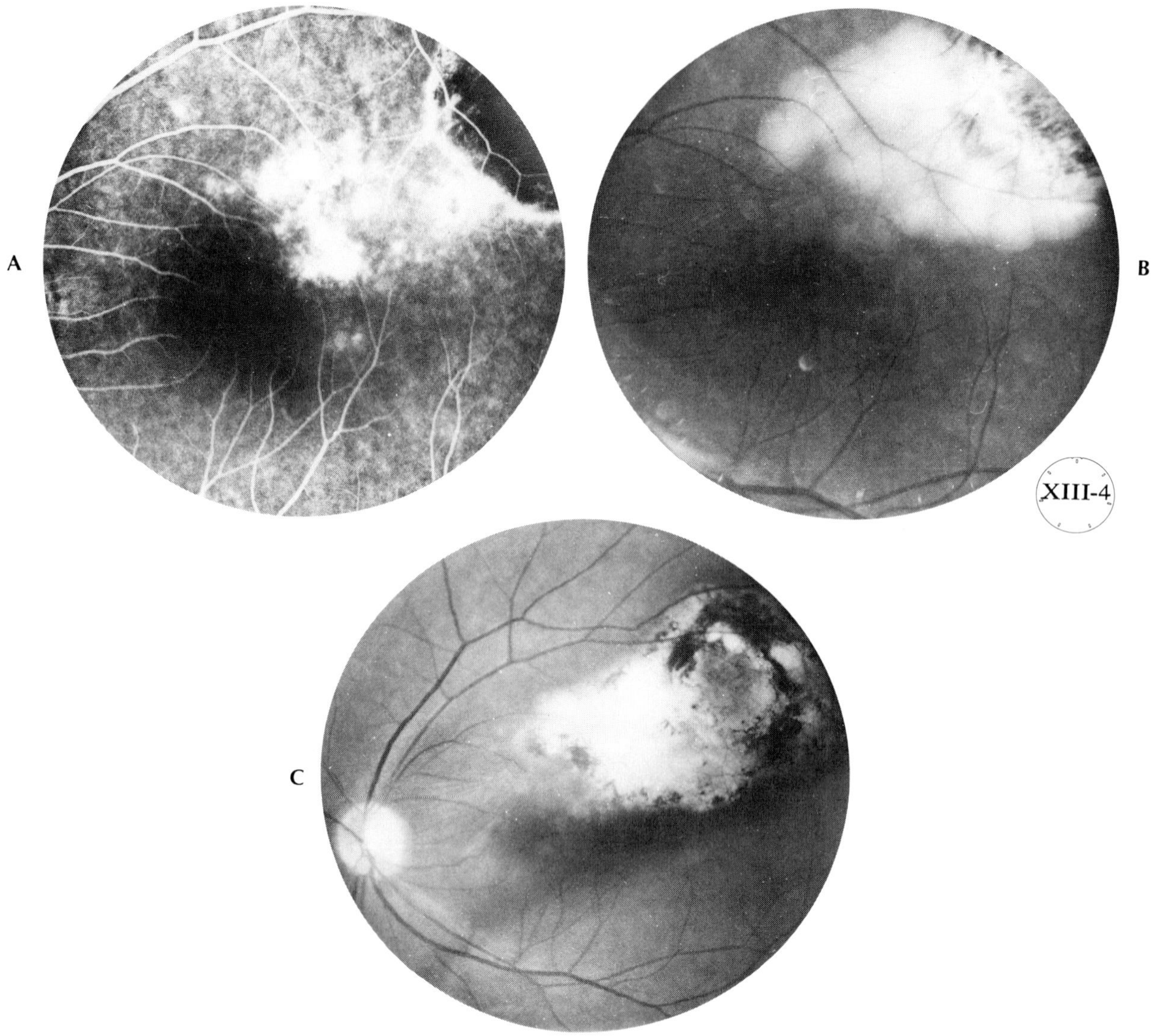

Fig. 12-7. A, Fluorescein angiogram showing macular edema secondary to reactivation of a superotemporal toxoplasmosis scar. Vision was reduced to 20/100. **B,** Contiguous barrage-type photocoagulations were employed to obliterate the area of reactivation on the periphery of the toxoplasmosis scar. **C,** Wide-angle view of treated superotemporal paramacular region 12 weeks after photocoagulation, showing atrophy and scarring of the previously active area. Vision improved to 20/30.

The results of photocoagulation should be watched closely, and photocoagulation of any areas where the chorioretinal tissue has not been destroyed around the previous toxoplasmic scar should be repeated.

The treatment of choroidal or retinal neovascularization should be intense, as described in those particular sections (pp. 142 and 248, respectively).

Complications. Complications other than the formation of macular striae and hemorrhages from small choroidal or retinal vessels are few. It is possible to reactivate some lesions by photocoagulation, but this problem is extremely rare.

Follow-up. The healing procedure is monitored at 1-month intervals following photocoagulation. If fundus photography shows the photocoagulation scar or the toxoplasmic scar to be changing, fluorescein angiography should be used to determine if a neovascular response or any other unfavorable condition is evolving.

TOXOCARA CANIS OR *T. CATI* INFESTATION

Clinical symptoms. Blurred vision, metamorphopsia, haze over the entire visual field, and photopsia are some of the more common symptoms noted by individuals with *T. cati* or *T. cani* infestation.

A

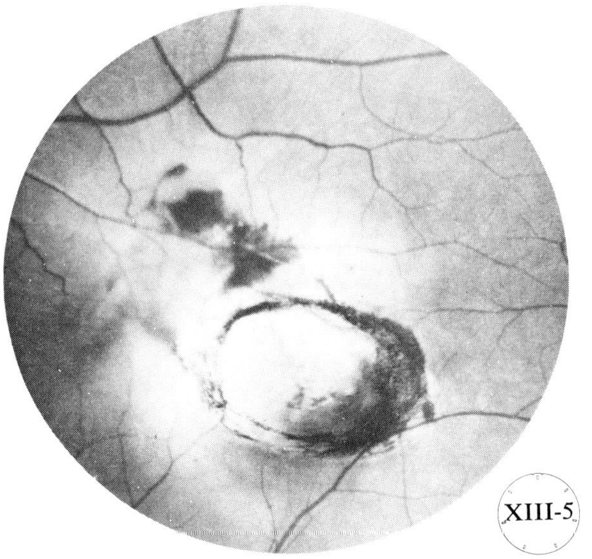

Continued.

Fig. 12-8. A, Neovascularization and subretinal hemorrhages at the margin (10 o'clock position) of a toxoplasmosis scar, involving the superotemporal macular region and reducing vision to 20/100. **B,** Fluorescein angiogram showing the development of early filling and staining of the new vessels in the fibrovascular membrane between the large scarred area and the fovea. **C,** Fluorescein angiogram showing more pronounced leakage from the subretinal neovascularization. **D,** Fluorescein angiogram during the venular phase, showing marked leakage from the neovascular membrane into the subretinal space and portions of the sensory retina. **E,** Argon laser photocoagulation was applied with Grade 4 intensity to the area of neovascularization in the macular region. **F,** Healed zone 5 weeks after photocoagulation, showing some residual hemorrhages, eradication of neovascular tissue, and glial proliferation. **G,** Late healed photocoagulated area, showing absorption of hemorrhages, destruction of neovascularization, and improvement of vision to 20/30.

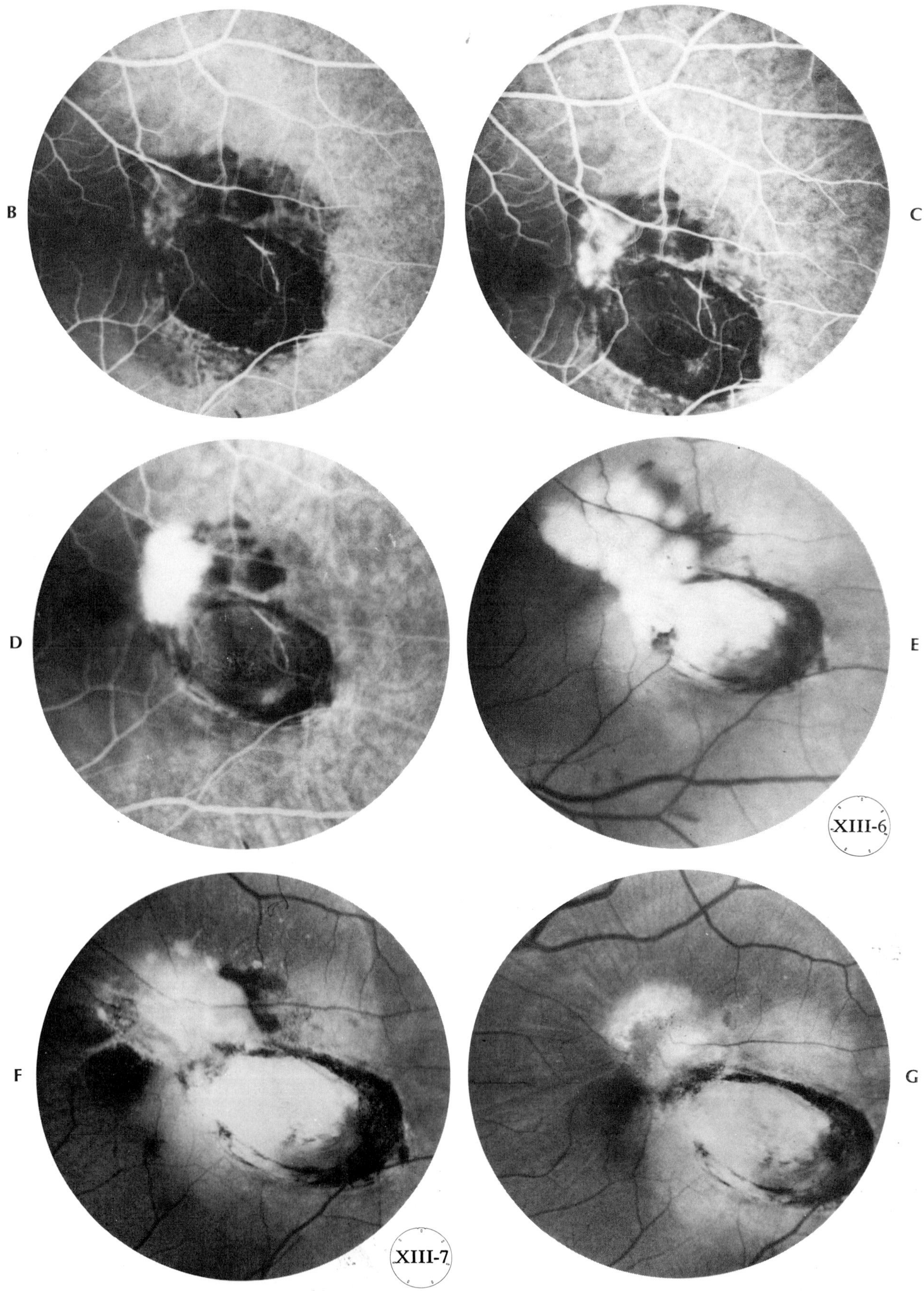

Fig. 12-8, cont'd. For legend see p. 239.

Ophthalmoscopic appearance. Patients with *Toxocara* infestation usually show a large granulomatous lesion in the choroid and retinal areas that extends into the vitreous. This large mass of glial tissue is nodular and may be surrounded by considerable vitreous haze. The base of the lesion may show pigmented areas in the choroid and retina. The lesion may involve the macular and paramacular regions.

Ancillary diagnostic examinations. Stereo fundus photography is used to document the course of the disease.

Fluorescein angiography may be helpful in determining the amount of leakage, disruption of surrounding chorioretinal tissue, changes following photocoagulation, and any residual chorioretinal blood vessels entering the tumor following treatment.

Indications for photocoagulation. If the lesion is growing in size, it can be photocoagulated directly, although this procedure usually is not helpful. Photocoagulation around the base may slow the progress of the ocular reaction to the larval protein and usually causes the lesion to diminish in size slowly. Supplemental direct photocoagulation can later be done in an attempt to destroy the antigenic tissue that is causing even further granulomatous reaction.

Photocoagulation approach. The xenon-arc source or argon laser is used for photocoagulation of the entire periphery of the base of the nodular glial outgrowth into the vitreous with an overlapping row of intense coagulations to destroy the choroidal and retinal blood supply into the granuloma. These coagulations are at least **300μ to 600μ** in diameter, although they can be smaller in areas close to the macular region. Exposures of **0.2 to 0.5 sec** are required for penetration into the depths of the choroid, and the entire periphery of the lesion is photocoagulated at a single session (Fig. 12-9). Photocoagulation directly to the tumor is not employed with this circumferential photocoagulation technique. The patient is prescribed moderate systemic doses of steroids during the 2 to 3 weeks following photocoagulation therapy (20 to 40 mg of prednisone taken orally daily).

The fundus is evaluated 3 to 4 weeks after photocoagulation, and if there is any sign of choroidal or retinal vessels entering the tumor, the periphery of the base of the growth is rephotocoagulated to destroy the choroidal input into the granuloma. Systemic doses of steroids are continued during this period. This process is repeated until the tumor itself has been rendered void of any peripheral chorioretinal vascular nourishment.

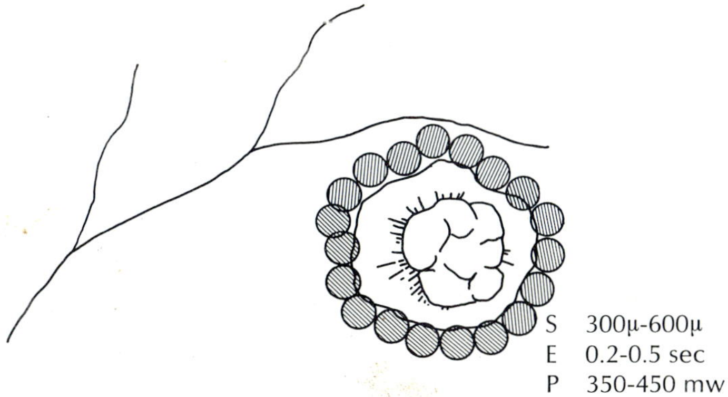

Fig. 12-9. Placement of 300μ to 600μ Grades 3 to 4 overlapping, linear, punctate coagulations around the border of the *Toxocara* granuloma to obliterate the choroidal and retinal blood supply to the lesion.

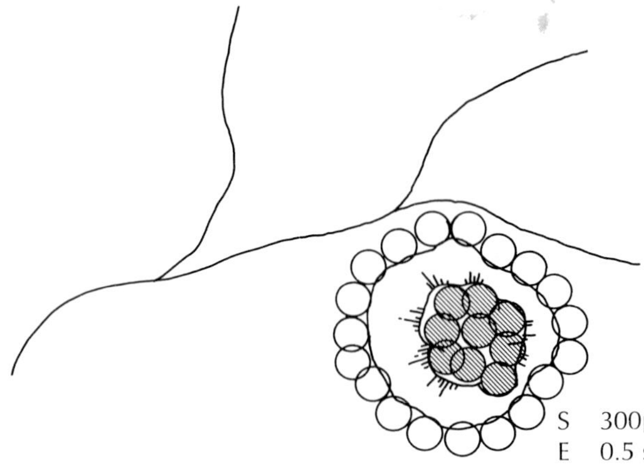

Fig. 12-10. Application of 300μ to 500μ punctate, overlapping, barrage photocoagulations to the granuloma mass to destroy the central vascular supply and tumor tissue.

When the peripheral vascular supply to the granuloma has been destroyed by photocoagulations to the border of the lesion, the tumor itself can be directly treated with **300μ to 500μ** argon laser coagulations or **450μ (1.5°)** xenon-arc coagulations at **0.5 sec** and a high intensity (**600 mw** with the argon laser or **Red II** with the xenon-arc source) (Fig. 12-10). A coagulum may appear on the surface of the granuloma, but it may not be prominent. Longer exposures and higher power inputs may be needed to affect tissues deeper in the tumor (Fig. 12-11).

Complications. The complications include gliosis of the macular region, macular striae, hemorrhage at the time of photocoagulation, and possibly reactivation of the granuloma with marked vitreous haze formation. It is most important that the administration of moderate systemic doses of steroids be continued and that atropine 1% be given with steroid drops at least twice daily for 2 to 3 weeks after photocoagulation.

Follow-up. The patient is seen at approximately 2-week intervals following photocoagulation, and the tumor mass usually will slowly shrink because of the decrease in blood available to the granuloma. Photocoagulation should be reapplied at any time that renourishment is suspected from the choroidal or retinal vessels. Direct rephotocoagulation to the tumor mass is recommended when the tumor mass has shrunk considerably and if the peripheral chorioretinal vessels are known by fluorescein angiography to be obliterated. Photocoagulation can then be used to destroy the remnants of the shrunken granuloma.

Fig. 12-11. A, *Toxocara canis* granuloma in a 52-year-old woman who had intermittent blurred vision for 4 months before the *T. canis* granuloma was recognized. Because of marked vitreous haze, vision in her right eye had decreased to 20/200. **B,** Overlapping 300μ argon laser photocoagulations were applied to the periphery of the granuloma. **C,** Additional xenon-arc photocoagulations were applied to the periphery of the tumor mass to decrease the retinal and choroidal vascular supply. **D,** *T. canis* granuloma 7 weeks after xenon-arc photocoagulation, showing a slight diminution in the total mass of the granuloma with no reactivation or increased vitreous clouding. **E,** Granuloma after four xenon-arc and two argon laser photocoagulation treatments, showing a 60% decrease in the tumor mass and elevation with no reactivation or worsening of the vitreous reaction.

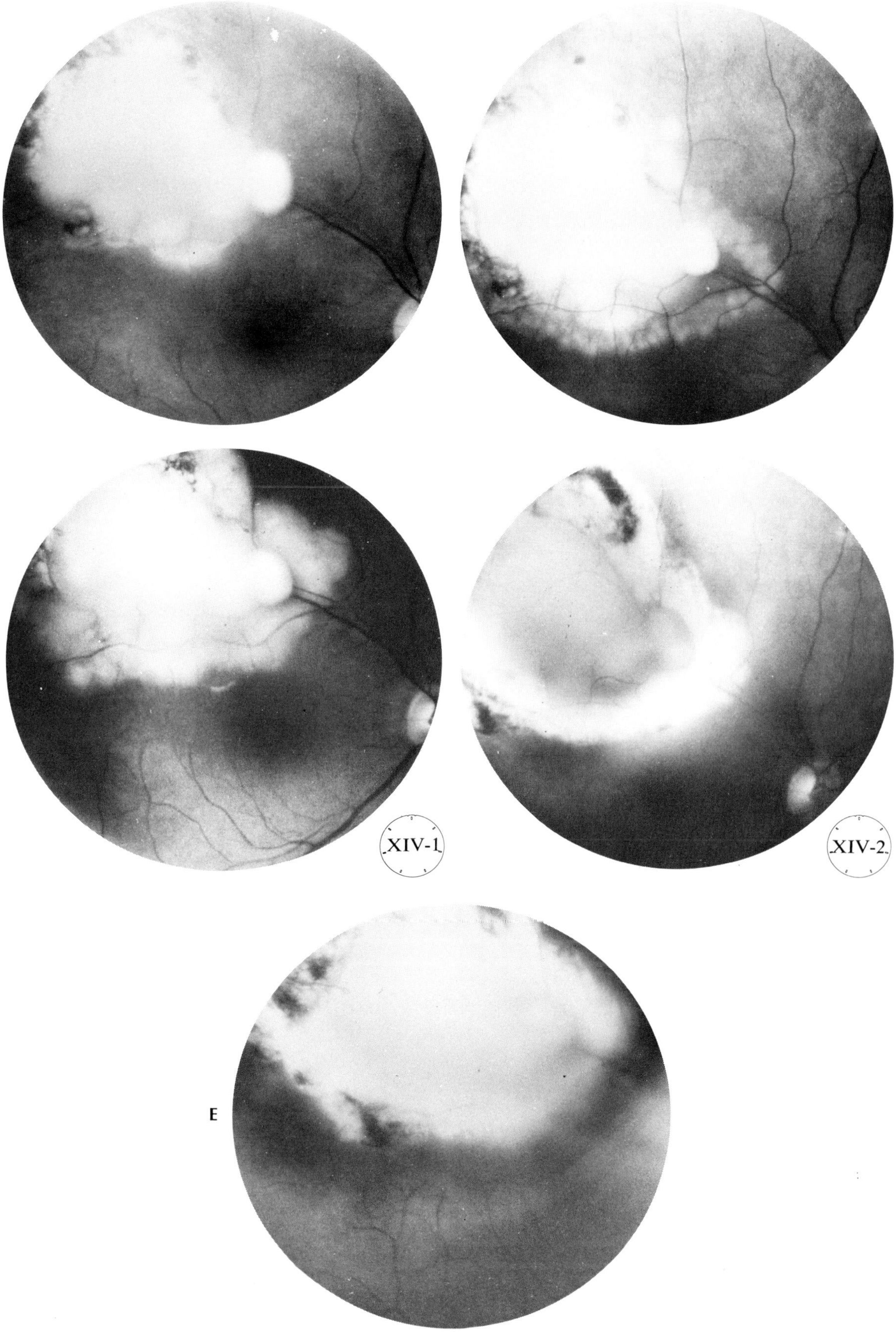

Fig. 12-11. For legend see opposite page.

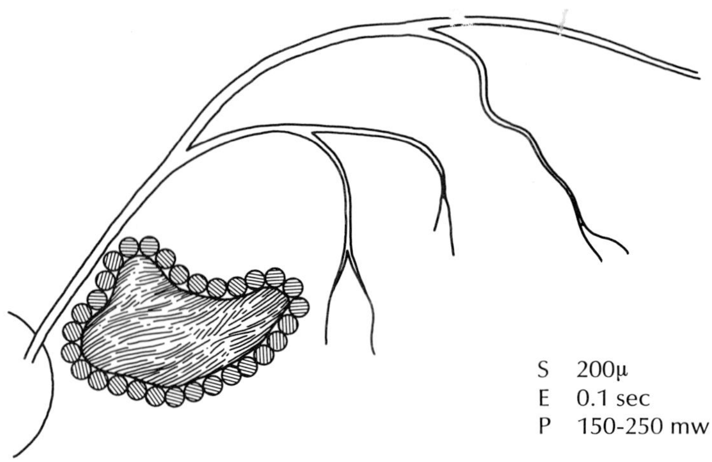

Fig. 12-12. Placement of initial punctate, linear, contiguous coagulations around the periphery of the diseased pigment epithelium in a manner designed to include normal retina.

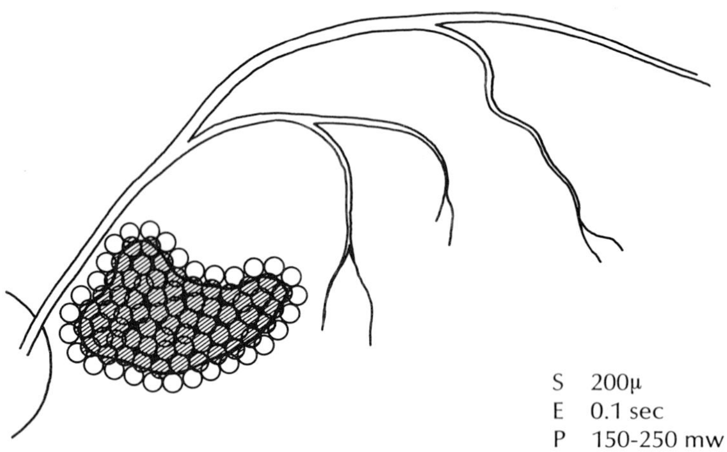

Fig. 12-13. Placement of 200μ Grades 2 to 3 punctate, barrage-type, overlapping coagulations in the central area of diseased pigment epithelium. Coagulations should be slightly less intense in the papillomacular bundle region.

Fig. 12-14. A, A slightly pale, irregular zone of pigment epithelial swelling and depigmentation superior to the foveal region in the left eye (arrow) of a 21-year-old man who had complained of blurred vision (20/60) of 2 months' duration. **B,** Fluorescein angiogram showing diffuse staining and leakage from the pigment epithelial defect. This staining and leakage is consistent with pigment epithelial disease (arrow). **C,** Overlapping, 200μ punctate coagulations were placed in the area of diseased pigment epithelium and extended a short distance into normal retinal tissue around the periphery of the lesion. **D,** Healed area 2 months after photocoagulation, showing a slight hypertrophy of the pigment epithelium and a thin layer of scar tissue at the level of the pigment epithelium (arrow). **E,** Fluorescein angiogram 2 months after photocoagulation, showing destruction of the diseased pigment epithelium and obliteration of the leaking areas. Vision improved to 20/25.

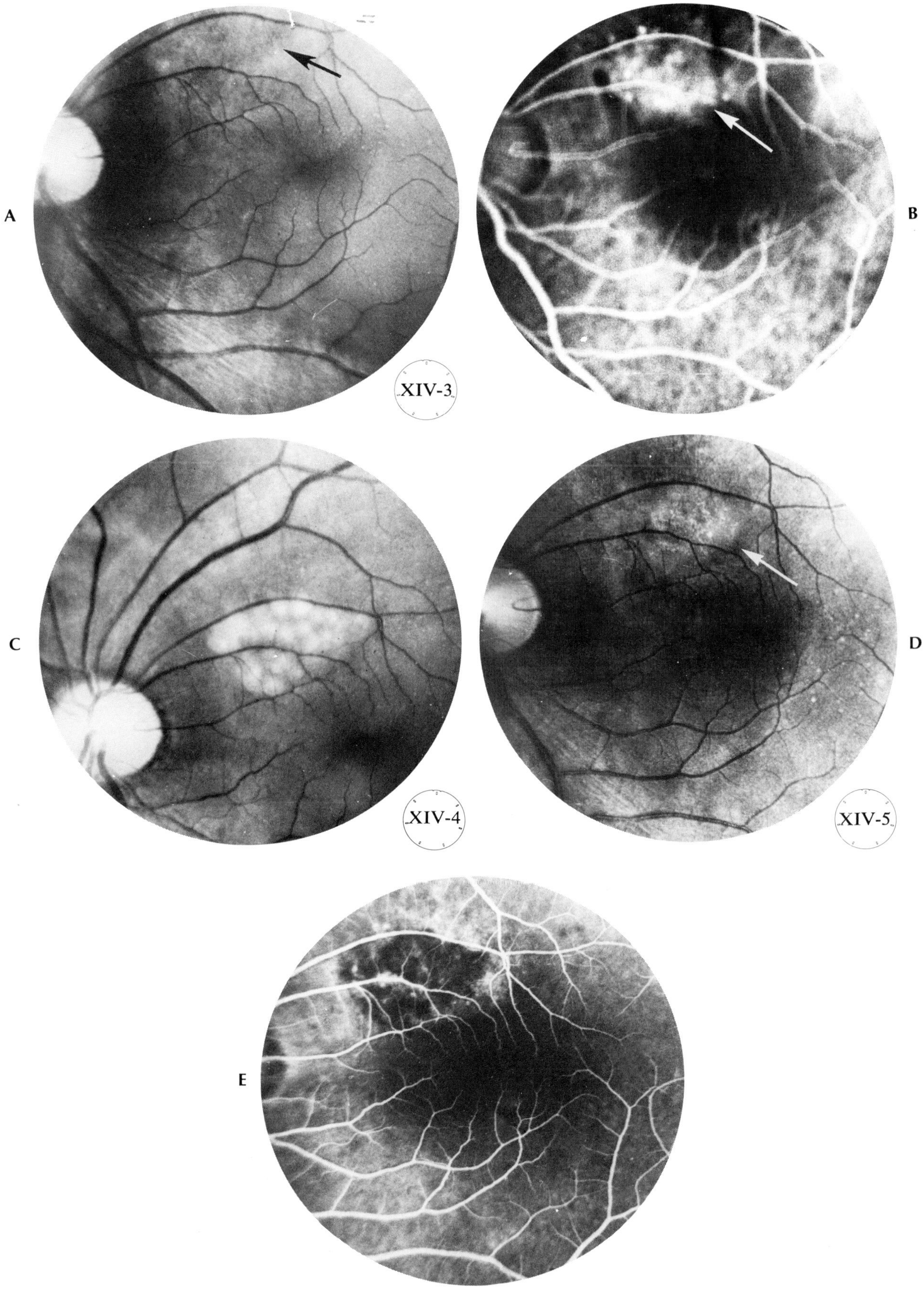

Fig. 12-14. For legend see opposite page.

PIGMENT EPITHELIOPATHY

Clinical symptoms. Because of involvement of the sensory retina, blurred vision, metamorphopsia, micropsia, and occasional photopsia are the prominent symptoms of pigment epitheliopathy.

Ophthalmoscopic appearance. A serous detachment of the sensory retina can be observed in the macular region, although the defect and leakage from the pigment epithelial and choroidal region cannot usually be detected during ophthalmoscopic examination. Occasionally, a yellow plaque can be seen in the pigment epithelial layer in the macular or paramacular area.

Ancillary diagnostic examinations. Fluorescein angiography will show an area of diffuse leakage from the pigment epithelium. This leakage and staining of the pigment epithelial lesion begins in the early choroidal phase and becomes more prominent later. Neovascularization cannot be seen, nor is there any evidence of pooling areas other than the weak fluorescein glow occasionally observed from the fluid in the subretinal space.

Indications for photocoagulation. Photocoagulation should be reserved for those cases where the pigment epithelial lesion is spreading and threatening foveal function by direct invasion or secondary indirect edema and degeneration. If the pigment epitheliopathy does not respond to moderately high systemic doses of prednisone (60 to 80 mg daily orally) over a 3- to 6-week period, photocoagulation of thc pigment epitheliopathy can be considered.

Photocoagulation approach. Moderately intense coagulations (Grade 3) are placed to completely surround, envelop, and cauterize directly the pigment epithelial staining area (Figs. 12-12 and 12-13). These coagulations are overlapping, usually **200μ** in diameter at a **0.1-sec** exposure and with power intensities in the range of **150 to 250 mw.** Slightly less prominent coagulations (Grade 2) are made if the lesion is in the papillomacular bundle. The patient continues to receive steroids systemically during the course of the photocoagulation and for approximately 3 to 4 weeks after the photocoagulation treatment (Fig. 12-14).

Complications. The possible complications of macular striae, reactivation of the pigment epitheliopathy, and overgrowth of glial tissue can be expected in rare instances.

Follow-up. Prednisone (10 to 20 mg orally) should be continued for at least 4 to 6 weeks after the photocoagulation treatment, and the patient is followed at weekly intervals. If the disease process worsens after photocoagulation, systemic doses of steroids should be increased. Destruction of the pigment epithelial lesion should decrease leakage into the subretinal space, decrease the overlying retinal edema, and alleviate the macular condition.

ANGIOID STREAKS

Clinical symptoms. The patient with angioid streaks may notice no particular problem with his vision unless a subretinal hemorrhage, proliferation of neovascularization, or retinal disruption occurs secondary to degeneration of the angioid streaks. In these cases blurred vision, metamorphopsia, photopsia, and lightning flashes can be observed.

Ophthalmoscopic appearance. Angioid streaks have a peculiar characteristic bilateral appearance in the fundus primarily because of degenerative changes affecting particularly the elastic lamina that constitutes the mesodermal component of Bruch's membrane. The condition can be described by a fairly uniform picture consisting of a network of streaks varying in color from reddish to dark brown; these streaks usually emanate from a more or less circular ring around the disc and radiate irregularly to the equator. They are sometimes associated with a mosaic of white spots. Whereas some cases remain stationary indefinitely, in most others lesions develop in the fundus in midlife and sometimes become visually incapacitating in their severity. The most common complications are macular hemorrhages, pigmentary deposits and patches of atrophy, and occasionally the proliferative changes of disciform degeneration; coarse granulation or mottling of large areas of the fundus by pigmentary deposits suggesting the appearance of peau d'orange; patches of choroidal atrophy resembling the cicatrices of a chorioretinitis and usually showing some pigmentary proliferation; and colloid bodies on Bruch's membrane, occasionally associated with hyaline bodies on the optic nerve.

Ancillary diagnostic examinations. Wide-angle and regular color fundus photography can be important for showing the progression of the angioid streaks. Stereoscopic photography is advantageous but usually not required.

A fluorescein angiogram should be taken at yearly intervals unless hemorrhagic activity is observed. If an area of the angioid streaks begins to leak fluorescein, the angiographic examinations should be performed at 1- to 2-month intervals.

Indications for photocoagulation. An obvious area of neovascularization in a region of the angioid streak that is more than 750μ (½ DD) from the umbo should be considered for photocoagulation.

An area of intense fluorescein leakage from a region of the angioid streak should be watched closely and considered for photocoagulation if it increases in severity.

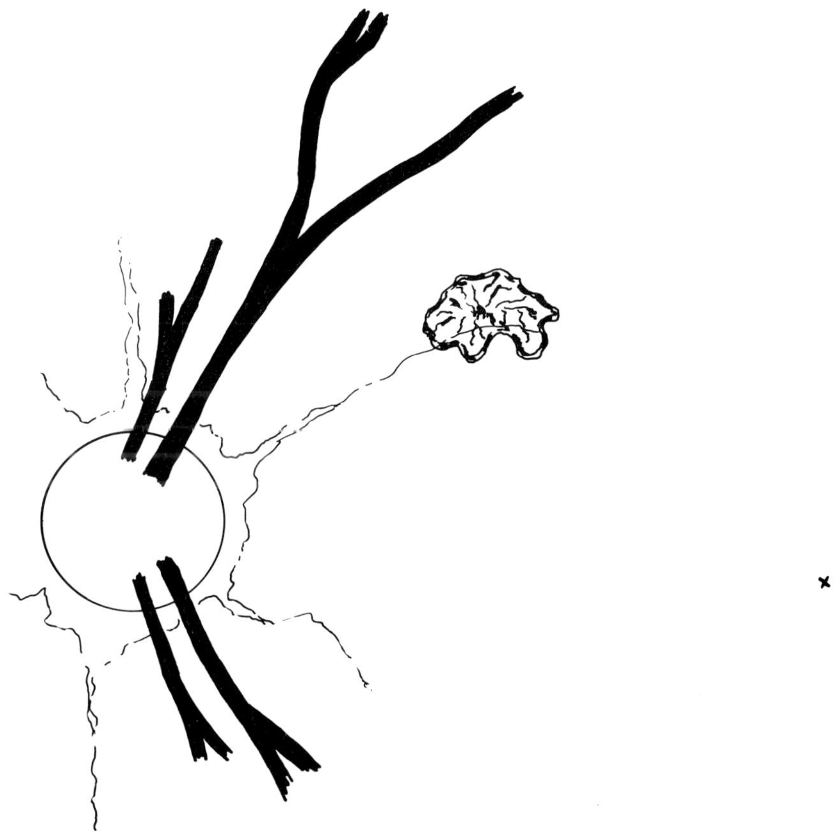

Fig. 12-15. Typical angioid streaks with early neovascularization in the form of a fibrovascular sheet at the point of disruption of Bruch's membrane.

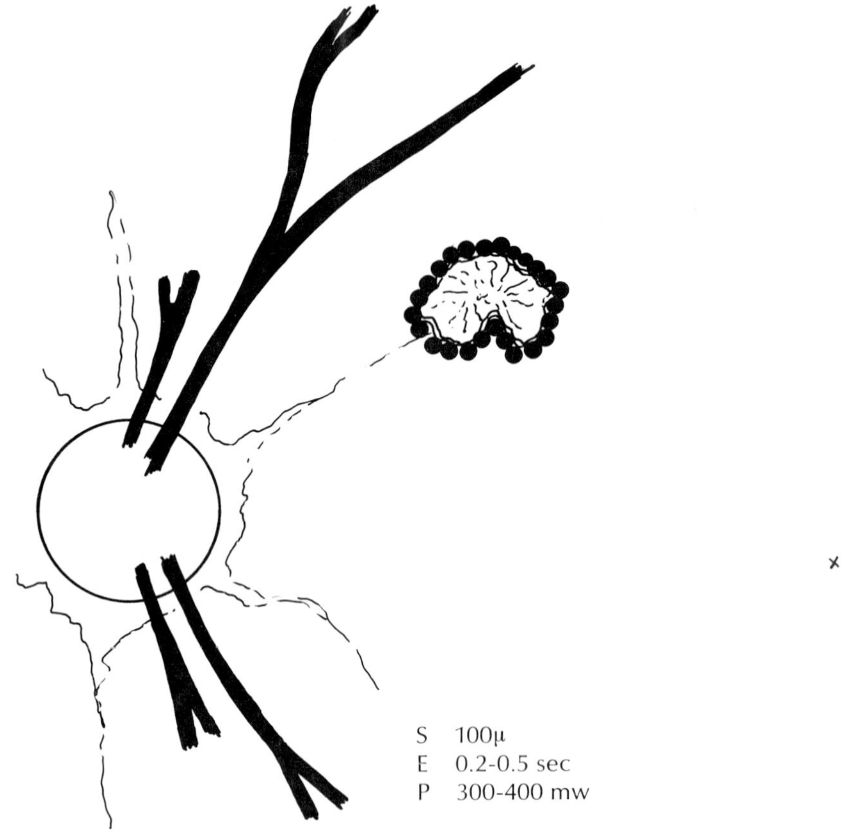

Fig. 12-16. Photocoagulation parameters and technique for placing a series of linear, contiguous, punctate coagulations around the periphery of the neovascularization into normal chorioretinal tissue.

Any area of the angioid streak that has ruptured, producing a subretinal or intraretinal hemorrhage, should be considered for photocoagulation if the area is at least ½ DD from the umbo. Photocoagulation should not be attempted within this 750μ radius of the umbo.

Areas of neovascularization or hemorrhage in the papillomacular bundle should be photocoagulated only if they are less than ½ DD in extent and positioned away from overlying edema or glial tissue, so that the neovascularization can be effectively coagulated. Other areas of neovascularization or Bruch's membrane rupture outside the papillomacular bundle can be coagulated with higher power intensities and with less concern for the overlying nerve fiber layer.

Photocoagulation approach. A topical anesthetic and a retrobulbar anesthetic are required for stabilization of the eye and for elimination of the minor discomfort experienced by the patient during photocoagulation. A plano–low-vacuum contact lens, the central portion of a three-mirror Goldmann lens, or the Goldmann fundus contact lens can be used for photocoagulation of the lesion.

The portion of the neovascular membrane closest to the fovea should be photocoagulated initially with chalk white (Grade 4) coagulations. Coagulations of **100μ** diameter produced by power intensities of **300 to 400 mw** at exposures of **0.2 to 0.5 sec** are usually adequate for coagulation of the fibrovascular membrane (Figs. 12-15 to 12-17).

The periphery of the fibrovascular sheet is coagulated entirely. An additional ring of

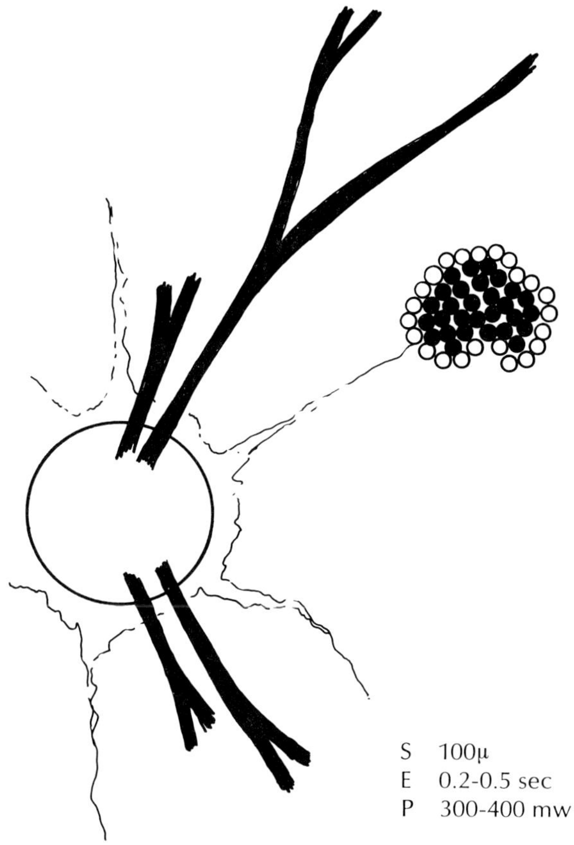

Fig. 12-17. Argon laser photocoagulation of the subretinal neovascularization central to the previously placed, surrounding rim of coagulations. All coagulations should be of Grade 4 intensity and should overlap centrally.

100μ coagulations is produced around the border of the neovascularization into normal retina.

Coagulations applied with similar argon laser dosages are then used to coagulate the fibrovascular membrane more centrally. At the end of the coagulation session the entire fibrovascular membrane should be covered with contiguous or overlapping coagulations so that no viable neovascular tissue remains untreated (Figs. 12-18 and 12-19).

Complications. The most common complication is hemorrhage from the fibrovascular membrane at the time of treatment. The utilization of a centripedal photocoagulation approach, where the periphery of the neovascular sheet is coagulated initially and more central photocoagulations follow, appears to minimize the possibility of hemorrhage from the neovascularization. Although the coagulations should be chalk white, it is recommended that the exposure interval be longer than 0.2 sec so that the energy not be applied too rapidly to the delicate neovascular tissue. If hemorrhage occurs from the area of neovascularization, the coagulations should be extended more peripherally around the area of hemorrhage to cauterize and obliterate the choroidal afferent channels.

The intense photocoagulations required for adequate treatment of the fibrovascular membrane occasionally will cause irreversible damage to the nerve fiber layer. The disastrous condition that can result from proliferation of the neovascular membrane and the concurrent hemorrhages definitely outweighs the possibility of nerve fiber damage from the photocoagulation during destruction of the neovascular process. It is certainly advisable to sacrifice portions of the nerve fiber layer, even in the papillomacular bundle, to preserve partial function of the macular region.

When additional photocoagulation is needed to eliminate untreated areas of neovascularization, it is advisable to commence treatment within the week following the initial photocoagulation session. During this time the retinal edema will cause the nerve fiber layer to be farther away from the neovascular sheet, so that the heat conducted from the subretinal membrane to the nerve fiber layer will be minimal. If photocoagulation is required beyond 2 weeks after the initial photocoagulation treatment, the destruction of the outer retinal elements and hyperproliferation of the pigment epithelium will increase the chances of irreparable nerve fiber damage. Permanent damage to the nerve fiber layer in this situation can be caused by the proximity of the nerve fiber layer to the pigment epithelium and by a more severe coagulation, which may possibly occur in the hypertrophied pigment layer.

Dense glial overgrowth, macular striae, and damage to the foveal receptor elements can result from overtreatment or from treatment too close to the foveal area. The retina

A

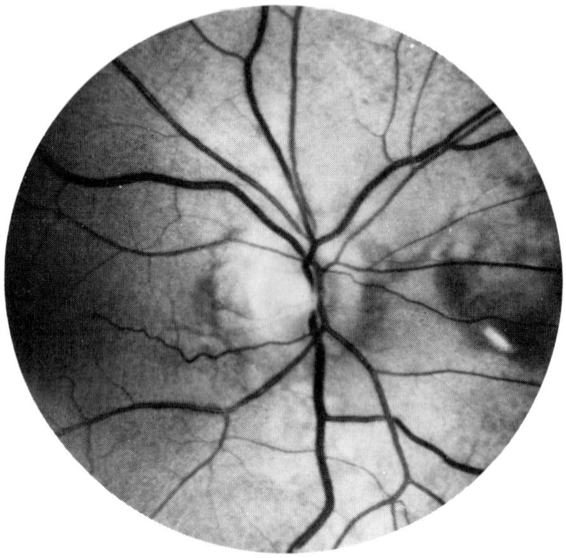

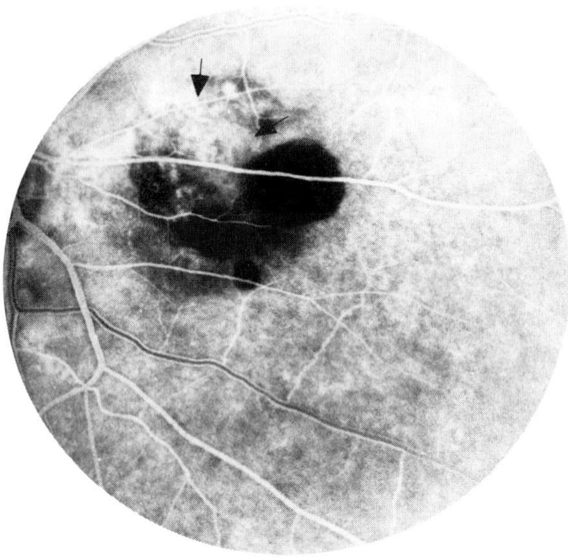

B

Fig. 12-18. A, A subretinal hemorrhage from an area of angioid streaks nasal to the optic disc in a 58-year-old man. **B,** Fluorescein angiogram during the late arteriolar phase, showing subretinal neovascular proliferation and leakage (arrows). **C,** Fluorescein angiogram during the late venular phase, showing increased leakage and staining in the region of the subretinal fibrovascular membrane (arrows). **D,** A barrage of 200μ, overlapping Grade 4 argon laser coagulations were placed in the region of the angioid streak and neovascularization. **E,** Wide-angle view of the posterior polar region 1 month after photocoagulation, showing complete destruction of the subretinal neovascularization. Note the residual subretinal hemorrhage and the peripapillary angioid streak formation. **F,** Treated area 8 weeks after argon laser photocoagulation, showing partial disappearance of the nasally located blood and complete destruction of the neovascularization. **G,** Fluorescein angiogram during the arteriolovenular phase, showing complete obliteration of the subretinal fibrovascular sheet and no evidence of staining or leakage. **H,** Photocoagulated area 3 months after photocoagulation, showing no evidence of neovascularization or hemorrhagic activity.

C D

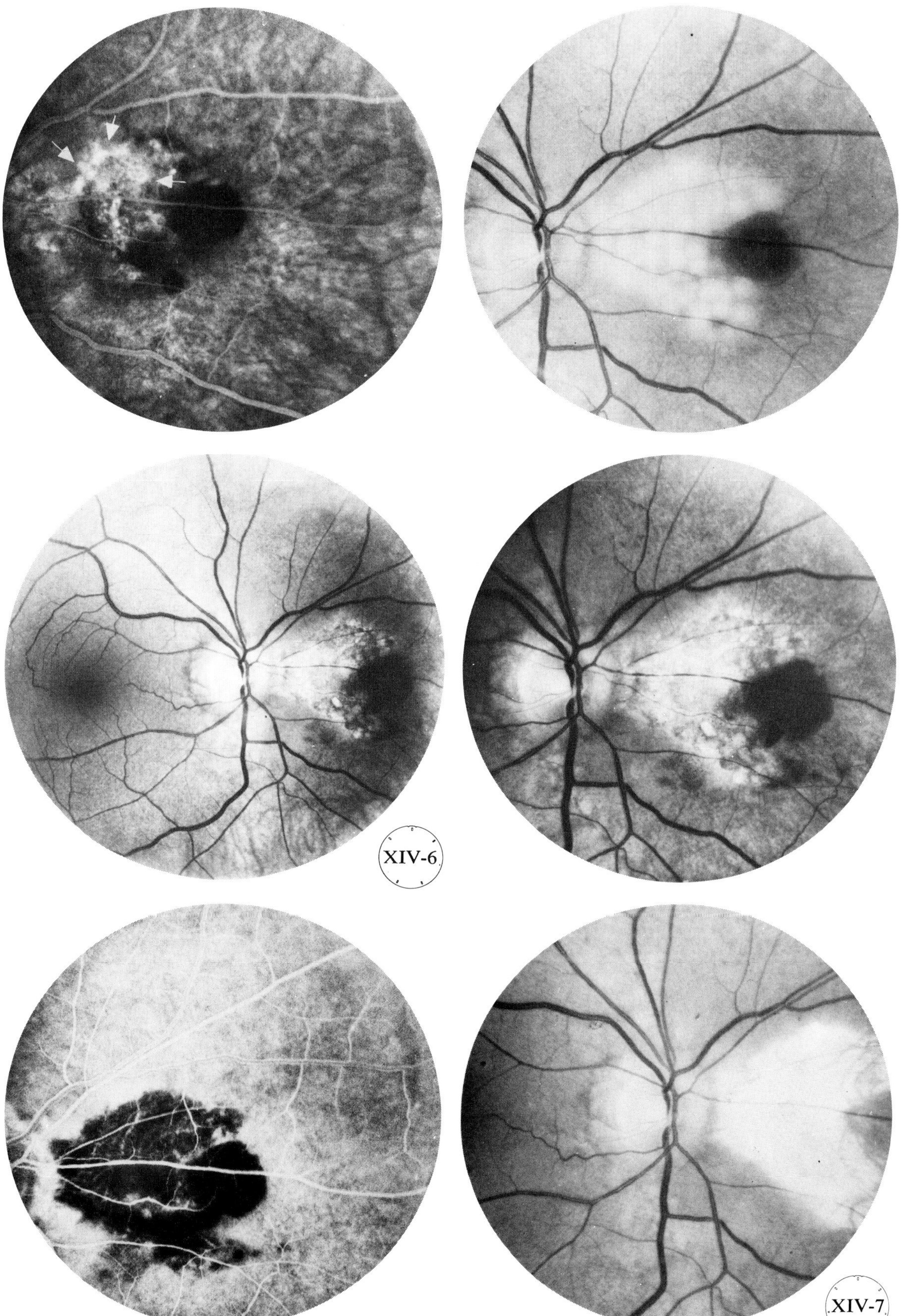

E F

G H

Fig. 12-18, cont'd. For legend see opposite page.

overlying the neovascular sheet should be clear of glial tissue proliferation so that the minimal amount of laser energy can be employed. Retinal edema can usually be reduced by the systemic administration of large doses (60 to 80 mg daily) of prednisone or similar steroid preparations.

The stimulation of the neovascular membrane, resulting in the rapid growth of the fibrovascular sheet around the area of treatment, can be produced by inadequate photocoagulation. The neovascularization must be treated and coagulated completely, and a surrounding rim of normal tissue should be cauterized during the photocoagulation session. The treatment intensities must be sufficient to obliterate the neovascularization deep in the retinal and superficial choroidal region.

Follow-up. The patient should be seen approximately 5 to 7 days following photocoagulation, and fluorescein angiography should be performed at this time to detect any areas of neovascularization that have inadvertently not been photocoagulated. If they can be found, they should be treated at this time. All neovascularization must be completely obliterated to prevent stimulation and further proliferation of the neovascular sheet.

A fluorescein angiogram should be taken approximately 3 weeks following the initial postphotocoagulation visit and examined carefully for evidence of any further neovascularization or other leakage defects. After the process has been stabilized, the patient should be examined at 3-month intervals, and fluorescein angiograms should be taken at approximately 6-month intervals.

CHOROIDAL (SUBRETINAL) NEOVASCULARIZATION

Clinical symptoms. The patient with choroidal neovascularization usually notices a gradual blurring of vision caused by the overlying retinal edema and occasional exudate formation. However, a sudden loss of vision can be caused by a hemorrhage beneath the sensory retina in the macular region. Metamorphopsia and micropsia have also been documented.

Text continued on p. 258.

Fig. 12-19. A, A subretinal hemorrhage in the foveal area and extensive edema of the fovea and macular region between the optic nerve and fovea in a 23-year-old woman who had developed blurred and distorted vision 13 years after having been struck with a tennis ball in her left eye. Circumferential scars representing healed choroidal ruptures can be seen around the optic nerve, and a grayish membrane similar to that developed with angioid streaks is located at the distal end of the healed choroidal rupture in the papillomacular bundle area. **B,** Fluorescein angiogram revealing extensive wormlike neovascularization in the region of the ophthalmoscopically visible grayish brown membrane, which represents a sheet of fibrovascular proliferation from the distal portion of the healed choroidal rupture line. **C,** Argon laser photocoagulation was directed to the area of subretinal neovascularization, forming overlapping coagulations of Grade 4 intensity in the papillomacular bundle zone in such a manner as to envelop completely the neovascularization and a small portion of surrounding healthy chorioretinal tissue. **D,** Photocoagulated zone 7 weeks after treatment, showing complete destruction of the neovascularization, elimination of retinal edema, and preservation of foveal vision (fixation pointer). **E,** Fluorescein angiogram 3 months after photocoagulation, during the arteriolar phase, showing no evidence of neovascularization or filling from the choroidal circulation in the area of photocoagulative obliteration of the subretinal neovascularization. **F,** Fluorescein angiogram during the late venular phase, showing staining of the choroidal rupture sites and glial tissue formed at the site of photocoagulation. Vision has improved from the prephotocoagulation level of $20/80^{-2}$ to 20/25.

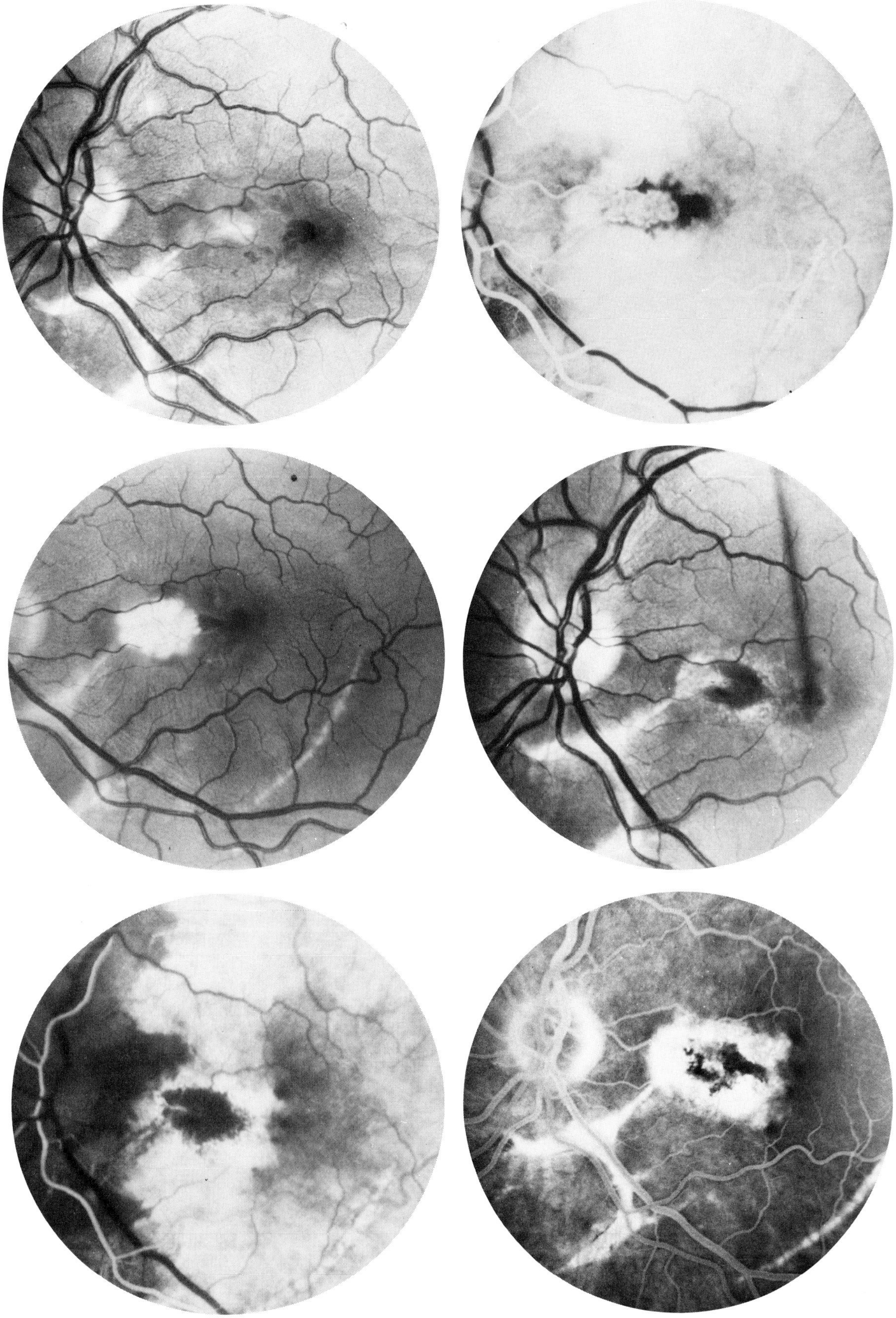

A B C D E F

Fig. 12-19. For legend see opposite page.

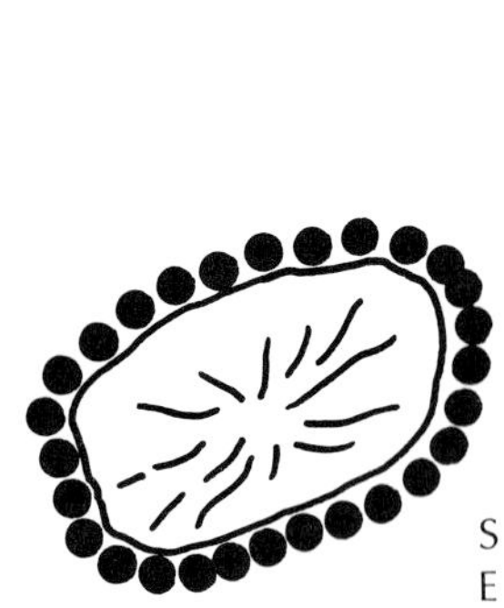

Fig. 12-20. Placement of punctate, contiguous or overlapping, linear argon laser coagulations around the circumferential perimeter vessel ("bicycle wheel") of the choroidal neovascular fibrous sheet. These coagulations must be of Grade 4 intensity and must impinge on normal retina.

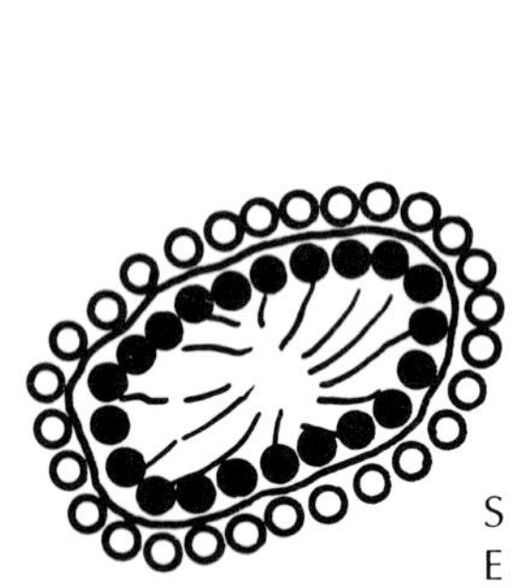

Fig. 12-21. Placement of a second contiguous row of intense coagulations inside the previously placed delimiting coagulations.

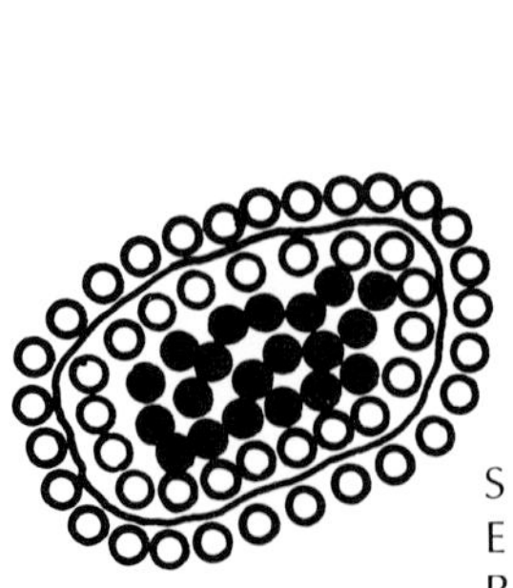

Fig. 12-22. Placement of overlapping Grade 4 argon laser coagulations in the central region ("bicycle spokes and hub") of the choroidal neovascularization. The entire neovascular area must be intensely treated to eradicate the deeply located neovascularization.

A 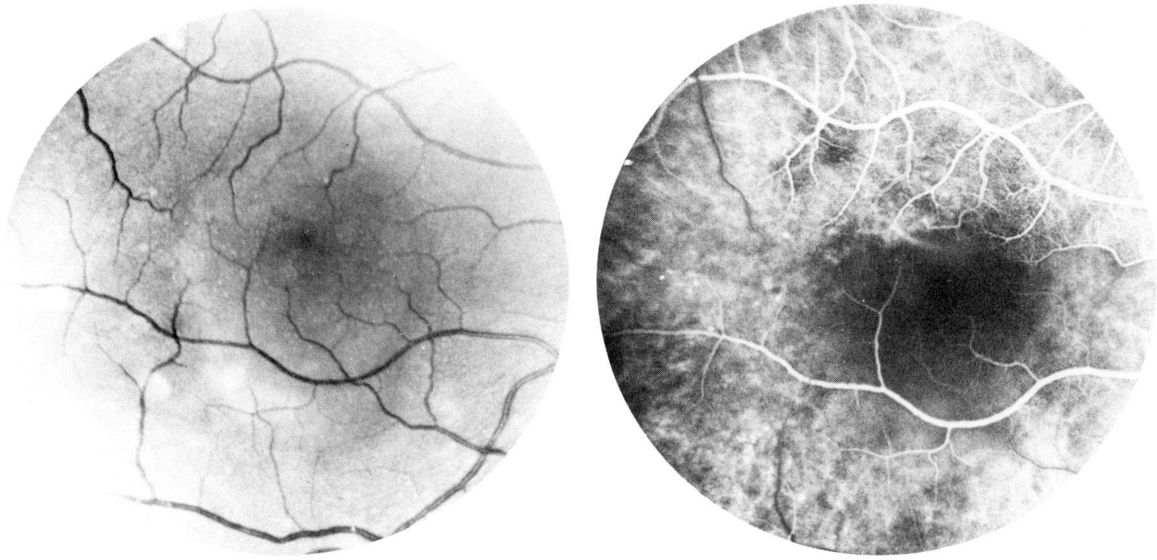 B

Continued.

Fig. 12-23. A, Macular and paramacular retinal edema with no hemorrhagic or exudate activity in a 48-year-old woman who had complained of rapidly blurring vision over a 2-month period. Vision was 20/70 with correction. **B,** Fluorescein angiogram during arteriolar phase, revealing a slight disturbance of the pigment epithelial region in the superotemporal perifoveal zone. **C,** Fluorogram during the arteriolovenular phase, showing some staining and slight leakage from the area of decompensated pigment epithelium (arrow). **D,** Fluorogram during early venular phase, showing progressive leakage from the pigment epithelial region in the superotemporal area of the macula. The patient was not photocoagulated at this time but was advised to return in 1 month for reevaluation. **E,** One month after the previous fluorescein angiographic examination the visual acuity had decreased to 20/100, the retinal edema had become more prominent, and a dirty gray fibrovascular membrane could be seen in the subretinal space in the region of the previously diseased pigment epithelium (arrows). **F,** Fluorogram during the early arteriolar phase, showing the appearance of a typical bicycle wheel choroidal neovascular configuration (arrow). **G,** Fluorogram during the arteriolovenular phase, showing more pronounced leakage from the wheel or periphery of the subretinal fibrovascular sheet and a typical surrounding area of hypofluorescence (arrow) of the fluorescein dye. **H,** Fluorogram during the early venular phase, showing intense leakage from the choroidal neovasular sheet into the subretinal space. **I,** The entire region of the choroidal neovascularization was treated as outlined in Figs. 12-20, 12-21, and 12-22 with Grade 4 coagulations to cauterize as deeply into the choroidal vasculature as possible. **J,** Fluorescein angiogram approximately 16 days after photocoagulation, during the late arteriolar phase, showing a small tuft of neovascular tissue (arrow) in the central fibrovascular sheet. **K,** Fluorescein angiogram during the arteriolovenular phase. The small area of choroidal neovascularization leaked more intensely, and the neovascular tufts can be seen more definitely. **L,** Fluorescein angiogram during the late venular phase, showing a combination of leakage from the central neovascular tufts and staining of the glial tissue in the coagulation site (arrow). **M,** Intense argon laser photocoagulation was directed to the remaining areas of suspected neovascularization. **N,** Healed area 2 months after argon laser photocoagulation, showing complete destruction and obliteration of the choroidal neovascularization. There was an eventual improvement in vision to 20/30 6 months following the final photocoagulation session.

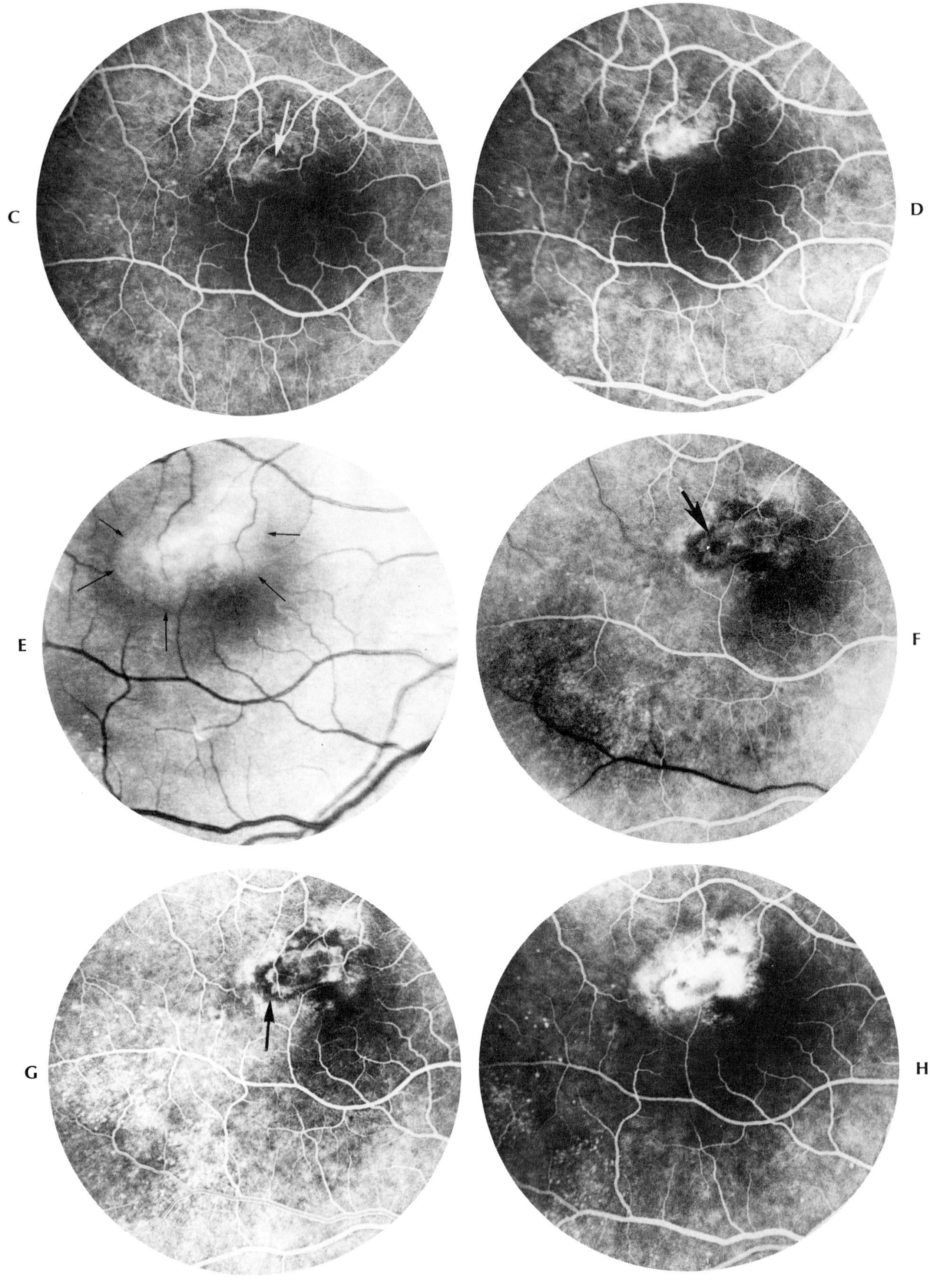

Fig. 12-23, cont'd. For legend see p. 255.

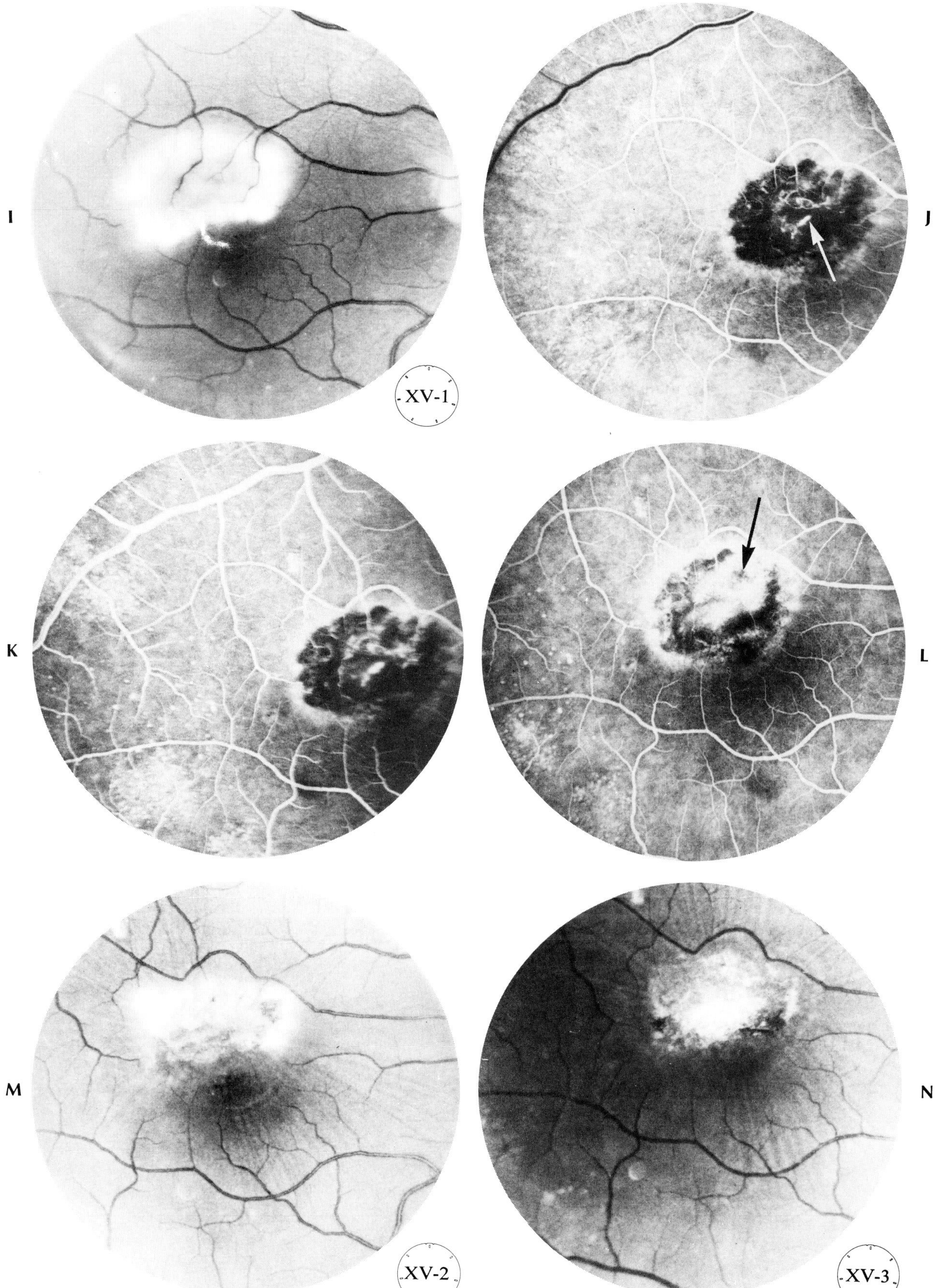

Fig. 12-23, cont'd. For legend see p. 255.

Ophthalmoscopic appearance. Choroidal neovascularization can occur with angioid streaks, with dehiscences in Bruch's membrane, with atrophy of the choriocapillaris and pigment epithelial regions secondary to choroidal scarring (histoplasmosis), with hemorrhagic or serous detachment of the pigment epithelium, and in the region of a previous choroidal rupture. The most common type of choroidal neovascularization arises from a degenerated area of the macular region where apparent atrophy and pigment proliferation of the outer retinal and inner choroidal elements have been noted for an extended period of time.

As the neovascularization grows through the atrophic zone from the choroid to the subretinal space, the fluid leakage from the neovascularization can collect in the subretinal space beneath the sensory retina, or it can leak into the sensory retina itself. The overlying retina can become edematous, and in later stages hard exudates frequently are deposited around the edematous retinal area.

The fibrovascular sheet of neovascularization assumes a grayish brown, hazy, ill-defined appearance as it grows beneath the sensory retina, and it can usually be identified if the overlying sensory retinal edema is minimal. As the membrane progresses, hemorrhages commonly occur beneath the sensory retina, and the full-blown triad of clinical observations, strongly indicating choroidal neovascularization, can be present. This nearly pathognomonic triad includes extensive sensory retinal edema, hard exudates surrounding the edematous zone, and subretinal hemorrhages intermingled with the exudates and edema. If the membrane can be visualized ophthalmoscopically or by fluorescein angiography, the diagnosis of choroidal neovascularization is definite.

As the hemorrhagic activity progresses and glial repair proceeds, the entire macular and paramacular zone can become degenerated into an elevated gliotic fibrous tissue mass. This area of organized tissue resulting from the extensive gliosis and degraded blood products usually remains stable but can demonstrate hemorrhagic activity.

Ancillary diagnostic examinations. Stereoscopic color fundus photography can be extremely useful for documenting the progress of edema, exudates, hemorrhages, and fibrovascular membrane.

The most useful diagnostic technique is fluorescein angiography, which shows the formation of a typical "bicycle wheel" sheet of neovascularization that becomes apparent in the late part of the choroidal flush phase. This neovascularization becomes more prominent during the retinal arteriolar and venular phase. The circumferential vessels of the neovascularization, representing the bicycle wheel, can be seen to be fed from multiple spokelike feeder vessels emanating from a central hub. Surrounding the bicycle wheel leakage is a zone of relative hypofluorescence caused either by avascularity or blockage resulting from glial and pigment tissue proliferation. The entire area of neovascularization will leak and fluoresce brightly during the early and late venular phases. The neovascularization must be identified during the early retinal arteriolar phase so that the limits of the neovascularization may be determined for the purpose of photocoagulation.

Tangent screen campimetry will show the progression of the macular changes. Amsler grid evaluations will also be helpful in determining any change in the central visual field, as well as the recurrence of any macular symptoms following photocoagulation therapy.

Photocoagulation approach, complications, and follow-up. The photocoagulation approach, complications, and follow-up are identical to those outlined under the section on Angioid Streaks (p. 248) (Figs. 12-20 to 12-23).

SECTION THREE

Anterior segment photocoagulation

Chapter 13

Iris abnormalities

PHOTOCOREOPLASTY FOR DISPLACED PUPILS

Indications for photocoagulation. The displacement of the pupil away from the visual axis due to congenital, traumatic, or postsurgical causes can be corrected by photocoagulation. A portion of the pupil can be brought into the area of the normal, centrally placed visual axis by appropriate argon laser photocoagulation of the intact iris. With displaced pupils an optical coreoplasty is indicated if more central placement of the pupil will improve vision. Centering of the pupil can be achieved in phakic and aphakic individuals if sufficient iris tissue is available for photocoagulative retraction.

Photocoagulation approach. The pupillary aperture is moved more centrally by shrinking the fibers of the dilator muscle in the area toward which one wishes to move the pupil. Coagulations of **500μ** and a **0.1-sec** exposure are produced in the area just inside the outer limit of the collarette of the iris. Coagulation intensities (**250 to 450 mw**) sufficient to cause a demonstrable instantaneous shrinkage of the iris tissue at the moment of impact are used. A coagulum may or may not be seen, depending on the depth and density of the iris pigment. These coagulations should be contiguous in a single or double linear row and confined to areas of the iris that will produce retraction of the pupillary border in the desired direction after photocoagulation. With updrawn and displaced pupils this procedure usually involves placing linear coagulations in a 200° to 250° arc of iris toward which the pupil is meant to be displaced (Fig. 13-1).

A second linear row of contiguous coagulations of approximately the same dosage is then produced just peripheral to the previous coagulation line. This coagulation line lies between the previous coagulations and the outer border of the collarette and should include the outer collarette region. These coagulations usually produce further retraction of the pupillary border. Additional rows of coagulations can be placed peripheral to the previous coagulations to obtain a maximal amount of pupillary displacement and retraction (Figs. 13-2 and 13-3).

Subsequent photocoagulation sessions should be scheduled 3 weeks later if further retraction of the pupil is desired. The same routine of placing coagulations in the circumcollarette area and placing secondary coagulations more peripherally should be employed. At least 3 weeks should be allowed for healing of the photocoagulated regions if full displacement of the pupil is to be accomplished (Fig. 13-4).

Complications. Complications of corneal burns, iris hemorrhage, cataract formation, pigment dispersion in the anterior chamber, and glaucoma are possible with xenon-arc

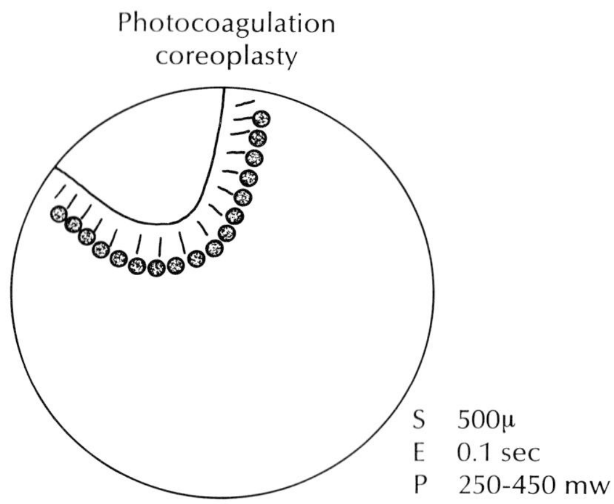

Fig. 13-1. Placement of 500μ punctate, linear, contiguous coagulations in the area of the iris sphincter, toward which the pupil is to be retracted.

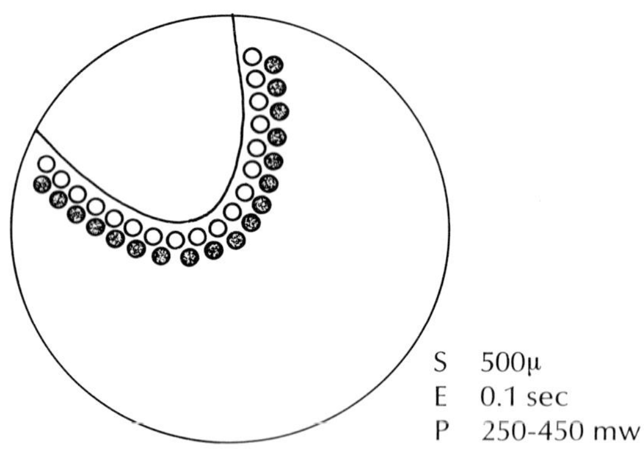

Fig. 13-2. Placement of an additional row of 500μ argon laser coagulations immediately peripheral to the previously placed coagulations to retract the iris.

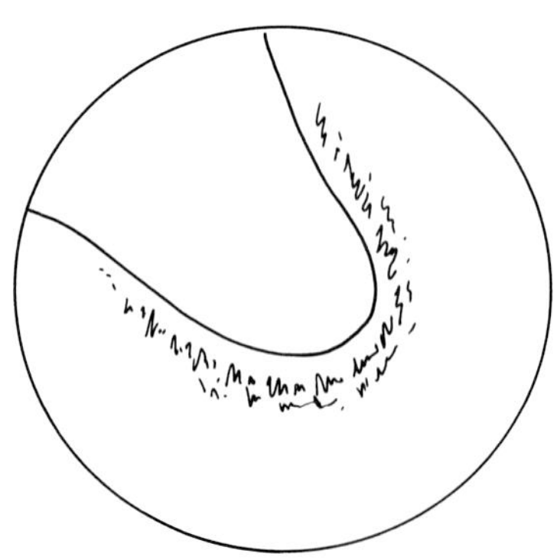

Fig. 13-3. Iris tissue retracted by argon laser photocoagulation.

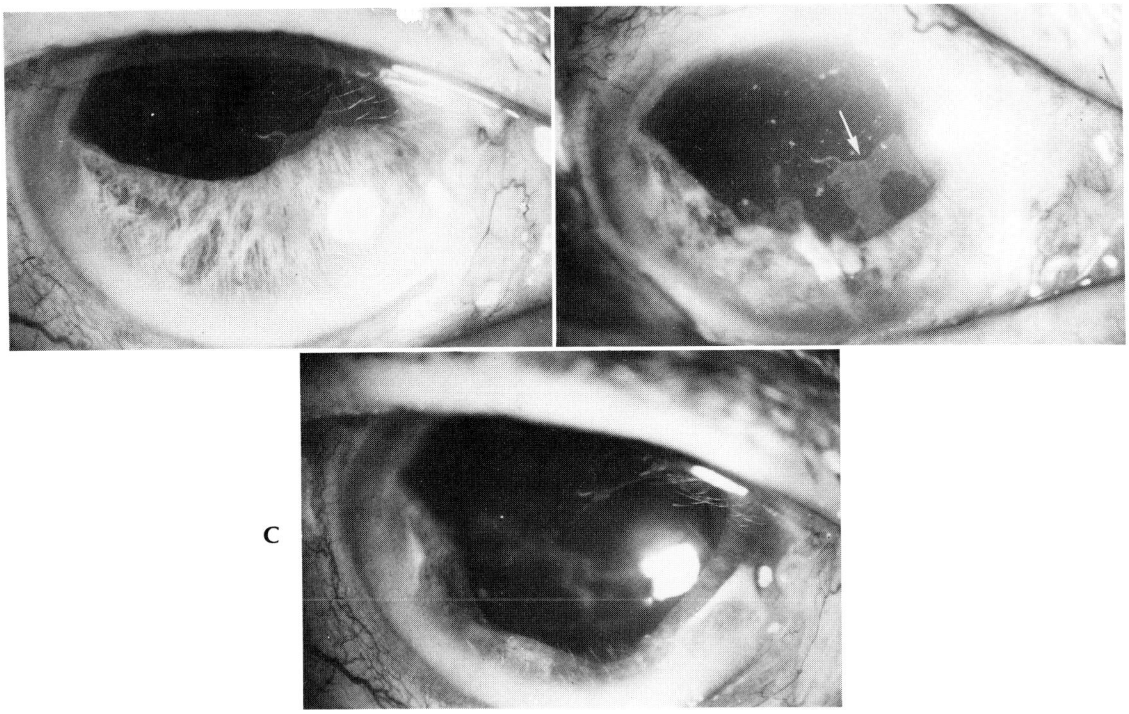

Fig. 13-4. A, An updrawn pupil in a 67-year-old man following cataract extraction resulting in vitreous loss. **B,** Marked retraction of the pupil following argon laser photocoagulation to the border of the iris. Note the pigmentation on the anterior hyaloid, signifying marked posterior synechia formation (arrow). **C,** Healed iris 2 months after photocoreoplasty.

photocoagulation but have not been observed with the argon laser. Careful titration of the energy to produce the desired effect is necessary if these particular complications are to be avoided.

Follow-up. The patient should be followed closely at 3- to 7-day intervals for the first several weeks to rule out the possibility of a rise in intraocular pressure. Further treatment may be given at these visits if necessary. Patients continue to apply cycloplegics and steroid medication topically for approximately 10 days following the final treatment.

PHOTOMYDRIASIS FOR DEBILITATING PUPILLARY MIOSIS

Indications for photocoagulation. With the use of stronger antiglaucoma miotics, individuals with moderately advanced nuclear sclerosis or cortical cataracts may complain of markedly decreased vision. Extreme miosis itself can be sufficiently debilitating, even without significant cataract formation. In such individuals photocoagulation can be considered for minimizing or eliminating the miotic effect of the medications administered topically. By doubling the pupillary diameter, the incoming light is increased by a factor of four. Small increases in pupillary size can thus significantly reduce symptoms related to miosis.

A pretreatment dilation with mydriatics administered topically is indicated for determining the possible benefit to be gained from photomydriasis. If such a trial dilation does not significantly improve the visual acuity because of retinal disease or extensive cataract formation, photocoagulation is not indicated.

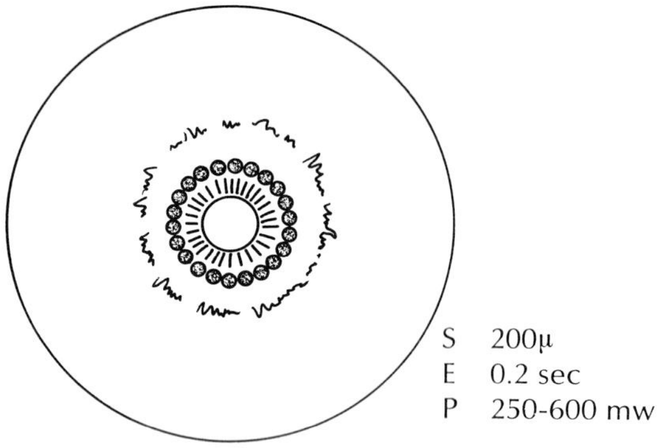

Fig. 13-5. Placement of 200μ linear, interrupted coagulations and retraction of the iris tissue immediately at the time of photomydriasis.

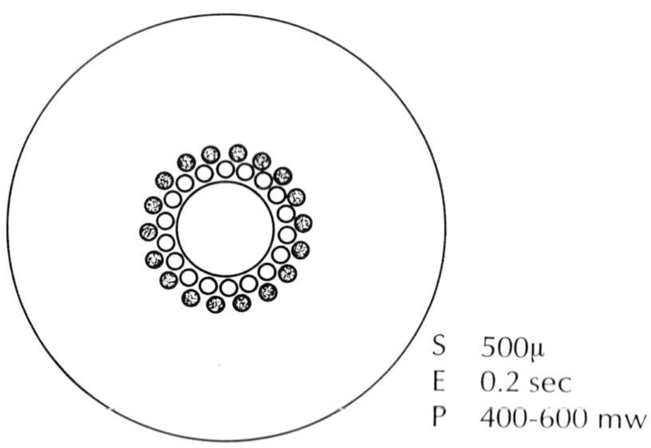

Fig. 13-6. Placement of secondary 500μ coagulations in a manner similar to that of Fig. 13-5, creating more extensive mydriasis of the pupil.

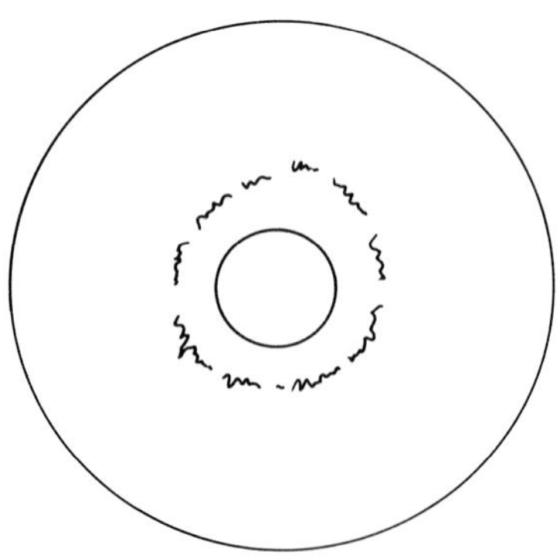

Fig. 13-7. Pupil several weeks after photomydriasis, showing a normal response to mydriatic agents administered topically and little or no response to miotic drops.

Eyes with narrow-angle glaucoma have not been treated, nor have eyes with advanced corneal endothelial disease. These considerations are discussed under Complications.

The primary desired result of photomydriasis is the mild dilation of the pupil to counteract the miotic effect of the patient's regimen for glaucoma. A secondary desired result is the preservation of topically induced mydriasis for the purpose of adequate ophthalmoscopic examination. In essence, the postoperative pupil should resist the miosis induced by the patient's medications but should still respond to dilation.

Photocoagulation approach. The treatment technique consists of treating the iris directly, using the slit lamp delivery system of the argon laser photocoagulator. Neither a contact lens nor a corneal bath is required, and a retrobulbar anesthetic is not necessary for

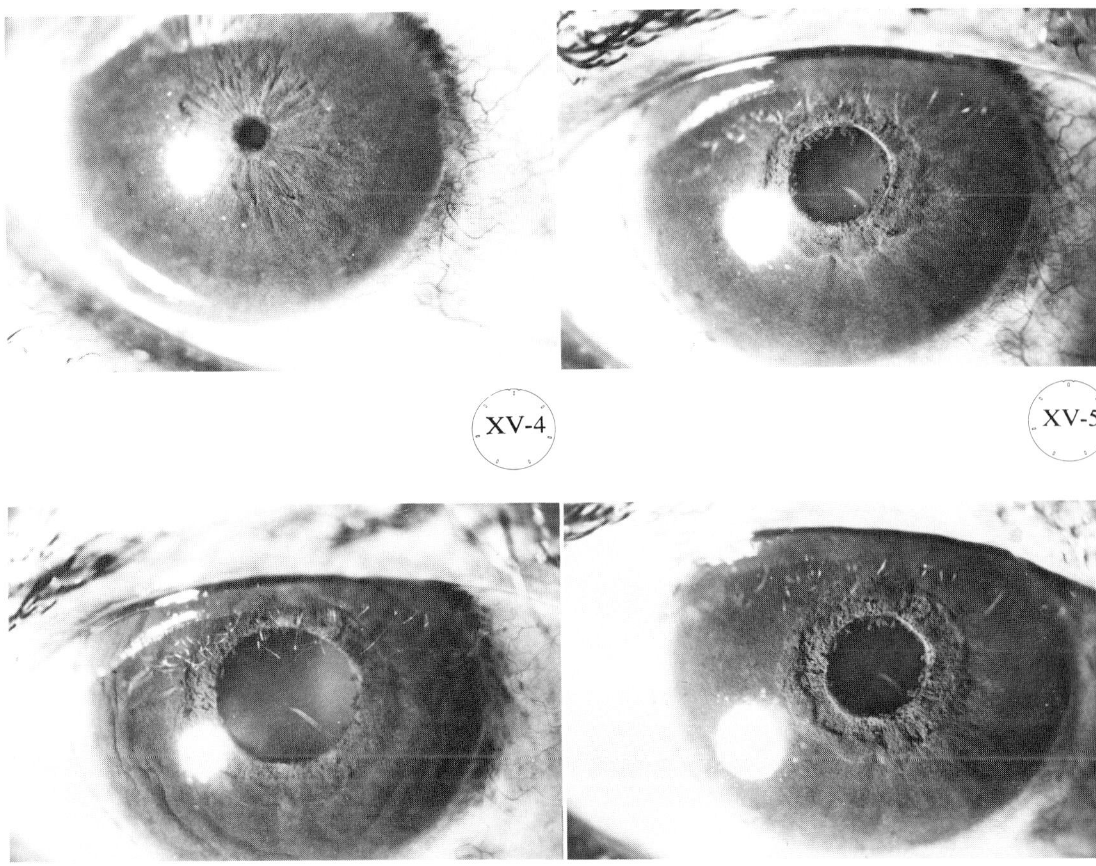

A B C D

XV-4 XV-5 XV-6

Fig. 13-8. A, The right eye of a 55-year-old man with moderately severe open-angle glaucoma who was treated by 4% pilocarpine hydrochloride administered every 3 hr. The miosis of the pupil in combination with moderately advanced nuclear sclerosis prevented him from obtaining a visual acuity better than 20/100. **B,** Pupil immediately after photomydriasis, showing moderate dilation of the pupil caused by weakening and retraction of the iris sphincter area. **C,** Pupil dilated with mydriatic drops 1 month after argon laser photomydriasis, showing retention of the mydriatic capability of the treated iris. **D,** Pupillary area after a topical course of 4% pilocarpine 2 months after argon laser photomydriasis.

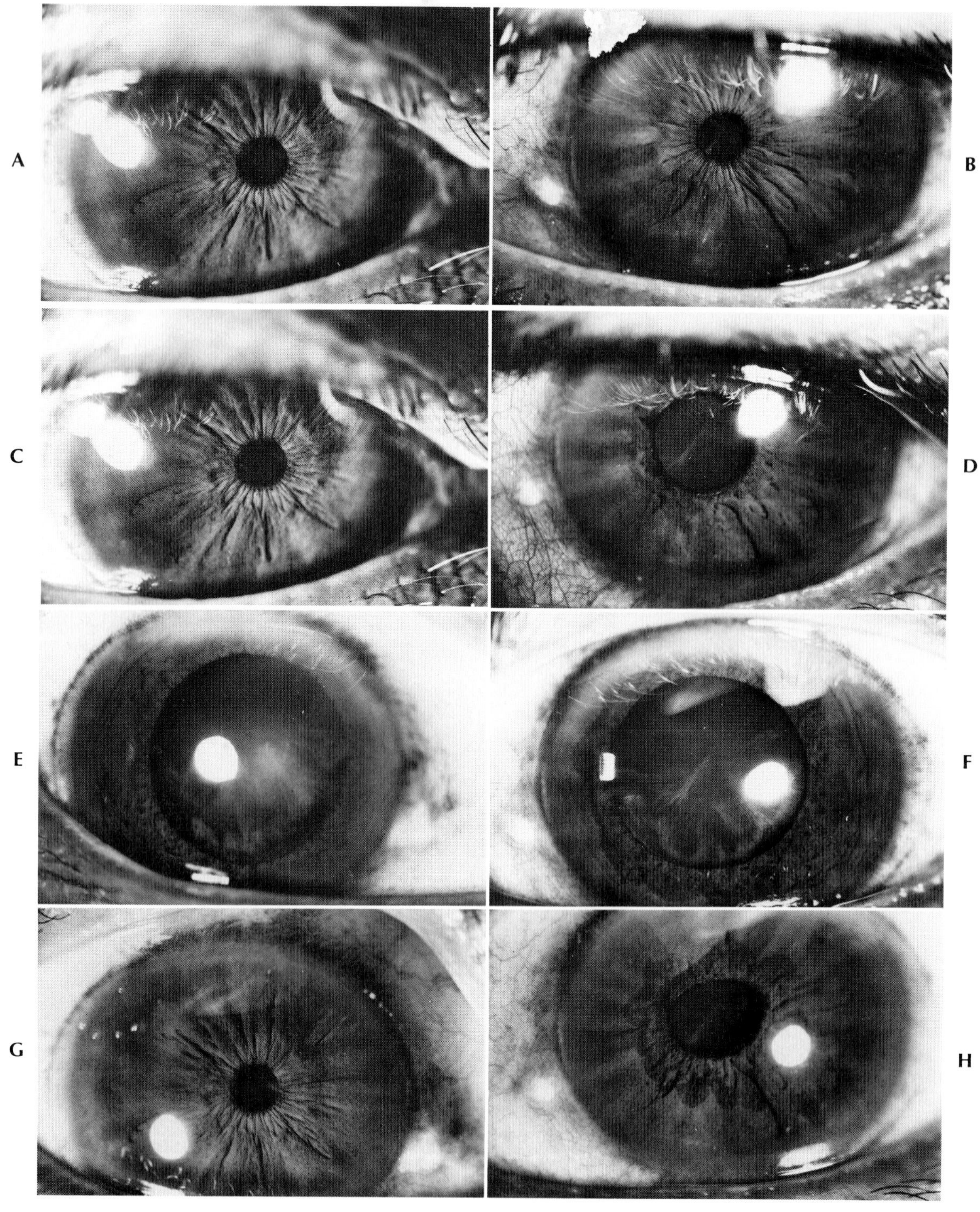

Fig. 13-9. Untreated right eye, **A,** and to-be-treated left eye, **B,** in a 50-year-old man with mild nuclear sclerosis and severe discomfort and blurring of vision during the miosis following 4% pilocarpine instillation. **C,** Control untreated right eye. **D,** Left iris immediately after argon laser photomydriasis with dilation of the pupil to approximately 3.5 mm. A slight flare and a few cells, which cleared within 1 hr after treatment, were noted at this time. **E,** Response of the untreated right eye to mydriatic drops. **F,** Similar response of the treated left eye to mydriatic drops. **G,** Response of the untreated right eye to the patient's normal regimen of 4% pilocarpine administered four times daily. **H,** Response of the treated left eye to the patient's normal regimen of 4% pilocarpine administered four times daily, showing lack of miosis after pilocarpine instillation.

most patients. The topical use of an anesthetic is helpful in reducing the patient's frequency of blinking.

Multiple **200μ** impacts are placed immediately adjacent to the pupillary border in a contiguous manner for 360° (Fig. 13-5). The desired effect is an immediate shriveling of the iris and moderate oozing of iris pigment and plasmoid aqueous, not a severe explosion. An exposure of **0.2 sec** and power settings in the range of **250 to 600 mw** have seemed ideal. The power setting must be adjusted to individual iris pigmentation. Lower power settings produce some immediate shriveling of the iris, but the resultant mydriasis is lost once the patient resumes his regimen of miotics. Higher power settings, especially with shorter exposures, produce bubbles and pigment explosions, and these effects are excessive.

Once the initial 200μ barrage has surrounded the pupillary border, an additional **500μ** treatment circle is made just outside the initial treatment circle (Fig. 13-6). The purpose of this second row of treatments is to reinforce the initial row and to cover thoroughly the region of the iris sphincter, which forms a broad 1-mm band surrounding the pupillary border. As the spot size is increased to 500μ the exposure is kept at **0.2 sec** and the power is increased to **400 to 600 mw.** The desired effect again is a moderate oozing of pigment and plasmoid aqueous, not a severe explosion. After the second row of treatments has been completed, the pupil will usually have doubled its original size (Fig. 13-7). These figures schematically summarize the treatment technique. Some pupils may lose a significant portion of their newly acquired mydriasis once the patient resumes his topical regimen of miotics. If so, retreatment should be instituted (Figs. 13-8 and 13-9).

Three methods of retreatment have been utilized. The first method is to repeat the original double-circle technique, treating the same area adjacent to the pupillary border. Enhancing the injury to the sphincter muscle until an appropriate amount of sphincter function has been obliterated, this method can produce satisfactory results.

Another retreatment method is the photocoagulation of a more diffuse area of iris, even out to the iris periphery. This method does produce a sustained amount of mydriasis, but it injures the dilator as well as the sphincter muscle, and after treatment the pupil responds poorly to both miotics and mydriatics. Such a diminished response to mydriatics is not advantageous.

The third method of retreatment incorporates dilation of the pupil with mydriatics and then with treatment of the iris sphincter muscle, using the same double-circle technique. This method appears to be very effective and may be used not only as a retreatment technique but also as an initial technique for patients taking stronger miotics. Before laser treatment, however, the pupil should not be dilated to more than 3 or 4 mm. Further dilation, followed by photomydriasis, will result in an excessively large pupil.

After treatment all patients continue to take their usual medications for glaucoma. Acetazolamide 500 mg is taken orally as a single dose immediately following treatment, and steroids are prescribed to be applied topically 4 times a day for 3 to 7 days.

Complications. A mild iritis is the most common complication observed. All patients will have an immediate postoperative plasmoid iritis, but this problem will dissipate rapidly in the majority of the patients treated. A delayed iritis can occur several weeks after treatment, and these patients can be effectively treated with homatropine and steroid drops.

Corneal edema and a rise in intraocular pressure after treatment have been observed, especially with excessive treatment. The intraocular pressure rise can be easily controlled with acetazolamide and oral doses of osmotic agents. Overtreatment, resulting in liberation of excessive pigment, should be avoided. Patients with glaucoma under borderline control should be observed carefully. Exacerbation of an underlying glaucomatous condition has not been a significant problem in the patients treated, but one should be aware of this possible complication.

A small hemorrhage developed in one of my patients at an impact site of rather high intensity (600 mw). The hemorrhage was readily cauterized by further photocoagulation and presented no subsequent problem.

Inadvertent treatment of the macular region directly through the pupil remains a potential problem, particularly in the absence of a retrobulbar anesthetic. Patients unable to maintain a steady gaze should receive a retrobulbar injection. In the absence of an anesthetic, the patient should be asked to look in a temporal or nasal direction when treatment is being performed. This maneuver displaces the macula away from the line of treatment. An alternative technique is to reflect the laser beam through a three-mirror lens at an angle across the anterior chamber.

Patients with narrow angles have not been treated, because the postoperatively reduced miosis might induce an acute attack. A diminished response to miotic agents would seem, theoretically, to pose a problem for these narrow-angle patients. The effect of photomydriasis on eyes with narrow angles is under further study.

Follow-up. The patient should be seen at 3- to 7-day intervals following the photomydriasis procedure to ascertain whether further treatment is required and if there are any complicating factors. Patients continue to apply steroid medications topically for approximately 7 days following the final treatment.

PHOTOIRIDOTOMY

Indications for photocoagulation. Although peripheral iridectomy is a relatively benign procedure, there are circumstances where an iridotomy can be performed without surgical intervention. If a laser iridotomy can be performed with less trauma to the anterior segment, it could be indicated, rather than more extensive anterior segment surgery, as the primary approach. The technique of laser iridotomy may well substitute for a surgical iridectomy in certain ocular conditions.

Photocoagulation approach. For 1 hr before the iridotomy miotics (4% pilocarpine) are administered every 15 min to the eye to be treated.

A 2-ml retrobulbar injection of 2% lidocaine with hyaluronidase is administered to achieve anesthesia and akinesia. An injection may not be required but should be carefully considered, since the photocoagulation procedure may be uncomfortable and may result in a linear burn rather than a penetrating coagulation.

The anterior segment photocoagulation contact lens can be inserted and Ringer's solution allowed to run through the lens at a slow drip rate if the proposed iris coagulation area is peripherally located and near the posterior corneal surface. Usually, no contact lens is required.

An area approximately two thirds of the distance from the iris sphincter to the iris-corneal angle at the 9:30 or 2:30 position is then selected for the photocoagulation procedure. Precisely focused coagulations of **200μ** at **0.5-sec** exposure and a power intensity of approximately **300 mw** are placed in the form of a square in this region (Fig. 13-10). The distance between the four photocoagulations is approximately 400μ, and the effect of the coagulations is to raise a small mound of iris tissue into the anterior chamber away from the underlying lens surface. In this manner the iris is drawn taut and elevated away from the lens surface before the actual penetrating photocoagulation.

A **50μ** coagulation is then produced at an exposure of **0.5 sec** and intensities of

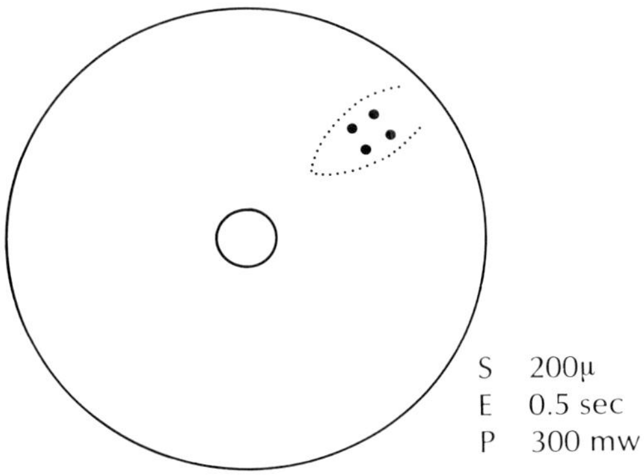

Fig. 13-10. Photoiridotomy. The four preliminary argon laser coagulations are placed in the form of a square 400μ from one another in the area of proposed photocoagulation penetration.

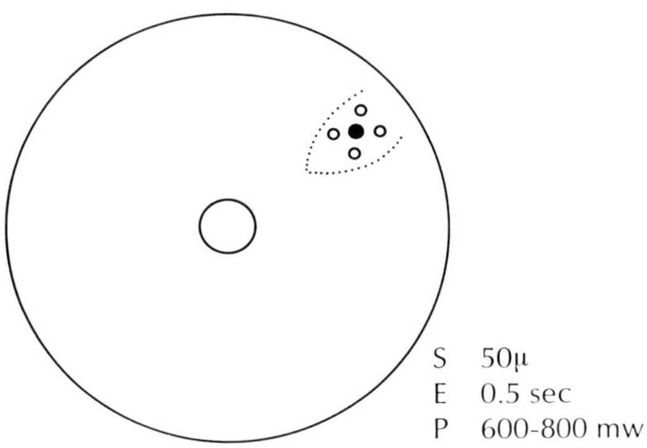

Fig. 13-11. Photocoagulation parameters for the penetrating photocoagulation in the previously prepared area.

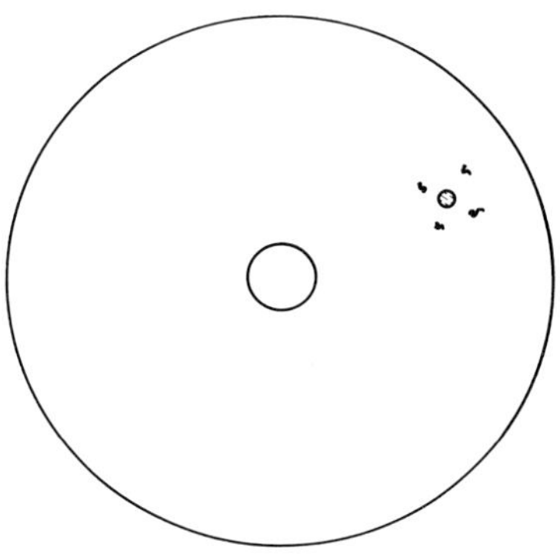

Fig. 13-12. Eventual atrophy of the area after penetrating photocoagulation to produce a patent photoiridotomy.

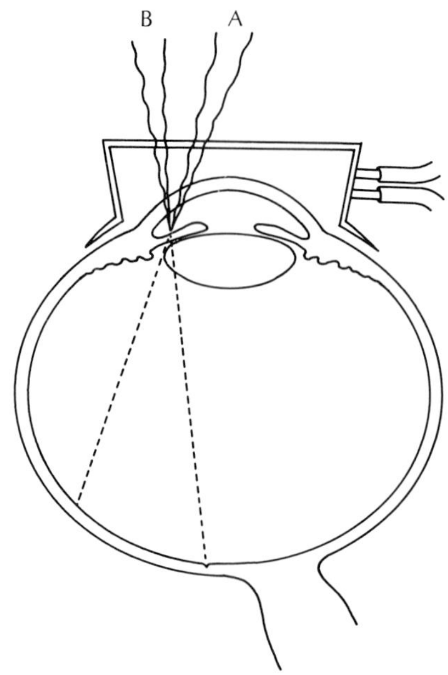

Fig. 13-13. Argon laser photocoagulation beam must be directed away from the visual axis *(A)* during any iris or anterior segment photocoagulation to avoid coagulation of the macular *(B)* and posterior polar region.

approximately **600 to 800 mw** inside the area bounded by the four previous coagulation spots (Fig. 13-11). The coagulations should be sufficiently intense to penetrate through the iris, resulting in subsequent development of a filtering iridotomy. The production of an iridotomy in brown-eyed patients usually requires higher power levels than in blue-eyed patients. Usually, the iridotomy site will not open for 1 to 3 weeks following this procedure but may be patent immediately (Fig. 13-12).

If these primary photocoagulations fail to produce a patent opening during the first 3 weeks, the procedure should be repeated within the previously treated site. Coagulations of **50μ** with an exposure of **0.5 sec** and intensities of **600 to 800 mw** should again be employed. If necessary, the procedure can be repeated for several weekly intervals. Each photocoagulation session produces some degree of iris atrophy, and the purpose of the repeated treatments is to create a sufficient opening in the crater formed by the previous coagulations (Figs. 13-13 to 13-15).

The photocoagulation beam should be angulated with reference to the iris surface at all times, so that any laser energy inadvertently penetrating the iris will strike the retina anterior to the equator.

Complications. Corneal burns have been observed following photoiridotomies but have resolved spontaneously. Punctate opacification of the lens in the area of the iridotomy has been noted, but only if high-intensity power levels have been utilized. Animal studies have shown these opacities to be very superficial, punctate, and nonprogressive. The use of the anterior segment contact lens with peripheral iris photocoagulation for cooling of the nearby corneal structure is advisable.

Follow-up. The patient is followed at intervals of 3 to 4 days for the first 2 weeks to determine the extent of the iritis and anterior chamber reaction. The patient continues to take steroid preparations and acetazolamide, if necessary, for at least a 2-week period following photocoagulation.

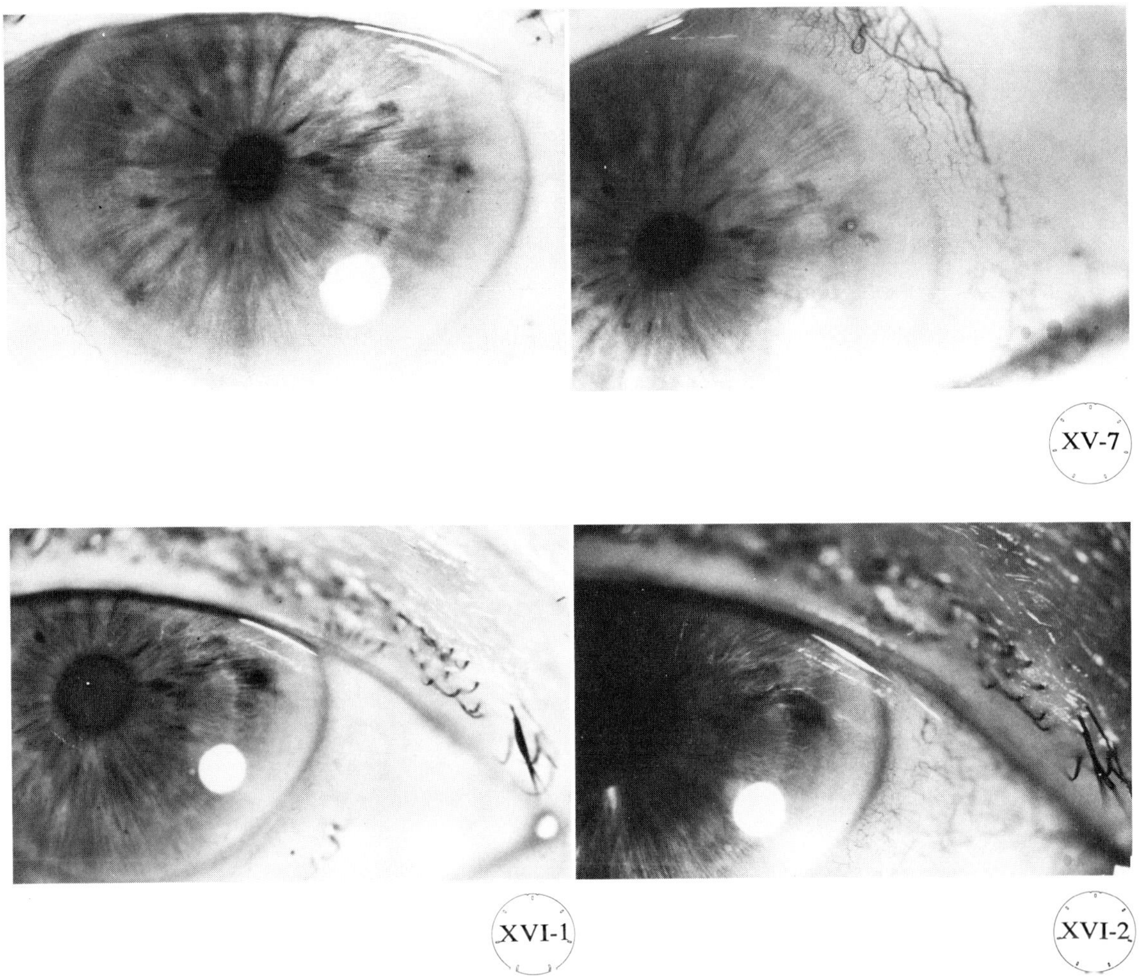

A B C D

Fig. 13-14. A, Left eye with extremely shallow angles and repeated episodes of increased intraocular pressure and associated pain in a 72-year-old woman. **B,** Four preparatory coagulations placed in the form of a square. The penetrating photocoagulation is in the center. A small bubble at the point of penetration can be noted as shown, at a power level sufficient for eventual production of the photoiridotomy. **C,** Photoiridotomy site 1 week after photocoagulation, showing an obvious opening through the iris. **D,** Site 2 months after photocoagulation. The photoiridotomy site has enlarged, and the lens surface is clearly visible through the iridotomy opening.

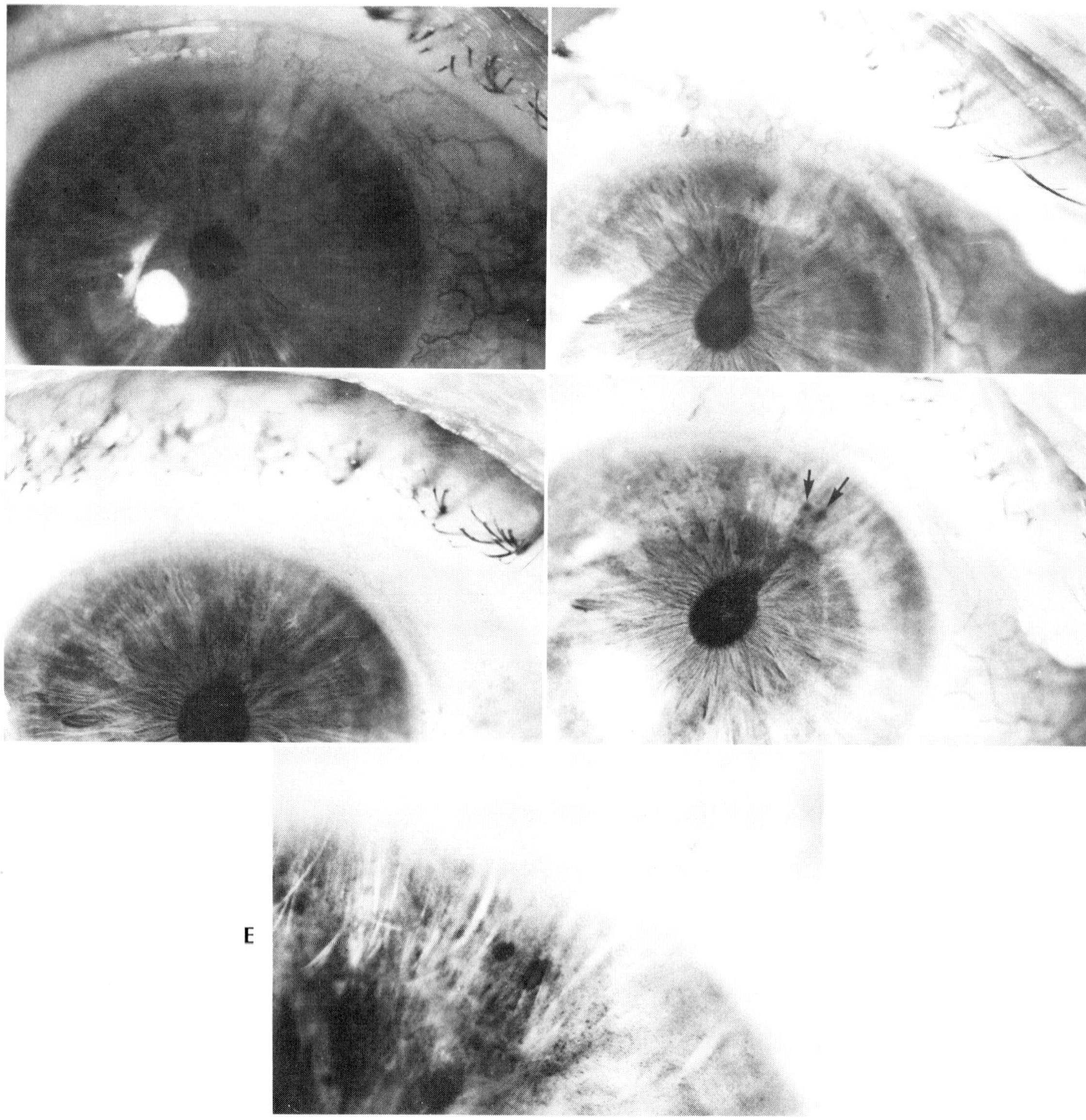

A B C D E

Fig. 13-15. A, Narrow-angle glaucoma, a slightly elevated pressure, and an extremely shallow chamber in a 57-year-old woman. **B,** A photoiridotomy procedure was performed at the 12:30 position, resulting in bubble formation at the iridotomy site and slight retraction of the pupil toward the photocoagulated region. **C,** Photocoagulated site 1 week after argon laser photocoagulation to the peripheral iris, showing thinning of the iris structure and tenting of the pupil but no obvious patent photoiridotomy. Photocoagulation was reapplied at this time with 50μ coagulations at a 0.5-sec exposure and a 600-mw power intensity. **D,** Photocoagulated site 10 days after treatment, showing two obvious photoiridotomy sites with complete penetration through the iris tissue (arrows). **E,** Magnified view of the two photoiridotomies 2 months following argon laser photocoagulation, showing discrete areas of atrophy and disruption of the iris tissue forming the patent iridotomy.

PHOTOCOAGULATION THERAPY OF IRIS CYSTS

Indications for photocoagulation. Iris cysts of a congenital or acquired nature can be treated by photocoagulation, particularly if they are enlarging, as documented by regular or stereoscopic anterior segment photography. The prognosis is particularly good if the iris cysts are exposed anteriorly, so that the inner areas of the cysts can be reached by the laser beam. Iris cysts behind the iris diaphragm cannot be treated effectively by photocoagulation.

Photocoagulation approach. Iris cysts on the anterior surface of the iris and away from the root of the iris can be treated, preferably with the anterior segment photocoagulation contact lens to ensure cooling of the cornea and neutralization of the corneal curvature power (Figs. 13-16 and 13-17). Iris cysts that involve the root of the iris or the area between the iris and the cornea can best be treated with the Goldmann three-mirror lens (Fig. 13-18), the anterior segment lens, or the Worst magnifying anterior segment lens. These lenses allow direct access to the chamber angle by the photocoagulation beam.

Photocoagulations are directed to the posterior wall of the iris cysts initially; the anterior segment photocoagulation contact lens or reflective contact lenses are used to visualize the anterior chamber angle for those cysts positioned at the base of the iris. Coagulations of **500μ** at a **0.2-sec** exposure and sufficiently intense (usually **200 to 300 mw**) to cause a moderate Grade 2 to 3 mucoid reaction are placed in a contiguous barrage fashion across the posterior cyst wall (Fig. 13-19). The biomicroscope is aligned so that the angle of coagulation is directed away from the macular area at all times.

The coagulation of the anterior wall of the cyst is then attempted, and mucoid white coagulations (Grade 2) are produced throughout the anterior cyst layer. A 1-mm area of iris tissue surrounding the iris cyst is also coagulated with similar coagulation dosages to produce complete atrophy and destruction of the cyst.

The photocoagulation impacts will create immediate shrinkage of the cyst wall and surrounding iris tissue, some bubble formation, and a marked dispersion of pigment, cellular debris, and proteinaceous material into the anterior chamber. Photocoagulation should be continued in the cyst area, despite clouding of the anterior chamber, to coagulate as great a surface area of the cyst as possible. Photocoagulation attempts may be

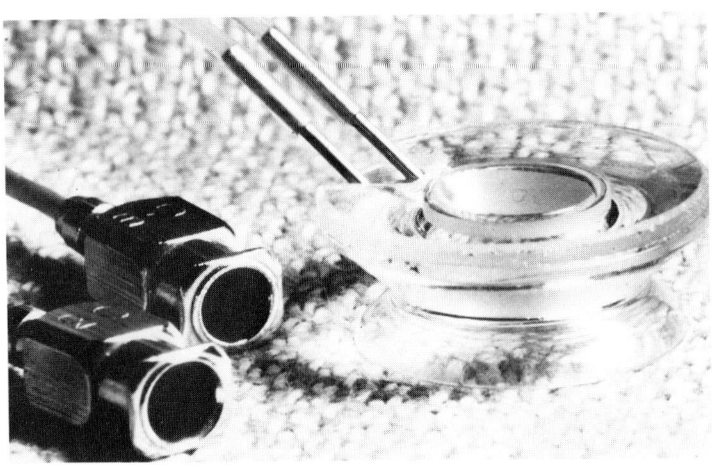

Fig. 13-16. Anterior segment photocoagulation contact lens with neutralizing front plano surface and infusion and exhaust ports with tubing.

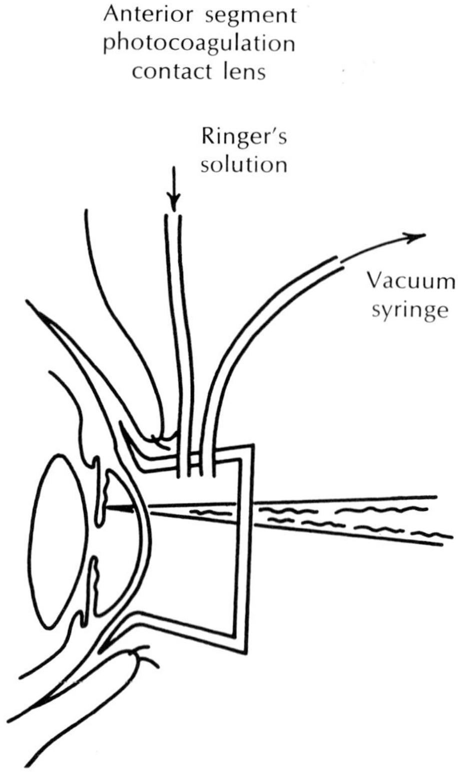

Fig. 13-17. Influx and outflow of Ringer's solution to cool the anterior segment region.

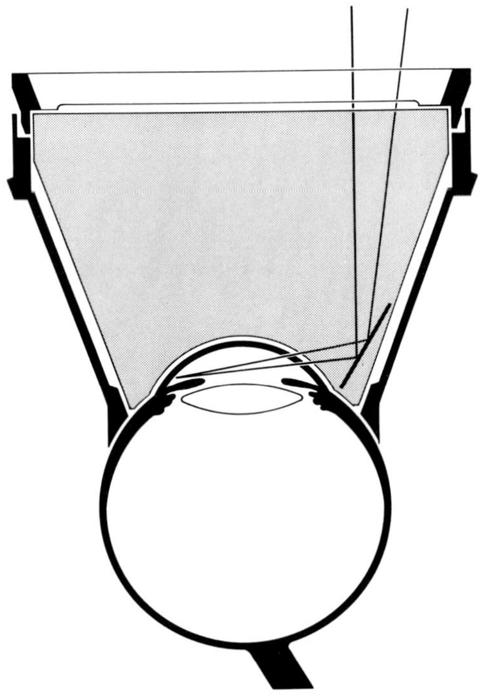

Fig. 13-18. Use of the three-mirror Goldmann contact lens to reflect the argon laser beam across the anterior chamber for photocoagulation of iris cysts positioned at the base of the iris.

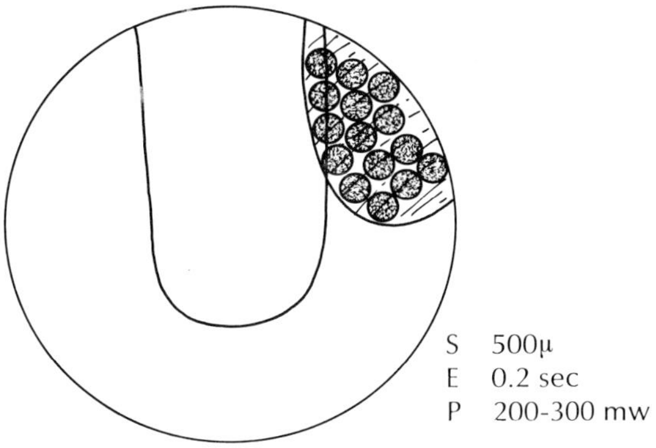

Fig. 13-19. Placement of argon laser coagulations in the anterior and posterior walls of the iris cyst.

A

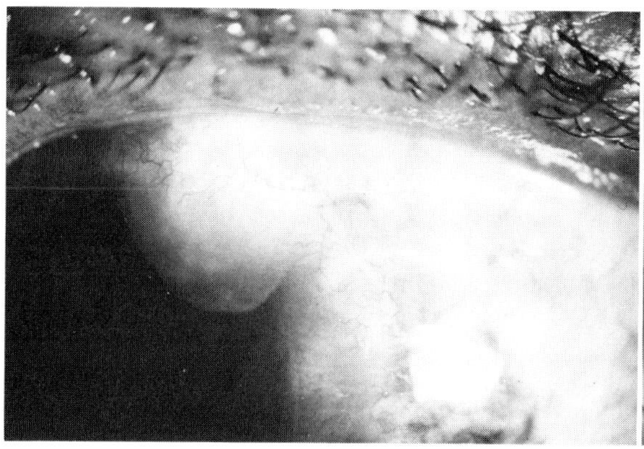

XVI-3

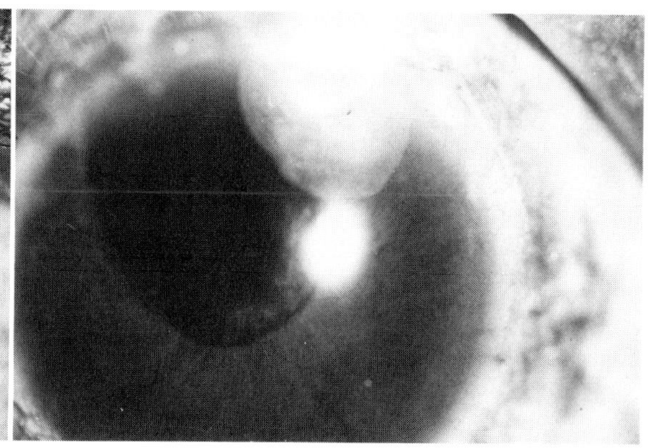

B

XVI-4

C

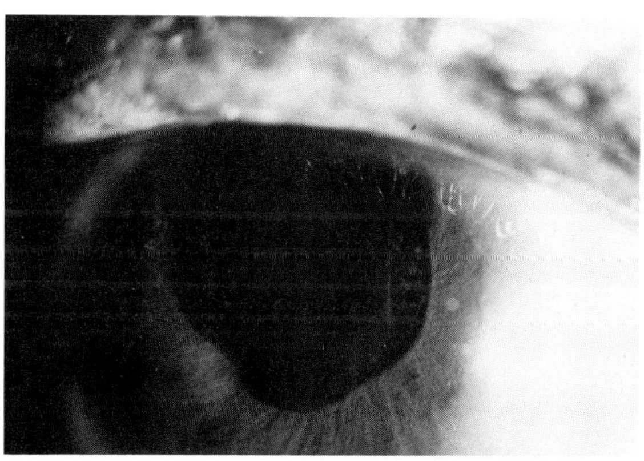

XVI-5

Fig. 13-20. A, An implantation iris cyst located superonasally in the anterior chamber 3 months after cataract extraction with a full basal iridectomy. **B,** Iris cyst immediately after argon laser photocoagulation to the posterior and anterior walls of the cyst. A Grade 2 coagulation intensity is required, and the entire surface of the cyst should be coagulated if possible. **C,** Photocoagulated area 6 weeks after treatment, showing complete disappearance and obliteration of the iris cyst.

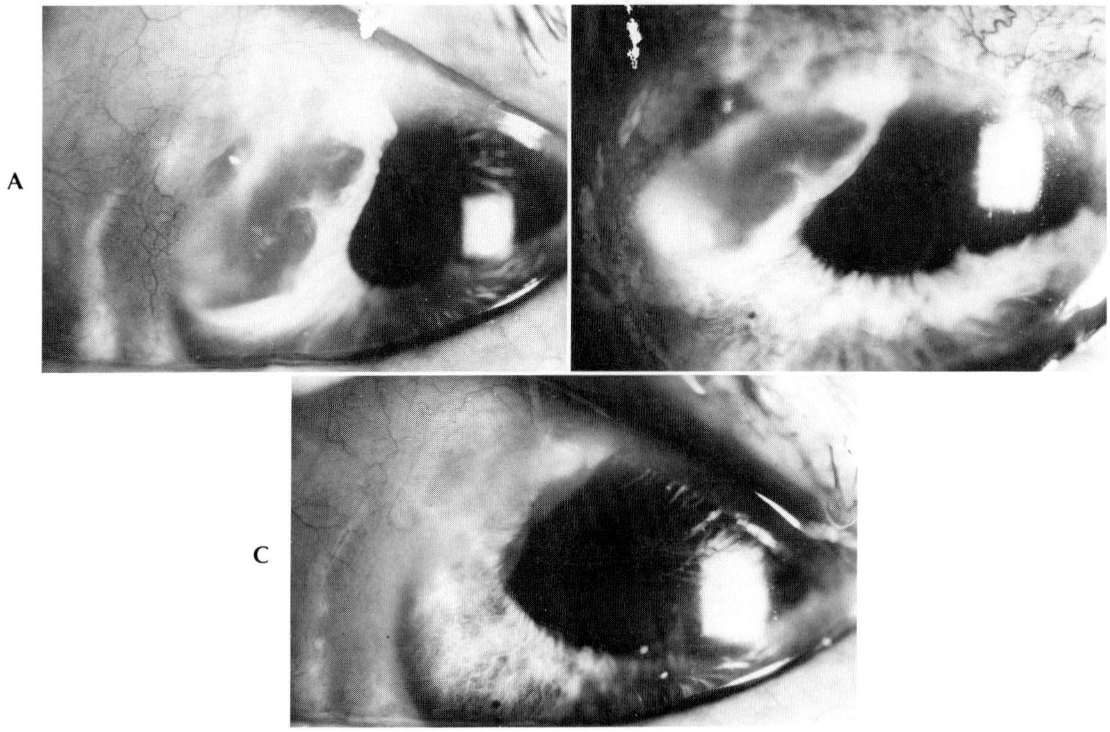

Fig. 13-21. A, An iris cyst occupying the superotemporal aspect of the angle of the right eye and a small subconjunctival cystic bleb 4 months after cataract extraction with a full-sector iridectomy. **B,** Iris cyst immediately after argon laser photocoagulation, showing the prominent coagulations of the posterior wall of the cystic structure. **C,** Photocoagulated area, showing complete obliteration of the iris implantation cyst and the small subconjunctival bleb 7 weeks after argon laser photocoagulation.

postponed for 3 to 7 days if visualization of the cyst becomes difficult. Clearing of the anterior chamber is usually accomplished during this interval (Figs. 13-20 and 13-21).

Corneal clouding may also occur during the photocoagulation procedure because of thermal injury to the stroma or endothelium. The anterior segment photocoagulation contact lens, with cooled Ringer's solution lavage, will help decrease this problem. Gravity flow at 1 drop every 2 sec with the IV bottle positioned 30 inches above the patient's head, or gravity flow plus mild suction with a syringe on the outflow line, will produce considerable corneal cooling and aid in avoiding this problem.

At the end of this procedure, the eye is photographed stereoscopically and patched for 12 hours; the patient is prescribed atropine drops 1% to be applied 2 times a day and steroid drops to be applied every 2 hours, for 10 days. The patient is asked to return in 3 days for reevaluation to determine the degree of iritis and involvement of the anterior segment.

Complications. The most common complication is a corneal burn caused by inadvertent refocusing of the beam into the level of the cornea. Denaturation or coagulation of the cornea can also occur because of the concentration of photon energy at the cornea that is required for treating closely approximated iris cyst walls. In some cases this iris cyst wall is adherent to the posterior cornea, and a corneal coagulation is inevitable. Most of these corneal burns disappear without residue or other corneal problems in 1 to 2 weeks. The photocoagulation angle must always be directed in such a way as to approach the iris cyst without being transmitted through the adjacent cornea. Furthermore, the beam must never be transmitted through the cornea along or near the visual axis.

Hemorrhage from the iris vessels is a possible complication, and the area of the iris cyst must be inspected thoroughly to determine if the vessels have grown along the walls of the cyst. These vessels must be avoided during photocoagulation. If a hemorrhage is produced, the surrounding area of cyst wall or iris or corneal tissue must be photocoagulated immediately with stronger power densities (increased power, continuous same exposure, and same spot size). If the hemorrhage occurs into the cyst, the increased absorption of the argon beam by the hemoglobin can be used advantageously to cause the destruction of the cyst. In these cases the blood film and the cyst wall are coagulated together, usually creating a Grade 3 to 4 coagulum, and results are uniformly good. The nearby structures should not be included in the treatment, if possible, because of the destructive nature of the process.

There is also a possibility that the photocoagulation beam can break through the cyst into the posterior segment, causing retinal damage. This complication has not occurred with my patients, but one must direct the photocoagulations away from the visual axis or macular area at all times in anticipation of such a problem.

A marked iritis can occur soon after treatment, and patients should be followed closely if this complication is suspected. All patients sustain some iritis after photocoagulation; the degree of iritis depends on the amount of iris tissue coagulated, the intensity of the burns, and the individual response of the patient. All patients should be seen 3 days following photocoagulation, or sooner if necessary. Cycloplegic and steroid medication administered topically is usually sufficient to relieve the inflammation and congestion of the anterior segment.

The dispersion of pigment and cellular debris, as well as the protein transudation into the anterior chamber following photocoagulation of iris cysts, can lead to temporary blockage of the trabecular meshwork and to secondary glaucoma. The glaucoma may be mild or severe, with intraocular pressures in the range of 40 to 60 mm Hg. Acetazolamide, 250 mg taken 4 times a day, should be prescribed, and the patient should be followed at 3-day intervals. Analgesics may be required in addition to patient reassurance. The glaucoma may cause a decrease in vision because of stromal or epithelial edema, but the glaucoma is temporary and will improve in 10 to 14 days. Acetazolamide therapy can be stopped, but tonometric and tonographic evaluation should be performed to assess the condition of the trabeculum.

Follow-up. Patients should be followed at 3-day intervals during the early post-photocoagulation period. The iris cyst will shrink over a period of 3 to 6 weeks, and if any of the cystic structures remain 2 months postoperatively, photocoagulation can be repeated. The same techniques that were employed initially are used.

PHOTOVASO-OBLITERATION OF IRIDOCYCLITIC MEMBRANES

Indications for photocoagulation. An iridocyclitic membrane may obstruct or occlude the passage of light to the posterior segment and retina. Frequently, attempts to incise these membranes can cause increased bleeding from blood vessels in the membrane, resulting in hemorrhage into the vitreous and anterior chamber. Each hemorrhage increases the amount of fibrin and glial response in the area of the membrane, compounding the overall problem. In those patients with a severe iridocyclitic membrane secondary to trauma, Still's disease, or other anterior segment problems, photocoagulation

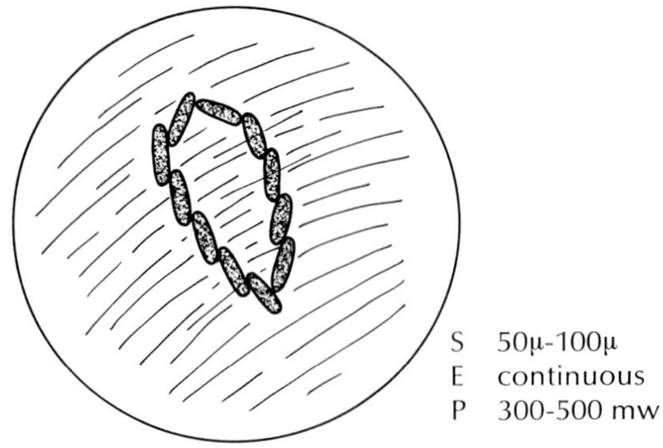

Fig. 13-22. Treatment of the periphery of the proposed discission zone with intense argon laser photocoagulation to destroy blood vessels that are deep in the iris or the cyclitic membrane and that might be ruptured at the time of discission.

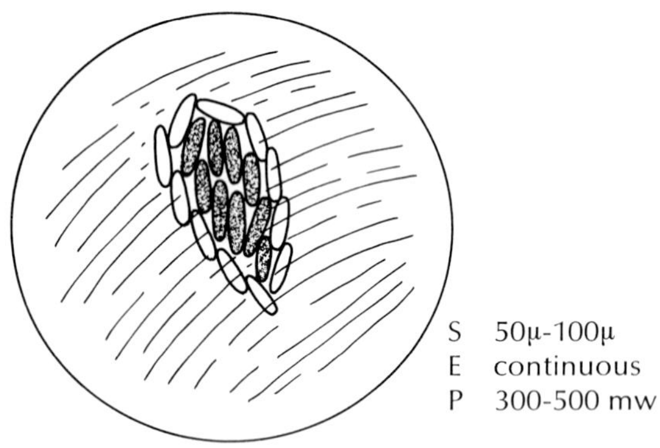

Fig. 13-23. Intense argon laser photocoagulations to the central proposed discission site; the beam is aimed away from the visual axis.

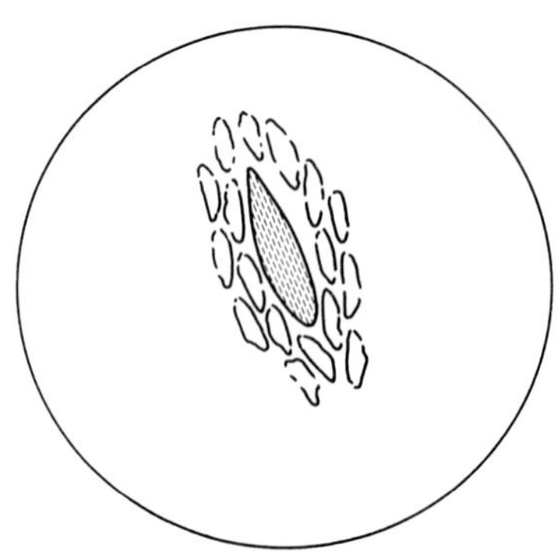

Fig. 13-24. Iridocyclitic membrane after discission of the membrane 3 days after photocoagulation.

can be of assistance, particularly if vascularization within the membrane can be visualized so that the membrane can be rendered avascular in the region of proposed discission.

Photocoagulation approach. The area of proposed discission through the iridocyclitic membrane is examined under high magnification by biomicroscopy, and areas of vascularization are noted in detail.

At the time of photocoagulation the anterior segment photocoagulation lens is placed on the cornea to decrease the retention of heat produced in the cornea by the photocoagulation. A **50μ to 100μ** beam is then utilized in a continuous fashion to paint over the area of proposed discission with sufficient intensities (**300 to 500 mw**) to cauterize or obliterate any vascularization (Figs. 13-22 to 13-24). The margins of the area to be photocoagulated are coagulated initially, to delimit the discission area and to obliterate the blood supply more centrally. The central iris area is then photocoagulated to a depth considered sufficient to obliterate any vessels along the proposed discission site. This obliteration can be monitored by observing the coagulum at the time of coagulation. An area of approximately 1 to 2 mm surrounding the discission zone should be made avascular by the photocoagulation.

The patient is then prescribed atropine 1% drops to be applied 3 times a day and steroid drops to be applied every 3 hours while the patient is awake. In addition, the patient is prescribed steroid ointment to be used in the treated eye at bedtime.

A

B

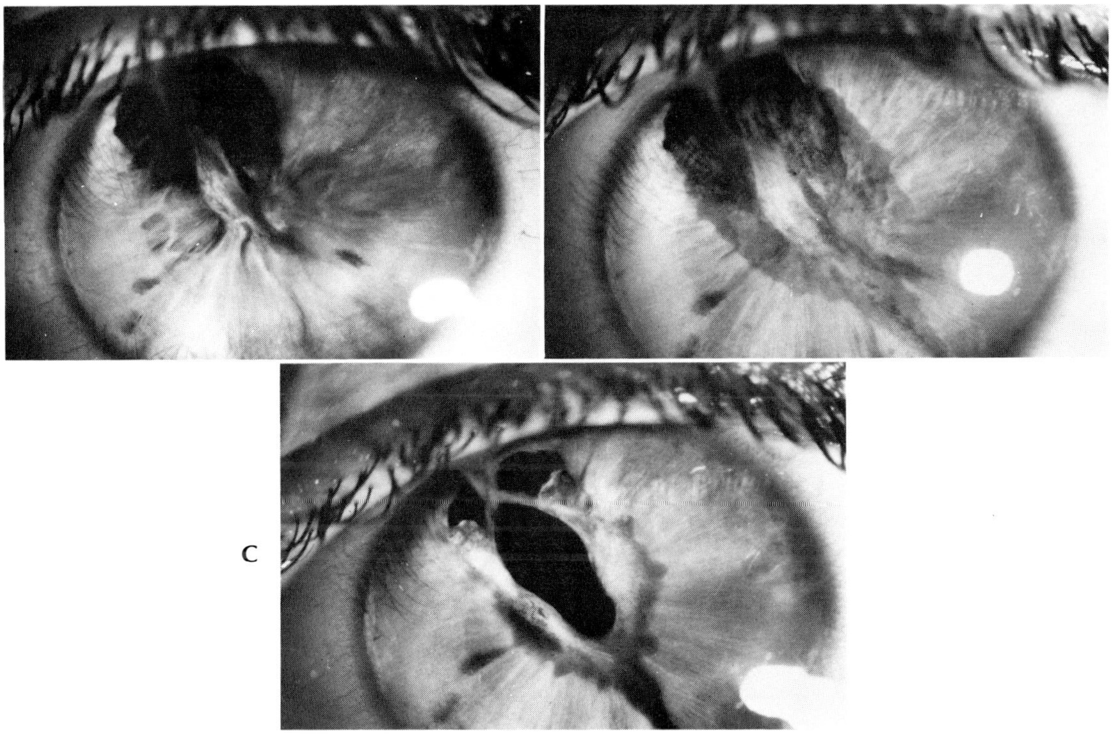

C

Fig. 13-25. A, A dense iridocyclitic membrane in the right eye of a 17-year-old girl who had had three attempted discissions resulting in hemorrhaging into the anterior chamber. **B,** Right eye immediately following photocoagulation, showing obliteration of iris vessels and coagulation of the iris tissue surrounding the entire proposed discission area. **C,** Right eye of the same patient 2 weeks after surgical discission of the avascular iridocyclitic membrane. Vision has improved from a counting-fingers acuity before the discission to $20/20^{-2}$ with a contact lens.

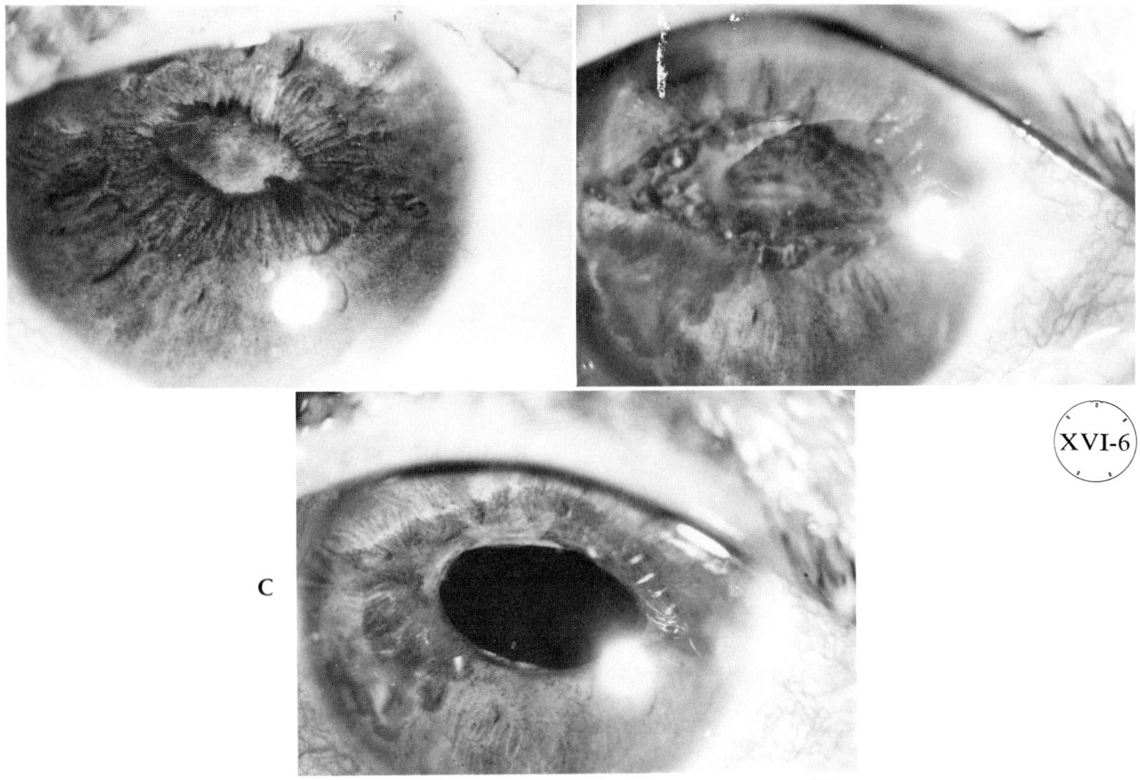

A B C

XVI-6

XVI-7

Fig. 13-26. A, Iridocyclitic membrane with pupil and iris completely bound down to underlying vascularized cyclitic membrane. **B,** Area immediately after argon laser photocoagulation of the proposed discission site, showing complete obliteration of the vascular portion of the iridocyclitic membrane. **C,** Area 4 weeks after discission through the photocoagulated avascular portion of the iridocyclitic membrane, showing a wide pupillary aperture. Visual acuity has improved from light perception to 20/40 with a contact lens.

The patient is observed within 3 days and is retreated at that time, if necessary, to close any remaining blood vessels. When these vessels have been cauterized, usually with short painting coagulation strokes, there should be no evidence of any vessels in the proposed discission site. The patient is then scheduled for discission of the iridocyclitic membrane 2 days following this examination. The patient continues to use cycloplegic and steroid drops (Figs. 13-25 and 13-26).

When the patient is admitted to the hospital for discission, the exact location of the discission site is discussed with the operating surgeon, so that he is directed to the precise zone of avascularity. The discission is then made, creating an adequate pupillary opening for visual purposes and for ophthalmoscopic visualization of the posterior pole.

The patient continues to use cycloplegic and steroid medication for a period of at least 1 month following discission.

Complications. The most common complication is the production of a marked iritic response in the anterior chamber. This response can lead to elevation of the intraocular pressure over a period of several days to several weeks; this elevation in pressure can be controlled by adequate topical cycloplegic and steroid therapy and carbonic anhydrase inhibitors.

Hemorrhage into the anterior chamber or vitreous at the time of photocoagulation has not occurred but is possible because of the high power density that must be used for coagulation of the vessels within the membrane. Photocoagulation surrounding the hemorrhage site is advised if any hemorrhage occurs at the time of initial treatment.

One must be careful not to perforate the membrane during photocoagulation and thereby transmit the energy to the posterior segment of the eye. The photocoagulation beam should intercept the iridocyclitic membrane at an angle directed away from the macular region.

Corneal burns and disruption of the endothelial surface have been noted, either from direct coagulation by the laser beam or from the heat conducted from the iris to the endothelial surface. The cooling anterior segment photocoagulation contact lens will help to minimize these particular problems.

Follow-up. The patient must be evaluated during the immediate postphotocoagulation period for exacerbation of his iritis or regrowth of blood vessels into the treated iris area. During the immediate postphotocoagulation period, all patients should apply frequent doses of cycloplegics and steroids topically and possibly should be given steroids systemically. Discission should be performed within 1 week following photocoagulation because of the possibility of regrowth of the vessels into the membrane. Topical cycloplegic and steroid therapy should be continued for at least 3 weeks following the discission, and the patient should be seen at biweekly intervals to ensure stabilization of the eye.

Part III

COMPLICATIONS OF OCULAR PHOTOCOAGULATION

Chapter 14

Complications

Ocular photocoagulation, like many special procedures in the practice of medicine, is not without the potential for various types of complications. The complications resulting from photocoagulation can occur relatively infrequently and assume little importance when the proper therapeutic approach is used. Some complications cannot be avoided, but the great majority can be the result of improper diagnostic evaluation of the eye and faulty photocoagulation technique. Complications of argon laser photocoagulation in the various anatomical areas are listed below.

Lids and adnexa: ecchymosis, muscle paresis, retrobulbar hemorrhage, subconjunctival hemorrhage

Cornea: opacification

Iris: sphincter damage, contraction, rupture

Lens: opacification

Vitreous: opacification, contracture

Retina: hemorrhage, contracture, striae, receptor layer damage, nerve fiber layer damage

Optic nerve: neuritis (thermal and ischemic), nerve fiber damage

COMPLICATIONS BY ANATOMICAL AREA

External

Argon laser photocoagulation usually requires no anesthetic other than one used topically, such as proparacaine. In certain patients the proximity of a macular lesion to the fovea, the location of a tuft of neovascularization next to a large retinal vessel, the inability of the patient to maintain fixation, the use of xenon-arc photocoagulation, or the lack of immobility of the eye usually necessitates the use of an injection of 2% lidocaine into the retrobulbar space and the extraocular muscles. Having the patient under adequate akinesia and anesthesia in situations such as these can be most important.

Hemorrhages into the lid, subconjunctivally or intraconjunctivally, can occur and can be minimized by the avoidance of areas with large amounts of vascularity during the actual penetration of the skin or conjunctiva. A retrobulbar hemorrhage or permanent paresis of an extraocular muscle has not been experienced by any of the 2,500 patients treated by this technique, but these complications are possible. The patient is usually warned that ecchymosis of the lid, subconjunctival hemorrhages, and chemosis of the conjunctiva may occur after photocoagulation, but no treatment for these conditions is advocated during the period after treatment.

Cornea

The cornea frequently undergoes punctate erosion of the epithelium during the photocoagulation procedure because of inadvertent abrasion by the plano-suction or three-mirror contact lens and by slight epithelial drying if the contact lens has not been used. Epithelial edema may occur when the contact lens has been used for an extended period, and this edema may interfere with photocoagulation because of the increased beam scatter at the epithelial surface. The problem is not significant, and epithelial repair takes place within 2 days; patching or medication is not required. Because of the potential for epithelial erosion or abrasion during the photocoagulation procedure, photocoagulation should not be considered when a slight conjunctivitis is present.

Defects in the epithelium, embedded foreign bodies, and opacities in the tear film such as mascara, flecks of dust, and face powder can act as nidi for the conversion of light to heat when trapped beneath the contact lens. Severe coagulations of the outer cornea can be produced if these foreign particles are irradiated, and caution should be exercised in this regard.

Stromal cauterization and opacification cannot occur under ordinary circumstances of chorioretinal photocoagulation unless the focus of the beam and the biomicroscope are inadvertently retrofocused on the corneal structures. Corneal burns during retinal photocoagulation have been reported, but these burns were observed only with an experimental instrument. Small corneal coagulations can be observed with the treatment of iris lesions close to the cornea (Fig. 14-1), but this problem can be minimized by the use of the anterior segment photocoagulation lens.

Endothelial damage to the cornea can occur rather easily if the cornea is not examined by biomicroscopy immediately before argon laser photocoagulation. Occasionally, flecks of pigment or tiny blood clots can be deposited on the posterior corneal endothelium, and these particles can absorb sufficient amounts of the argon laser beam to cause focal coagulation of the endothelium and the nearby corneal stroma. Defects in the endothelium that might cause scattering of the laser beam should be noted, since these defects may require the use of much higher energy levels for chorioretinal coagulation. If the laser beam is moved and an area of the cornea without endothelial haze is penetrated, the high power density then impinging on the retina could be sufficient to produce a choroidal or retinal rupture.

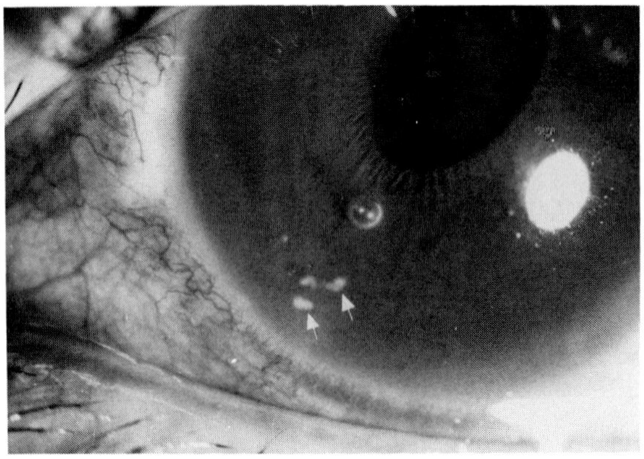

Fig. 14-1. A small corneal coagulation (arrows) observed during the production of an iridotomy by argon laser photocoagulation. The small area of corneal edema cleared within 3 days.

Anterior chamber

The anterior chamber should be free of abnormal amounts of protein (less than 2+ flare) and cells. Particulate matter will scatter the argon beam and requires higher energies for chorioretinal coagulation. Small amounts of heat could be generated in the anterior chamber. In general, photocoagulation should be postponed until any flare, cells, or other anterior chamber accumulations can be reduced or eliminated.

Iris

The excellent visualization systems that have been developed for argon laser photocoagulation and the small diameter of the argon laser beam make it difficult to unintentionally photocoagulate the iris structures. This inadvertent photocoagulation can happen, however, with direct photocoagulation of the more peripheral retinal areas or with the use of the mirror contact lens. Miosis of the pupil usually occurs rather rapidly if the sphincter is struck by the laser beam, and photocoagulation efforts may need to be curtailed. Usually, a 3 × 10 mm ribbon of gelatin sponge (Gelfoam) soaked with phenylephrine 10% and cyclopentolate 2% and placed inside the lower conjunctival cul-de-sac will redilate the pupil in 20 to 30 min. If dilation does not occur, the patient must be rescheduled for several days later and is prescribed homatropine 5% drops and dexamethasone (Decadron) 0.1% drops, both to be put in the affected eye 3 times a day during the interim.

Hemorrhage from the iris usually does not occur with an accidental iris coagulation unless a large amount of rubeosis iridis is present. In this case the hemorrhage can be extensive, delaying further photocoagulation attempts for several weeks. Topical treatment with cycloplegics and steroids is required for these patients. Fig. 14-2 shows a hemorrhage near the iris border that occurred during photomydriasis; it was absorbed within 2 days after treatment.

Lens

The argon laser photocoagulation biomicroscopy delivery system, or any other biomicroscope, should be used to evaluate the patient immediately before photocoagulation so that it can be determined whether cataract formation is present. The type of lenticular opacification should be documented with drawings, since the various types of

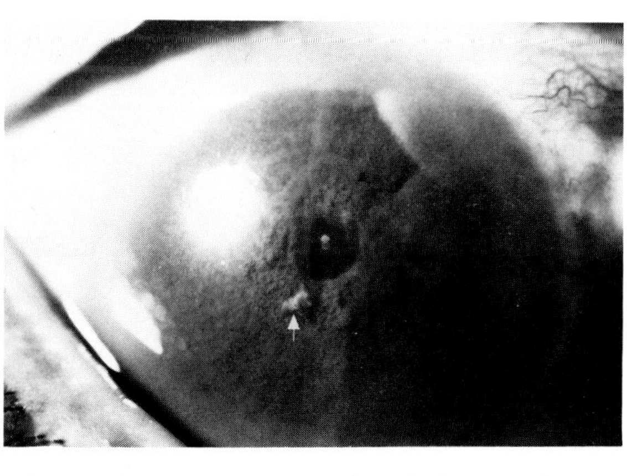

Fig. 14-2. A small iris hemorrhage (arrow) produced during photomydriasis. The region around the iris hemorrhage was coagulated, and the hemorrhage disappeared completely within 48 hr.

cataracts affect the argon laser beam differently. For instance, a peripheral cortical lenticular wedge opacity could diffuse a portion of the argon beam, creating a wedge of darkness in the image of the argon laser beam on the chorioretinal surface. For this reason the appearance of the argon target beam on the chorioretinal surface should be observed closely. Larger cortical wedge opacities may diffuse the laser beam completely, thereby thwarting photocoagulation attempts. However, the greatest hazard occurs when one fails to recognize this problem and increases the power so that a satisfactory chorioretinal coagulation can be made. If the beam is then moved off the cortical wedge and photocoagulation is applied, the tremendous increase in power striking the retina can cause a variety of complications, including a disastrous vitreal hemorrhage.

Nuclear sclerotic lenses tend to scatter the beam in a uniform manner and therefore require additional power for adequate retinal coagulation. This factor can usually be controlled and has not been hazardous. The lens itself, because of its yellow color, also absorbs a portion of the beam, but studies in my laboratory indicate that the formation of additional lenticular opacification from this absorption cannot be produced with corneal entrance powers less than **1.5 w** when used with spot sizes greater than **100μ** in diameter.

Blood, pigment, or other debris on either the anterior or posterior surface of the lens should be noted during the initial examination. These areas should be avoided during photocoagulation since small localized opacifications of the lens can occur, and have been produced in animal studies, because of the marked conversion of light to heat by these absorbent particles.

Vitreous

The vitreous body should also be examined thoroughly by biomicroscopy and ophthalmoscopy before argon laser photocoagulation. The location of clumps of pigment or blood and the diffuse infiltration of erythrocytes, leukocytes, or other debris should be noted carefully. Leukocytes and debris usually scatter the beam or deflect it sufficiently to require higher powers for retinal coagulation. Once the beam has been moved off the

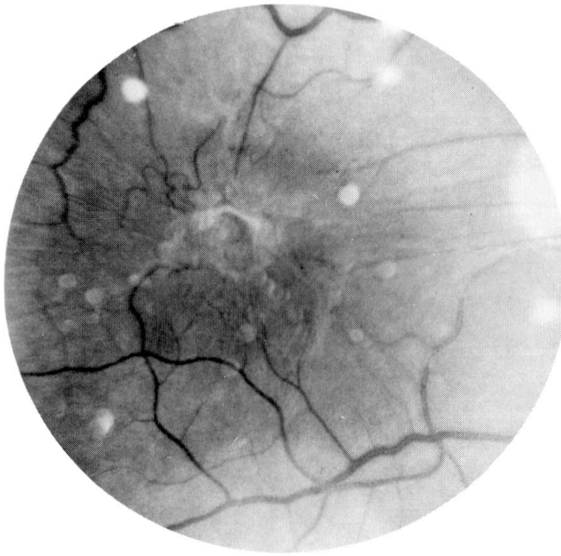

Fig. 14-3. A typical macular pucker occasionally observed after extensive xenon-arc photocoagulation.

opacification, a much larger power density is then available for chorioretinal coagulation and possibly extensive destruction. Clumps of blood in the vitreous will absorb the beam and create a small intravitreal coagulation around the nidus of absorption. These clumps of blood can hinder future photocoagulation efforts and contribute to generalized vitreous contraction.

Diffuse vitreous blood will also absorb the argon laser beam and may contribute to degradation of the vitreous structure. Photocoagulation should not be attempted if the lesion to be photocoagulated cannot be seen well by direct ophthalmoscopy. Photocoagulation should be deferred until the vitreous body has cleared sufficiently for this observation, so that the possibility of vitreous contraction is minimized.

Vitreous traction on the macula, producing macular pucker, has not been observed in my series of patients, but it has been mentioned by some observers (Fig. 14-3). The judicious use of argon laser energy for patients whose eyes have been thoroughly evaluated in regard to vitreous opacification should result in no complications in most patients because of the extremely small amount of argon energy usually necessary for the proper

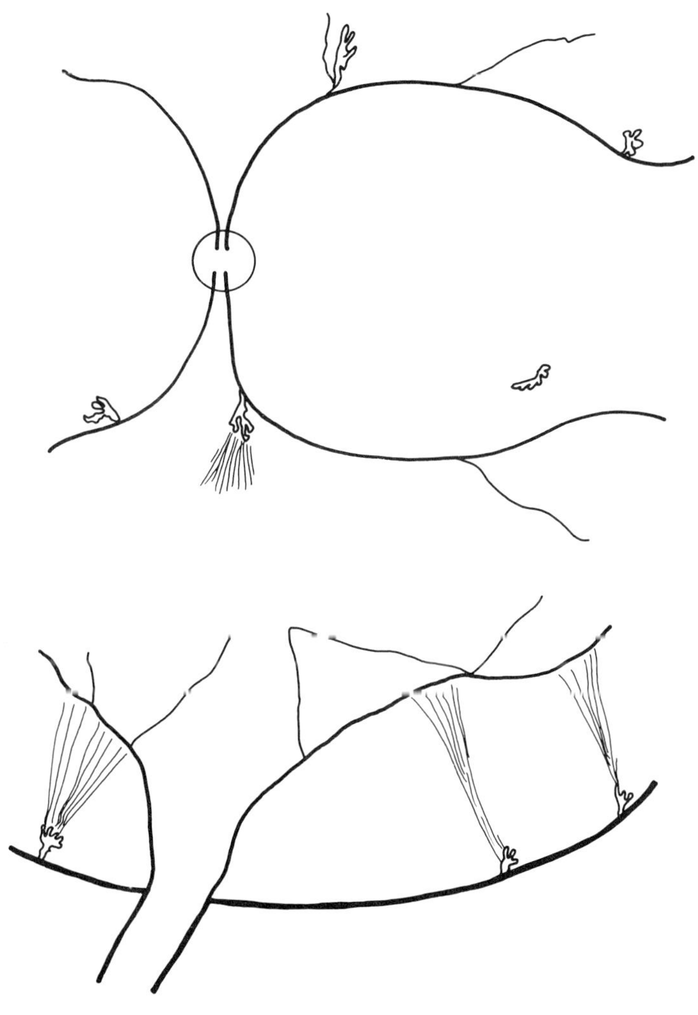

Fig. 14-4. Sagittal and direct appearance of the posterior hyaloid membrane highly detached from the retinal surface. Small neovascular growths extend from the retinal surface toward the vitreous along the vitreoretinal footplates.

coagulation of chorioretinal lesions. The condition of the vitreous body in all photocoagulation cases, and especially in diabetic retinopathy, should be evaluated carefully. The presence of tenting of the vitreous base or retinal structures in the midperiphery or posterior polar region should alert the observer to the partial collapse and contraction of the vitreous body. The posterior hyaloid should be examined in relation to the internal limiting membrane, and an effort should be made to determine whether the posterior hyaloid is shallowly or highly detached from the retinal surface.

A highly detached posterior hyaloid can usually be identified, since the areas of neovascularization from the retina can be seen to climb directly toward the central vitreous along footplates from the posterior hyaloid to the retinal surface (Fig. 14-4; see also Fig. 7-39). Similarly, neovascularization from the optic nerve usually grows along the lattice work provided by the posterior hyaloid into the central vitreous (see Fig. 7-36). Photocoagulation directly to the neovascularization can be attempted in these patients without large amounts of refluxed heat affecting the posterior hyaloid surface.

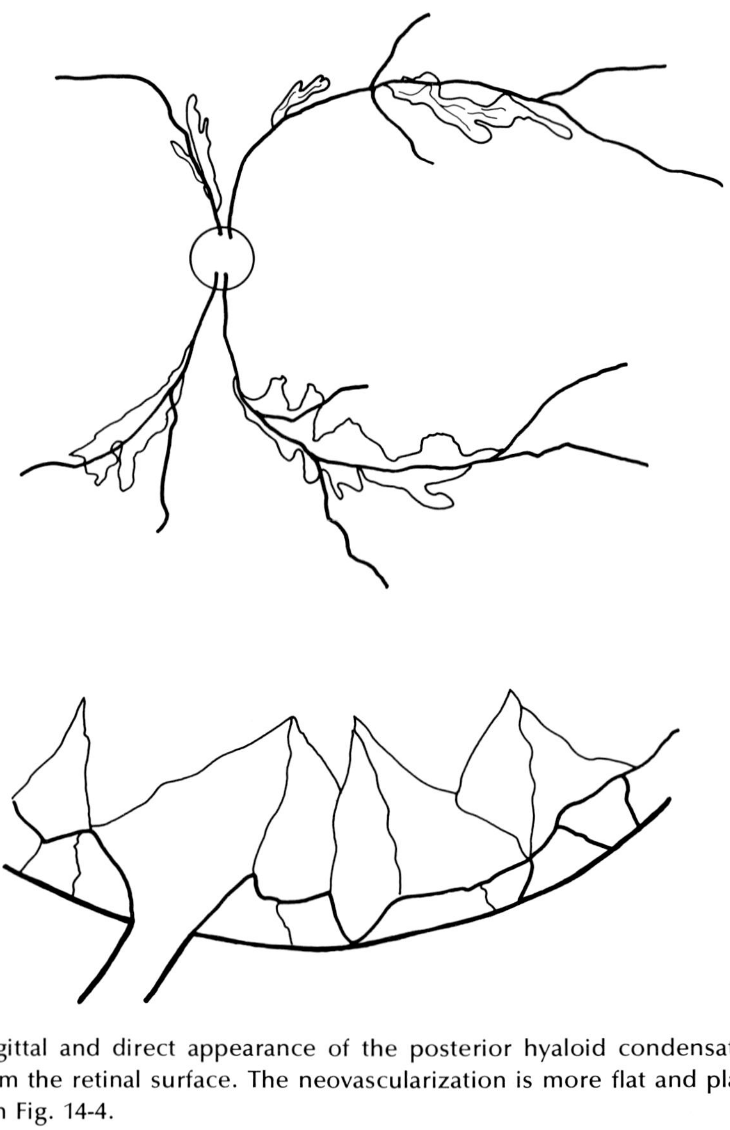

Fig. 14-5. Sagittal and direct appearance of the posterior hyaloid condensation shallowly detached from the retinal surface. The neovascularization is more flat and plateaulike than that shown in Fig. 14-4.

A shallowly detached posterior hyaloid is usually present with the peripapillary type of neovascularization and with the type of retinovitreal or surface neovascularization that can form a shelf or plateau along the vascular arcades (Fig. 14-5). This plateau of neovascularization may be closely approximated to the retinal surface and may curl into the vitreous at its most distal margins (Figs. 14-6 to 14-8). Photocoagulation of this type of neovascularization can seriously affect the nearby posterior hyaloid, causing additional contracture and

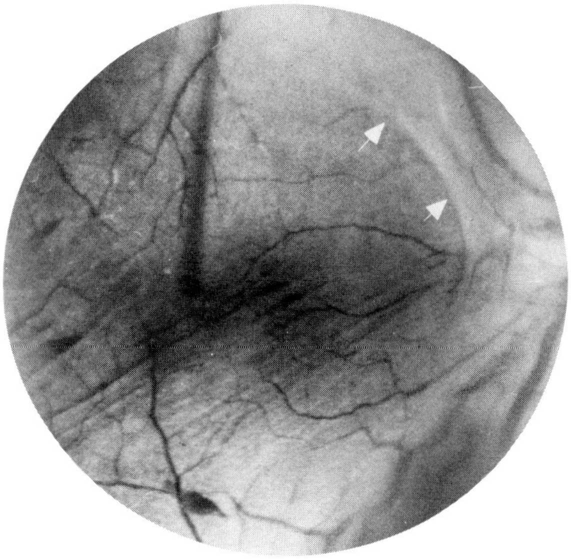

Fig. 14-6. Early crescent-shaped glial proliferation (arrows) along a shallowly detached posterior hyaloid extending a short distance from the optic disc. Note marked macular striae.

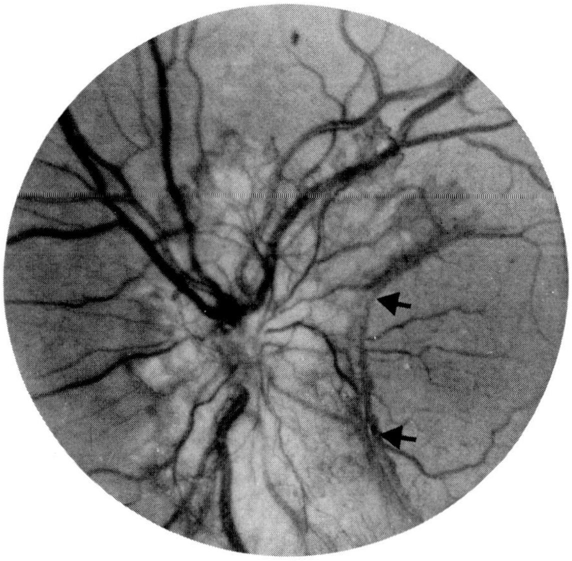

Fig. 14-7. More extensive neovascularization than that shown in Fig. 14-6 and early gliosis (arrows) of a shallowly detached posterior hyaloid extending from the optic disc region in a scepter-shaped crescent.

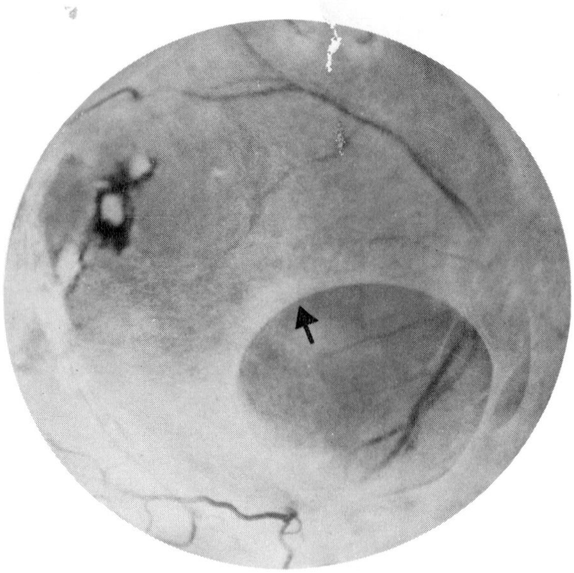

Fig. 14-8. Marked glial overgrowth and proliferation along the shallowly detached posterior hyaloid over the surface of the retina, obscuring many retinal details and preventing photocoagulation intervention. The macular region is blocked by a glial canopy (arrow).

possibly sufficient traction to precipitate a generalized retinal detachment. Photocoagulation should not be attempted in these particular cases because of the strong possibility of severe damage to the posterior hyaloid structure.

Retina

The most common complication of retinal photocoagulation is hemorrhage from small or large retinal vessels (Fig. 14-9) and occasionally from the choroidal vasculature (Fig. 14-10). Large-vessel rupture from the primary arteriole or venules along the arcades has not occurred in several years, because these vessels have been treated with lower power densities. The treatment of small nests of neovascularization has resulted in the occurrence of occasional hemorrhages, but these hemorrhages have never been significant (see Fig. 7-45, **B**). The power level needed to obliterate these areas of small-vessel formation is usually higher than the individual tolerance of some of the smaller vessels, and rupture of these vessels does infrequently occur. Larger spot sizes minimize this problem because of the increased area of coagulation produced, but hemorrhages from the very small vessels may still be observed.

A traction retinal detachment can occur if areas of glial proliferation or vitreoretinal adhesion are incorrectly evaluated. An eye with Grade 3 or 4, and usually Grade 2, vitreoretinal traction should not be treated with photocoagulation. Similarly, eyes with Grades 3 and 4 glial proliferation should not be considered for photocoagulation. In these cases the small amount of heat generated by the photocoagulation energy passing through the ocular media could be sufficient to cause further shrinkage of the vitreous body and subsequent retinal detachment.

Retinal striae may occur when photocoagulation produces a large area of scar formation (see Fig. 7-45, **C**). This problem can be difficult to avoid, but in general, high power densities should not be employed in the macular and paramacular areas because of the possible formation of excessive scar tissue.

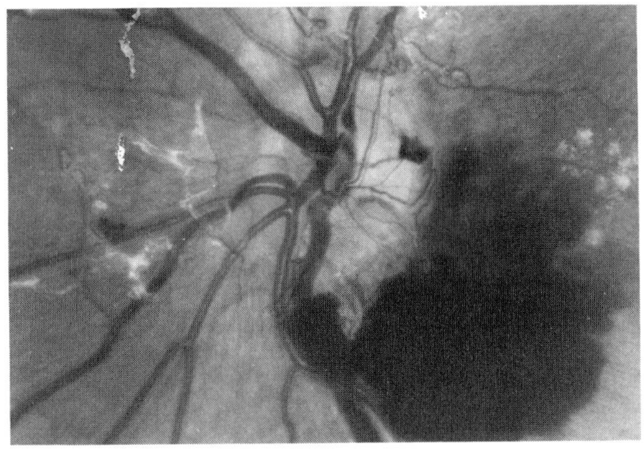

Fig. 14-9. A hemorrhage from the optic nerve region after inadvertent rupture of an area of neovascularization by argon laser photocoagulation.

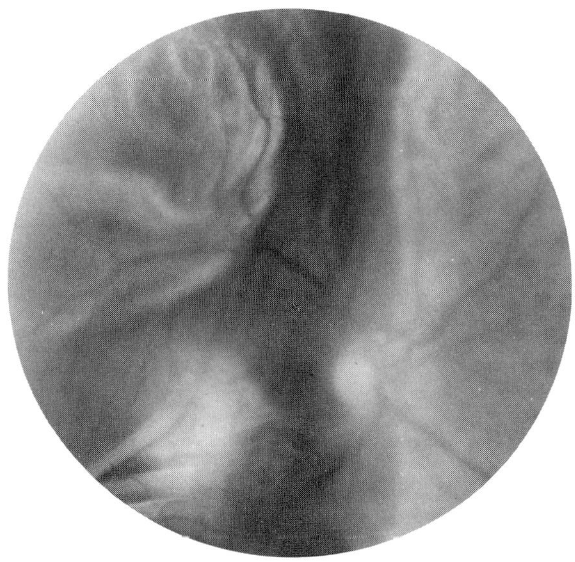

Fig. 14-10. A disastrous choroidal hemorrhage secondary to rupture of a choroidal vessel by an intense argon laser photocoagulation impact.

In general, photocoagulation into the macular area should not approach with 500μ of the umbo, because heat may be transmitted through the pigment epithelium or choroid into the central foveolar region. If blood occurs underneath the retina in the foveal region, photocoagulation should not be attempted within $1{,}000\mu$ (⅔ DD) of the umbo because of the distinct possibility that heat could be conducted easily through the blood layer to the foveolar zone. Preretinal clots and other areas of diffuse blood in the retrohyaloid space should also be avoided because of the localized production of heat and the possibility of increased conduction of the heat to the macular and perifoveal zone.

The photocoagulation of temporally located papillovitreal or retinovitreal fronds should be approached with great caution. The retinal areas lying behind the point of focus on the frond should be examined carefully to avoid the macular region. It has also been noted that the more highly developed frond extending far into the vitreous can be treated more safely

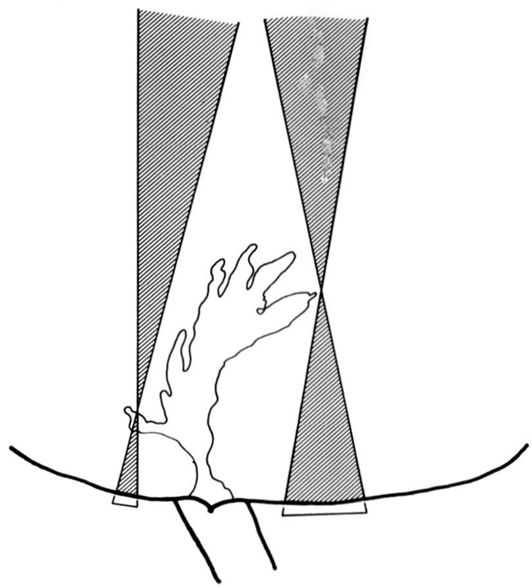

Fig. 14-11. Retinal areas behind highly extended fronds should be examined carefully for vital structures. The coagulating energy will expand over a greater area when the coagulation focus is farther into the vitreous, resulting in a decreased retinal power density.

because of the less hazardous background retinal absorption density of the stray energy. In these cases the divergence of the coagulating beam from the tip of the highly extended frond toward the retina is expanded over a greater area than with a frond closely approximated to the retina (Fig. 14-11).

Optic nerve

The optic nerve can be damaged in three ways: by thermal damage, by ischemic damage, or by an extremely high power flux density.

Thermal damage can occur when an attempt is made to photocoagulate a large vessel on the optic nerve head; this vessel absorbs the argon laser beam, producing a great amount of heat, which can cause coagulation necrosis of the nerve fiber layer. Furthermore, the peripapillary zone should not be treated if there are large accumulations of pigmented tissue or if there is choroidal or retinal neovascularization. These areas provide an effective nidus for the conversion of light energy to heat energy, resulting in possible secondary disruption of the overlying nerve fibers. It has been shown that the receptor elements usually are destroyed and the pigmented tissue proliferated in a previously photocoagulated area, so that a large amount of heat may be produced with additional photocoagulation, resulting in destruction of the much more closely approximated nerve fiber layer (Fig. 14-12). Argon laser photocoagulation can usually be applied in the peripapillary or maculopapillary bundle region without complication during the first photocoagulation, but a previously treated area should be avoided unless the procedure is done during a period less than 4 days after the initial photocoagulation. During this interval the previously produced retinal and pigment epithelial edema protects against the additional production of large amounts of heat.

The second way that damage to the optic nerve can occur is through the creation of an ischemic optic neuritis. A considerable portion of the blood supply to the optic nerve

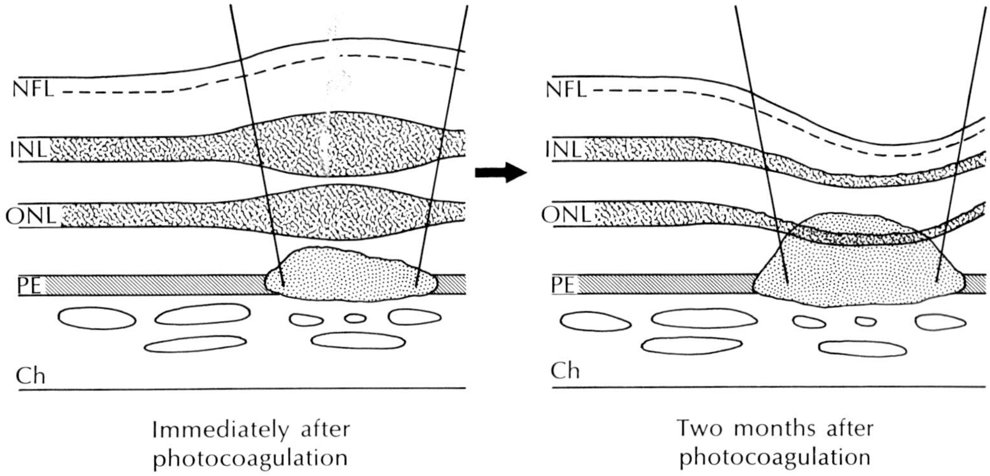

Fig. 14-12. Edema of the retinal layers during the period immediately after photocoagulation (left) protects the more distant nerve fiber layer from heat produced in the pigment epithelial layer during subsequent photocoagulation sessions within 4 days of the initial session. Two months after photocoagulation (right) the nerve fiber layer is much closer to the hypertrophied pigment epithelial layer because of the destruction of the outer retinal elements. Photocoagulation at this time under these circumstances could result in serious nerve fiber layer damage.

comes from the choroid and can be completely eliminated by heavy coagulations in the peripapillary region. The small amounts of nourishment coming from the retinal vessels in the anterior portion of the optic nerve can also be eliminated by direct and continual photocoagulation in this area. My experience has been that the optic nerve is resistant to repeated episodes of argon laser photocoagulation, but these factors must still be considered.

The third way that nerve fibers on the optic nerve head can be destroyed is through the inadvertent use of extremely small spot sizes with high power settings. The power density thus created at the photocoagulation site is sufficient to disrupt the nerve fibers, regardless of the presence of any absorbing substance. In my laboratory it has been possible to incise teeth and bone with focused argon laser beams of extremely high power density, and the same condition could possibly be reproduced by the inadvertent use of very high laser beam power densities on the optic disc region. Accordingly, input powers should not exceed 350 mw with a 0.1-sec exposure and spot sizes of **100μ** diameter or less.

GENERAL CONSIDERATIONS

It is most important to realize that a reduction of the diameter of the retinal impact spot size by one half while the corneal entrance power and exposure time remain constant increases the retinal power density by a factor of four (Fig. 14-13). However, since one is dealing with a biologic medium and since a smaller coagulation can be cooled more rapidly by conduction than a larger spot (see Fig. 2-13), the coagulative effect for a 4$\times$ increase in retinal power density may actually be less than 3$\times$. For example, the intensity of the coagulation produced by a 100μ diameter spot is usually less than 3 times that produced by a 200μ diameter spot with a similar power level and exposure. Therefore, when one reduces the spot size by one half, one should also reduce the corneal entrance power of the laser by at least a factor of three.

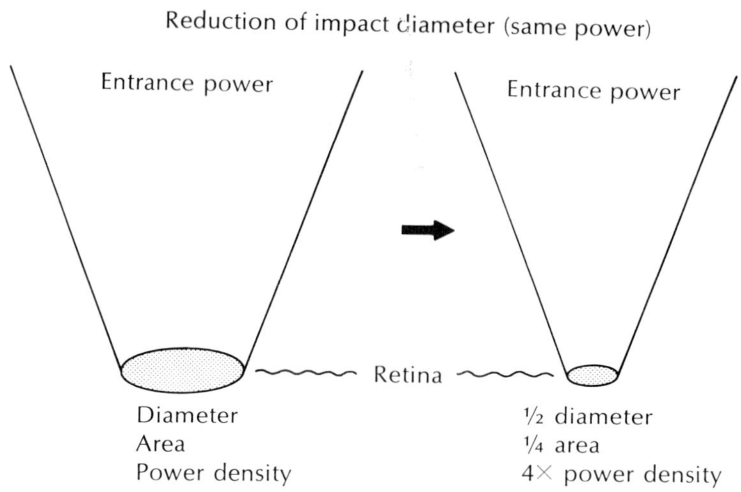

Fig. 14-13. A reduction in beam diameter by one half will increase the power density by a factor of four if the entrance power remains the same. When the spot size is reduced, the entrance power must also be reduced considerably to maintain the proper power density.

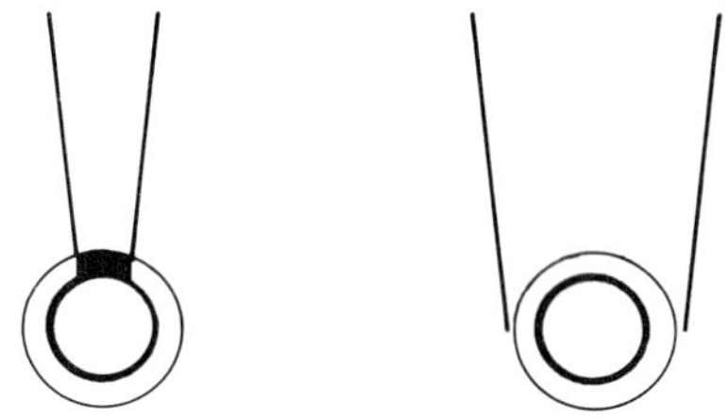

Fig. 14-14. Attenuated target beam size must be adjusted to be larger than the largest vessel to be treated (right) to obviate the coagulation necrosis of the vessel wall (left) that could result from a small localized impact.

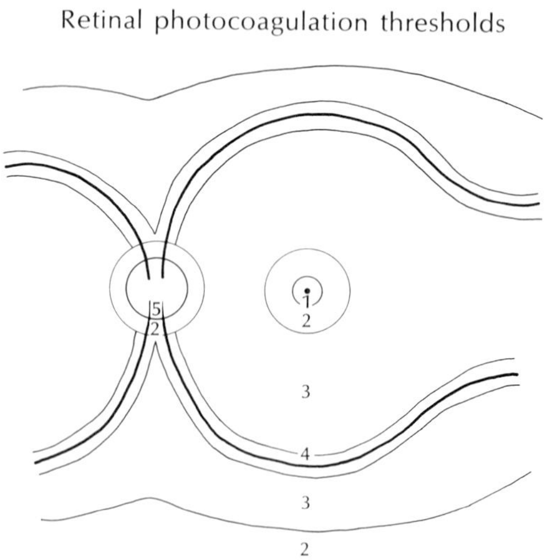

Fig. 14-15. Retinal areas of high *(1)* to low *(5)* sensitivity to ocular photocoagulation. Initial power settings must be adjusted accordingly in these various areas.

Retinal vessel rupture can also result from the treatment of the retinal vessel by a very small laser beam spot with a high power level. A portion of the vessel wall, rather than the entire vessel, can actually be coagulated, and rupture of that vessel wall can occur. It is therefore advisable to treat a vessel with a coagulation spot size that is slightly larger than the vessel (Fig. 14-14). This technique will create a more uniform blood column and vessel wall coagulation without spotty coagulation of the vessel wall itself.

Hemorrhages have resulted when photocoagulation has been directed from one point of the fundus to another area of greater pigmentation, thinner retinal tissue, thinner choroidal tissue, or decreased thermal diffusion capability. Fig. 14-15 gives the different degrees of sensitivity of the various retinal areas to ocular photocoagulation. Area #1 in the foveal and perifoveal area is most sensitive to laser photocoagulation because of less heat diffusion into the thinner overlying retina, the larger amount of pigment in the pigment epithelial cells, and the concentration of xanthophyll in the inner retinal layers. The macular region, area #2, is also quite sensitive to argon laser radiation because of the hyperpigmentation and increased heat-producing capability of the pigment epithelium. The peripapillary zone can also be markedly sensitive to the argon laser beam because of the proximity of the overlying nerve fibers to large clumps of pigment at the border of the optic disc; these clumps of pigment can provide an efficient nidus for the production of heat. The intermediate zones, #3, represent areas of average pigmentation and retinal thickness and usually allow a uniform coagulation. Variations in pigment density in the pigment epithelium and choroid should be evaluated, and appropriate adjustments of argon laser power should be made. The paravascular areas, #4, are moderately resistant to argon laser radiation because of the thickness of the retina in these zones. The most resistant tissue is the optic nerve itself, #5, which can resist relatively high power densities, provided that absorbing pigments such as blood and melanin are not present.

The possible complications that could be encountered during argon laser photocoagulation have been reviewed. Suggestions about argon laser photocoagulation technique and the evaluation process have been made so that the complication rate can be reduced and hazardous conditions that might be present can be avoided. The observance of anticomplication procedures and the compliance to previously described photocoagulation techniques should render argon laser photocoagulation a safe and effective method for the treatment of various ocular abnormalities.

Part IV

DIAGNOSTIC AND FUTURE THERAPEUTIC INSTRUMENTATION

Chapter 15

Adjunctive diagnostic examinations

FLUORESCEIN ANGIOGRAPHY

Intravenous fluorescein angiography has been available for the study of posterior segment diseases since its introduction in 1961. It has thus been possible to study chorioretinal diseases with the use of advanced photoelectrical devices and rapid sequential photography. This particular technique is a useful diagnostic aid in the evaluation of fundus diseases, particularly those involving the macular region. It has also served as a guide for the treatment of various chorioretinal vascular diseases affecting the posterior polar area. This section provides a classification of abnormal fundus fluorescence, as demonstrated in the fundus fluorescein angiogram, based on the work of Yannuzzi. Hyperfluorescence and hypofluorescence can be traced to the etiologic defect by utilizing the flow-sheet method devised by Schatz (Fig. 15-1).

Normal fundus fluorescein angiogram

The normal fundus fluorescein angiogram may be considered to consist essentially of two circulations, the retinal and choroidal, separated by a barrier of irregular density, the retinal pigment epithelium. The retinal pigment epithelium is most effective in the region of the macula as a barrier to the underlying fluorescence produced by the fluorescein-laden blood in the choroid. The relatively dark macular region present in the normal angiogram is caused by the macular pigment xanthophyll and the parafoveolar retinal capillary-free zone present in that region. In the normal fundus the choroidal vessels fill before the retinal vessels fill; therefore, the first change noticed in the angiogram after intravenous administration of fluorescein is a diffuse, patchy background fluorescence called the choroidal flush, which is followed almost immediately by the retinal vascular phases.

Abnormal fluorescence

Abnormal fluorescence can be classified in the following manner:

I. Blocked fluorescence
II. Transmitted fluorescence
III. Abnormal vascular fluorescence
   A. Permeability defects (leaks)
      1. Pooling
      2. Staining
   B. New and anomalous vessels
   C. Filling defects
IV. Pseudofluorescence
   A. Early pseudofluorescence
   B. Late pseudofluorescence

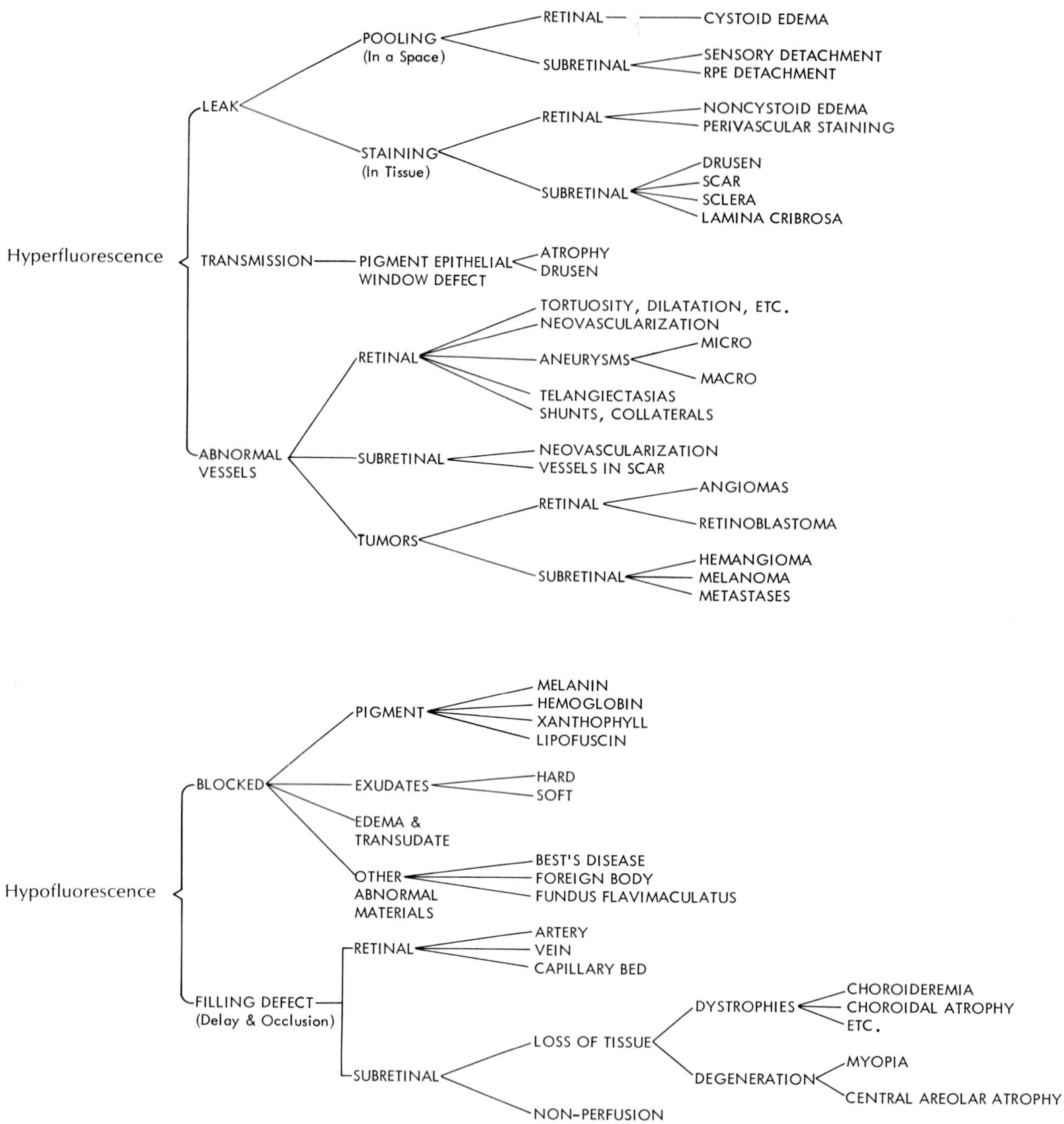

Fig. 15-1. Flow-sheet method to trace abnormal fluorescence to the etiologic defect.

A

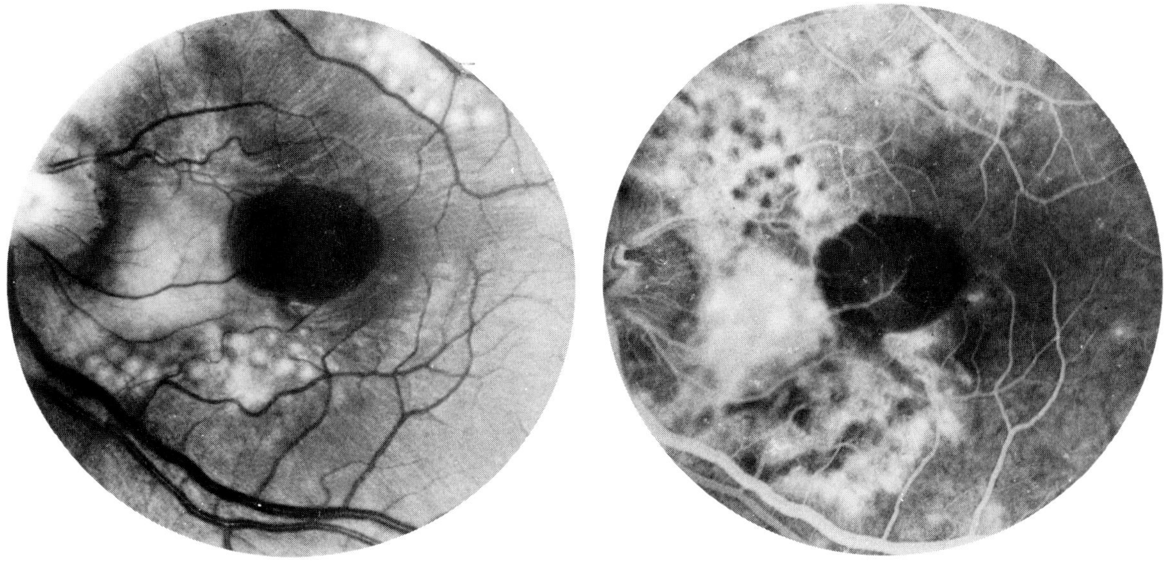

B

Fig. 15-2. A, Macular region of a patient with histoplasmosis, showing a subretinal hemorrhage and argon laser photocoagulations above and below. Considerable gliosis can be seen around the optic disc. **B,** Fluorogram showing blocked fluorescence by the central hemorrhage, areas of gliosis, and recent argon laser photocoagulations.

A

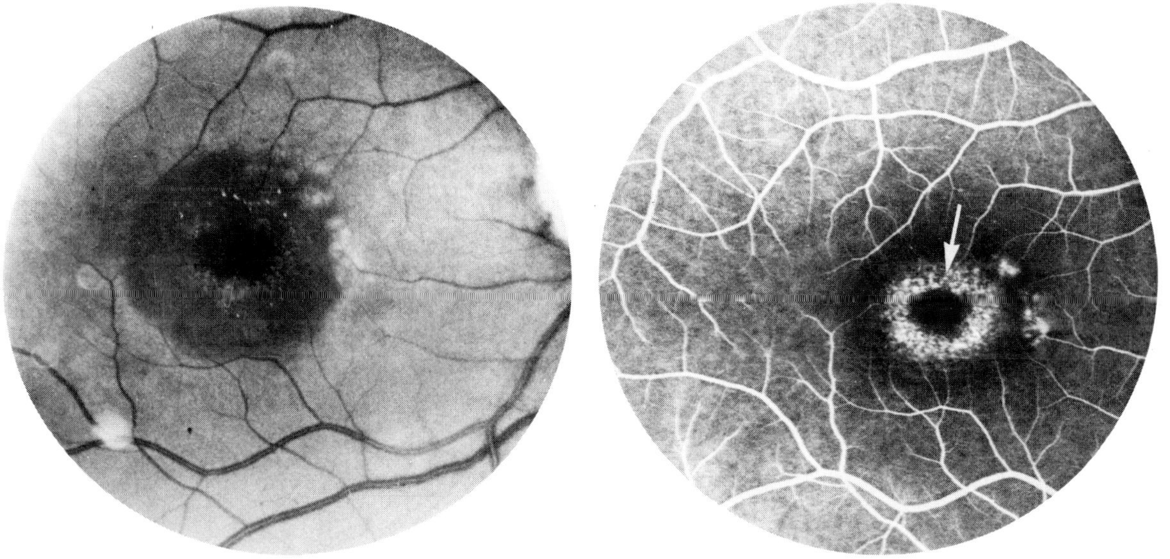

B

Fig. 15-3. A, Macular region of a 28-year-old man with chloroquine retinopathy, showing a typical bull's-eye pattern in the perifoveal region. **B,** Fluorogram showing obvious transmitted fluorescence from the choroid through the diseased pigment epithelium (arrow).

Blocked fluorescence

Blocked fluorescence occurs when tissue or fluid barriers lie between the fluorescing area and the film plane (Fig. 15-2). Hyperproliferation of the pigment epithelium or pigment in the retina, as well as tumors and blood, produce blocked fluorescence by obscuring the normal fluorescence produced by the choroidal or retinal circulation. Subretinal fluid, retinal exudates, and the coagulum from photocoagulation may also produce blocked fluorescence by obscuring the underlying choroidal pattern. Preretinal blood can block fluorescence, as can large vitreal opacities, particularly if they are lying close to the inner surface of the retina.

Transmitted fluorescence

Transmitted fluorescence occurs when there is a defect in the retinal pigment epithelium that allows fluorescence from the underlying choroidal circulation to be transmitted through the retina to the camera (Fig. 15-3). The characteristics of transmitted fluorescence are: (1) the appearance of fluorescence in the posterior pole coincidental with the initial choroidal filling, (2) persistence of the size and shape of the fluorescent region during the middle phases of the angiogram, and (3) disappearance of the fluorescent region from the angiogram when the fluorescein leaves the choroidal circulation (Fig. 15-4). The defects in the retinal pigment epithelium can occur from any inflammatory, traumatic, neoplastic, or other disease state that would affect the density of pigment and the thickness of the pigment epithelium.

Abnormal vascular fluorescence

Permeability defects (leaks). The retinal vasculature is normally impermeable to fluorescein and will conduct fluorescein through the retinal vascular channels without leakage into the retinal tissue. Choroidal vessels are normally permeable to fluorescein, but fluorescein does not enter the retinal tissue because of the impermeable barrier, the

A

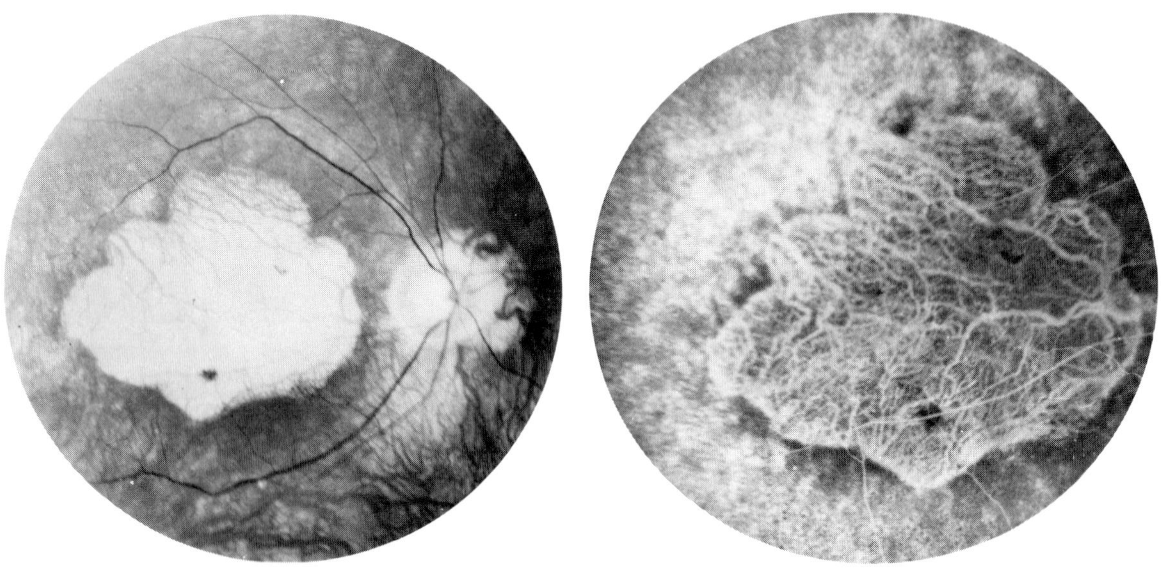

B

Fig. 15-4. A, A large pigment epithelial defect in the macular and paramacular region, showing the underlying choroidal vessels. **B,** Fluorogram showing the prominent choroidal vascular pattern transmitted through the absent pigment epithelial region.

retinal pigment epithelium. This layer prevents the fluorescence that freely flows from the choriocapillaris through Bruch's membrane from gaining entrance to the subretinal space or the retina, presumably because of the tight zonula occludens present between normal pigment epithelial cells. Primary disorders of the choroid or alterations in Bruch's membrane combined with defects in the retinal pigment epithelium, or both, serve to break down the normal chorioretinal barrier to fluorescein. When the fluorescein leaks into an anatomical space, such as the subsensory retinal or subretinal pigment epithelial region, it is specifically referred to as pooling.

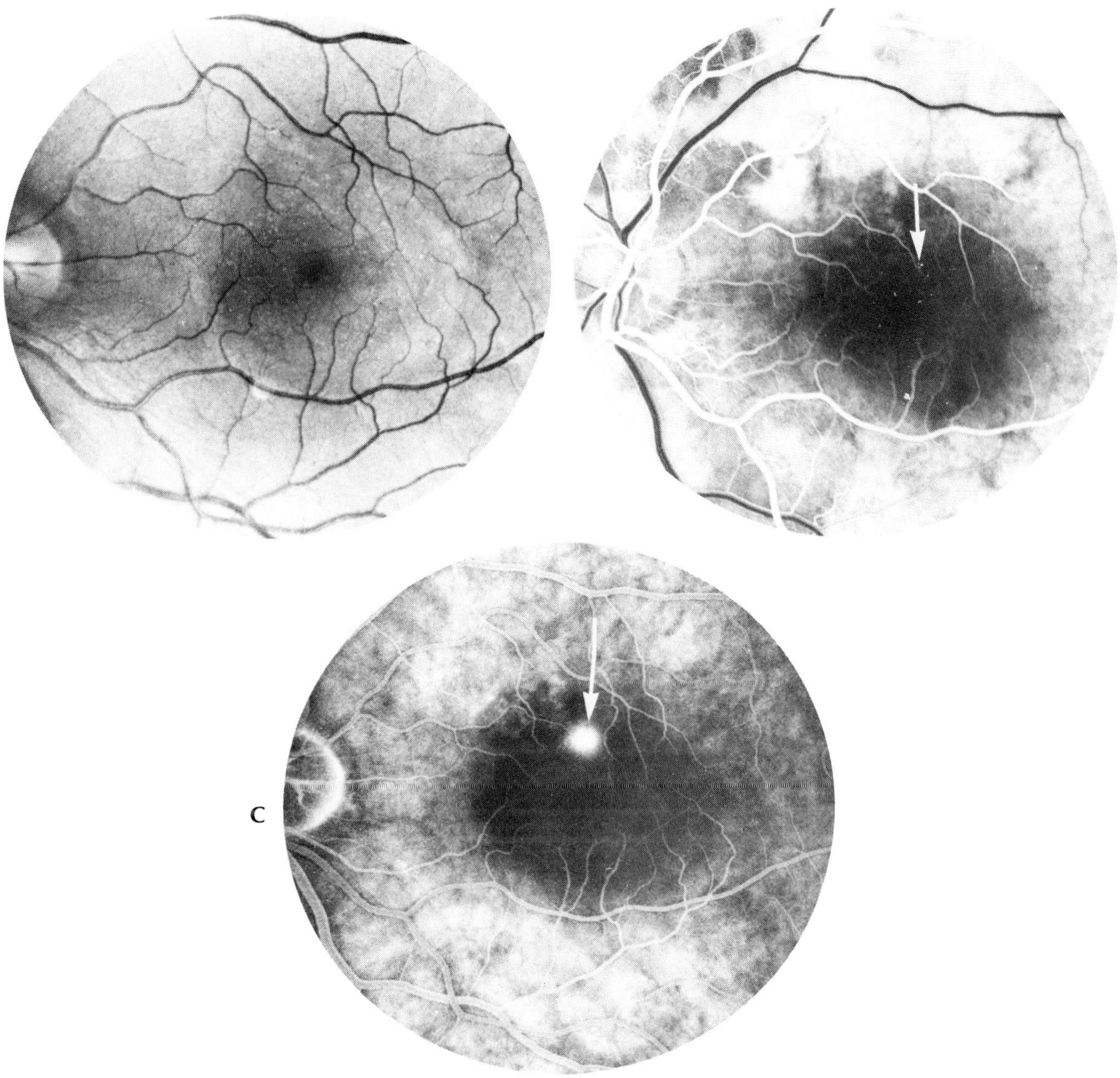

Fig. 15-5. A, A typical central serous choroidopathy and large serous detachment of the sensory retina in a 37-year-old patient. **B,** Fluorogram during the late arteriolar phase, showing very early leakage above the foveal region (arrow). **C,** Fluorogram during the venular phase, showing marked leakage of the dye from the pigment epithelial defect (arrow) and pooling in the subretinal space.

A 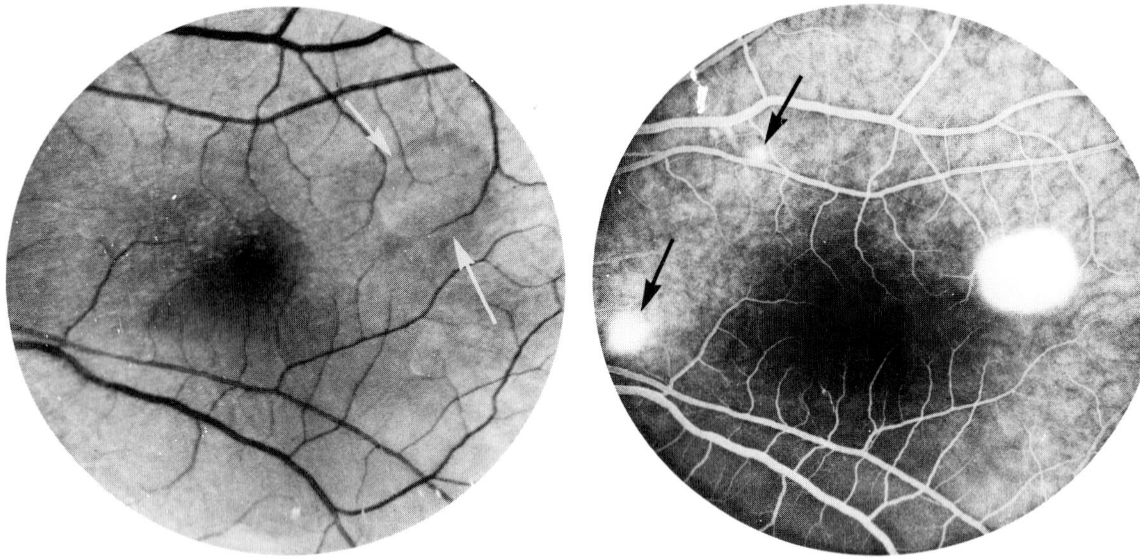 B

Fig. 15-6. A, Metamorphopsia and a serous detachment of the pigment epithelium temporal to the macular region (arrows) in a 42-year-old man. **B,** Fluorogram showing marked pooling of the fluorescein dye in the serous detachment temporal to the fovea and in the two other smaller serous detachments (arrows) in the nasal macular area.

A 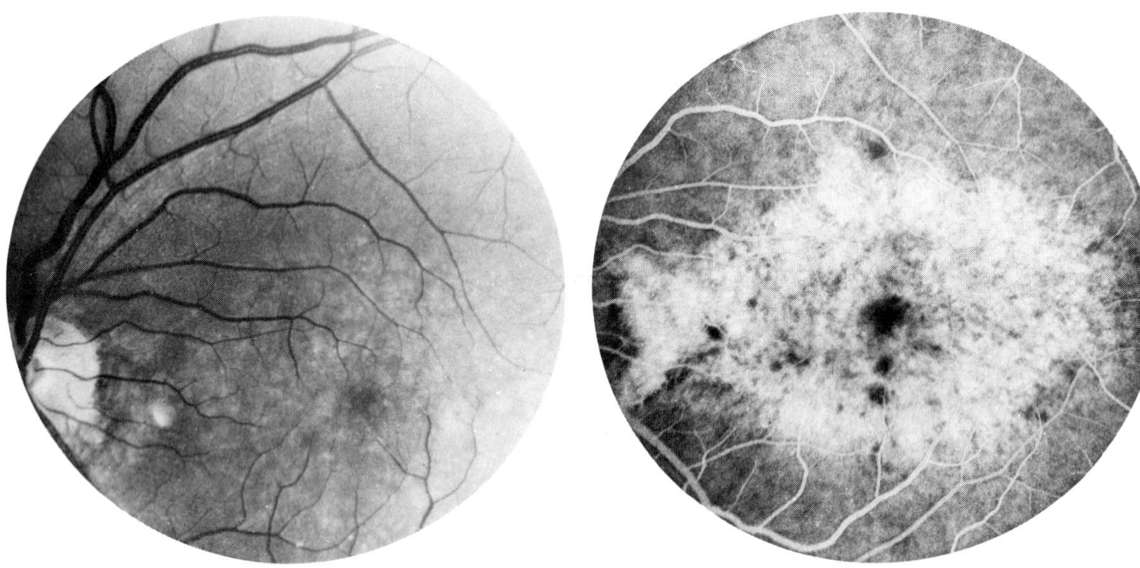 B

Fig. 15-7. A, Macular region of a 22-year-old man with Stargardt's maculopathy. **B,** Fluorogram showing areas of gliosis and marked fluorescein staining of the diseased pigment epithelial region.

A 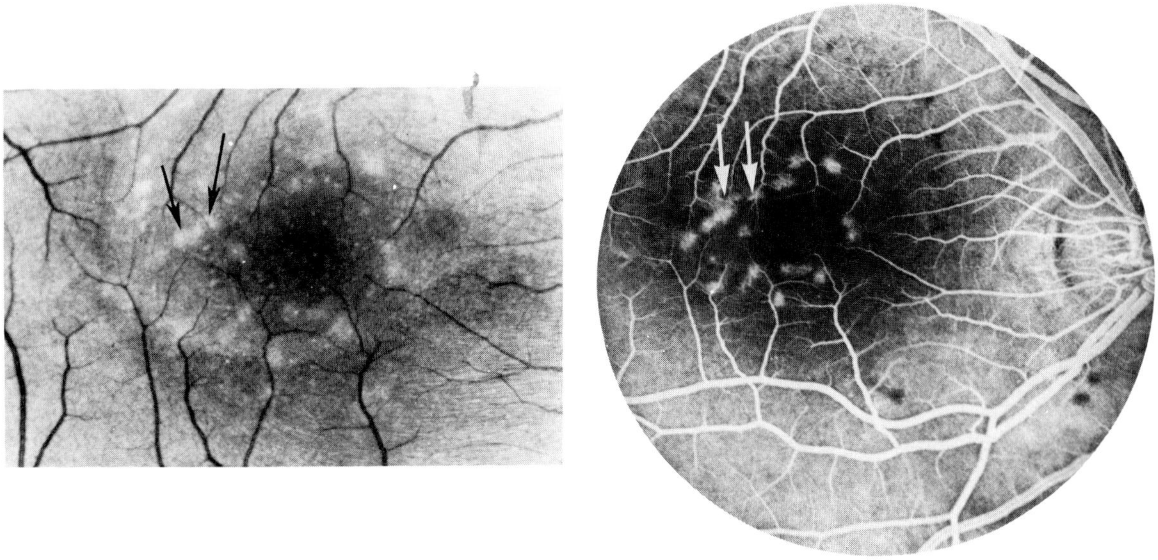 B

Fig. 15-8. A, Small photocoagulation scars in the perifoveal area (arrows) of a 27-year-old patient who was treated with ruby laser photocoagulation for multiple pigment epithelial defects and central serous choroidopathy. **B,** Fluorogram showing obvious staining of the small chorioretinal scars produced by the ruby laser photocoagulations (arrows).

A 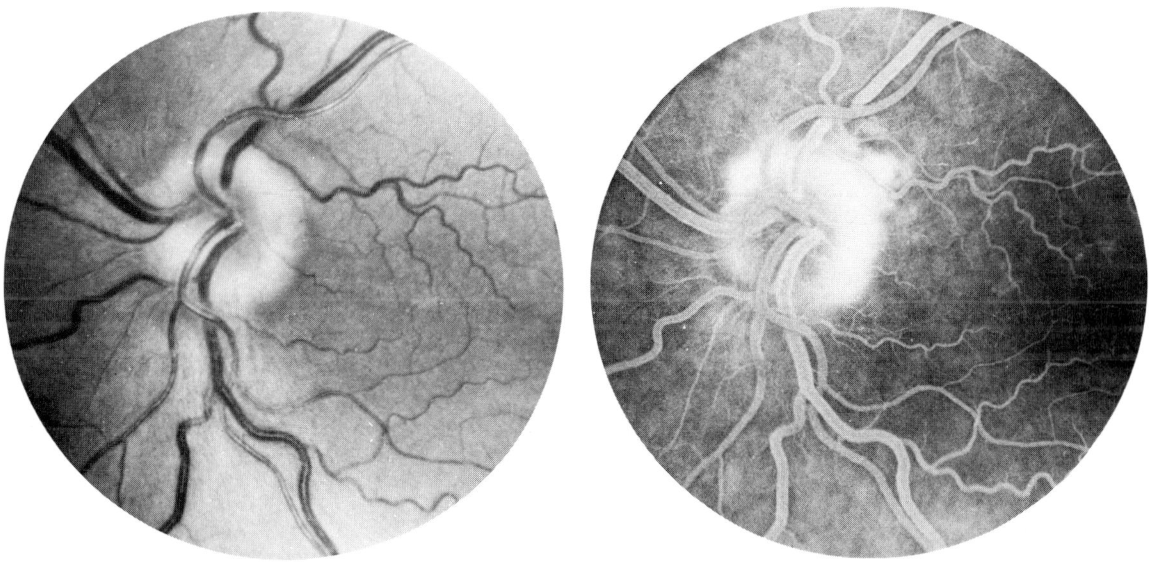 B

Fig. 15-9. A, Drusen of the optic nerve head associated with a small sector field defect in a 19-year-old man. **B,** Fluorogram showing staining of the drusen of the optic nerve region.

Pooling. Pooling is characterized by: (1) a minimal accumulation of the dye in the early phases of the angiogram because of the slow inflow of the fluorescein from the intravascular space to the pooling area; (2) an increase in the intensity of the fluorescence, and occasionally in the size and shape of the fluorescing region during the later phases of the angiogram as the concentration of the dye increases in the anatomical space; and (3) the persistence of fluorescence because of the fluorescein trapped in the pooling area after the choroidal and retinal circulations have been cleared of the dye (Fig. 15-5).

Areas of pooling may become poorly defined or smudged in the later phases of the angiogram. Solitary transmitted defects that do not change until their disappearance usually show sharply demarcated edges without the smudgy appearance noted with pooling defects (Fig. 15-6).

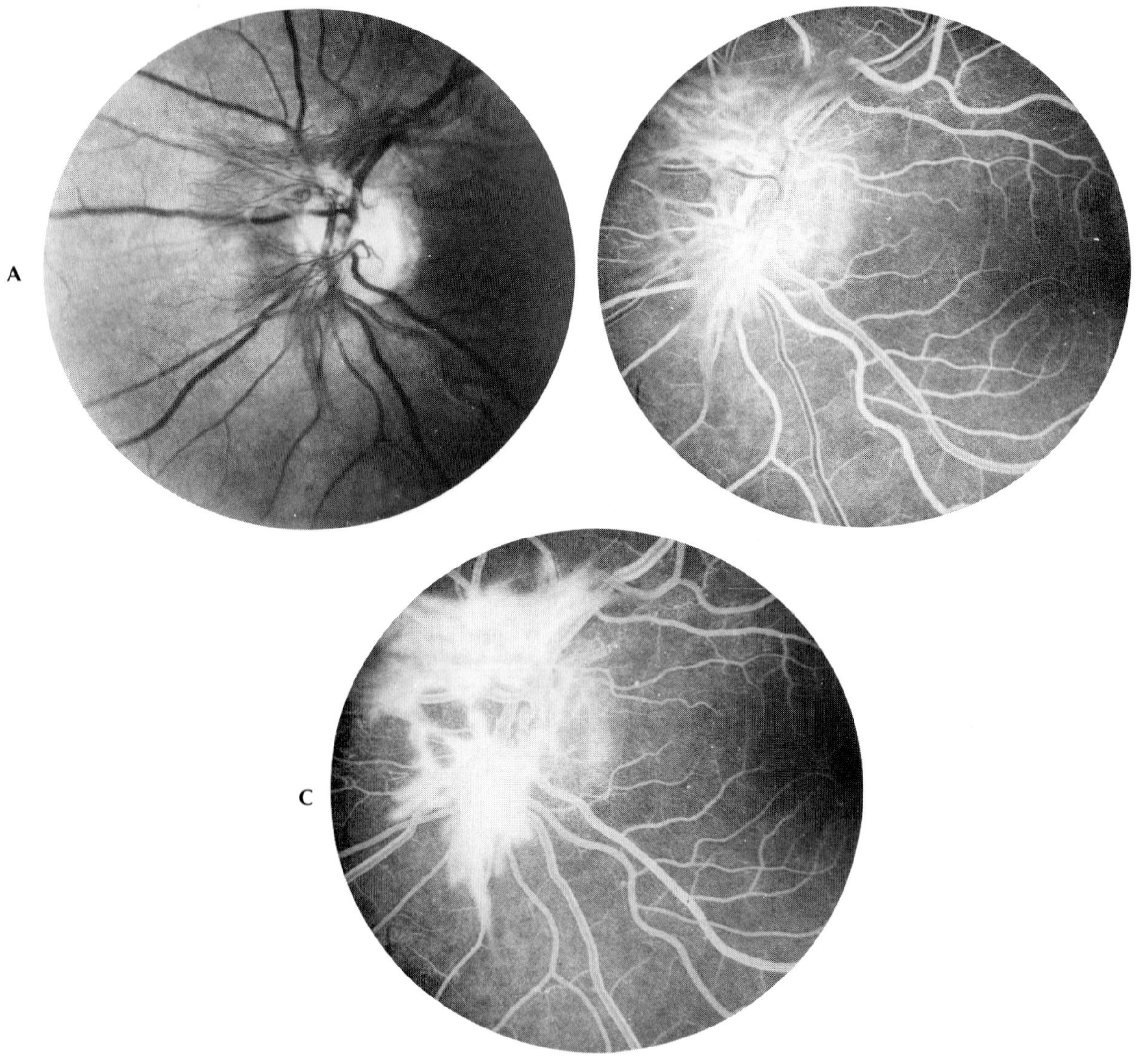

Fig. 15-10. A, A large confluent papillovitreal frond in a 36-year-old diabetic woman. **B,** Fluorogram during the late arteriolar phase, showing complete filling of the papillovitreal neovascularization. **C,** Fluorogram showing marked leakage of the fluorescein dye into the vitreous from the papillovitreal neovascularization.

Staining. The accumulation of fluorescein dye in a solid tissue, caused by leakage from a retinal or choroidal vessel, is referred to as staining. Retinal, gliotic, neovascular, or neoplastic tissue is stained by fluorescein dye leaking from a nearby abnormal vessel. The stained tissue may show considerable fluorescence for a long period of time, will show indistinct borders, will not grow in intensity when the leakage from the nearby abnormal vessel has decreased, and may show a configuration identical to the glial or pigment tissue proliferation seen in the Kodachrome fundus photographs (Figs. 15-7 to 15-9).

New and anomalous vessels. Any abnormality concerning proliferation or rechanneling of existing blood vessels can be observed by fluorescein angiography and is termed new or anomalous vessel formation (Fig. 15-10). Intraretinal vascular shunts, microaneurysms, and the various configurations of retinal and choroidal neovascularization can be seen dramatically as the fluorescein dye progresses through the vessels. Leakage beneath the retina, into the retina, and into the vitreous cavity can be easily observed.

Filling defects. Filling defects are characterized by the absence of fluorescein dye or a delay in its infiltration into an area of the choroid or retina. These defects include delayed filling, retrograde filling, and no filling of the retinal or choroidal vessels. Grade 3 and Grade 4 chorioretinal coagulations will produce a filling defect caused by scarring and obliteration of the vessels in the photocoagulation area. Peripapillary retinal pigment proliferation and atrophy, as well as other areas of chorioretinal atrophy, will also show delayed, and possibly retrograde, filling defects (Figs. 15-11 and 15-12).

Pseudofluorescence

Early pseudofluorescence. Early pseudofluorescence occurs when the excitation and barrier filters of the camera system do not have mutually exclusive transmission spectra, so that light emerging from the surfaces of high reflectivity in the fundus passes through the

A

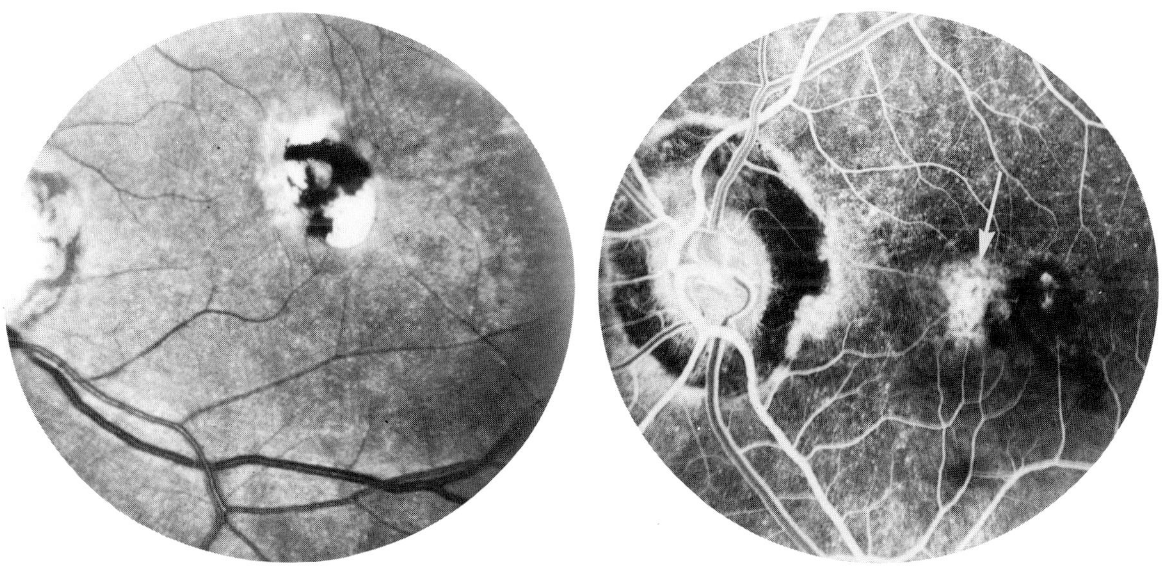

B

Fig. 15-11. A, An old toxoplasmosis defect in the macular region of a 26-year-old woman; inflammatory activity can be seen along the nasal border of the punched-out lesion. **B,** Fluorogram showing early choroidal neovascularization along the nasal border of the toxoplasmosis chorioretinal defect (arrow) and an obvious filling defect in the peripapillary space.

A 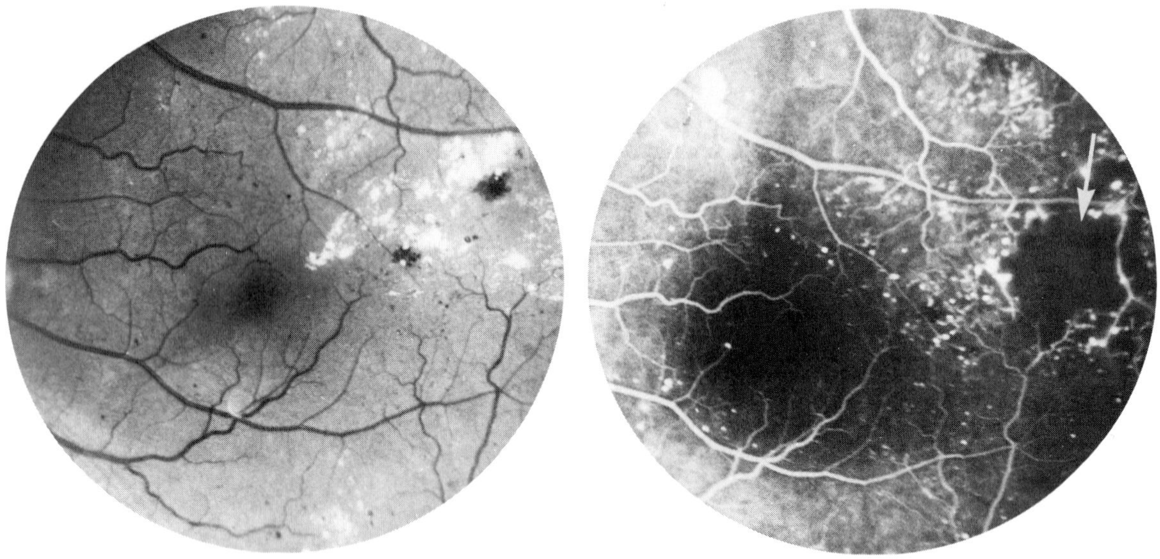 B

Fig. 15-12. A, Hemorrhagic activity, 2+ macular edema, and exudate formation, particularly in the temporal macular region, in a 27-year-old diabetic man. **B,** Fluorogram showing marked leakage from the temporally located vessels, microaneurysm formation, and a large retinal infarct (filling defect) (arrow).

A 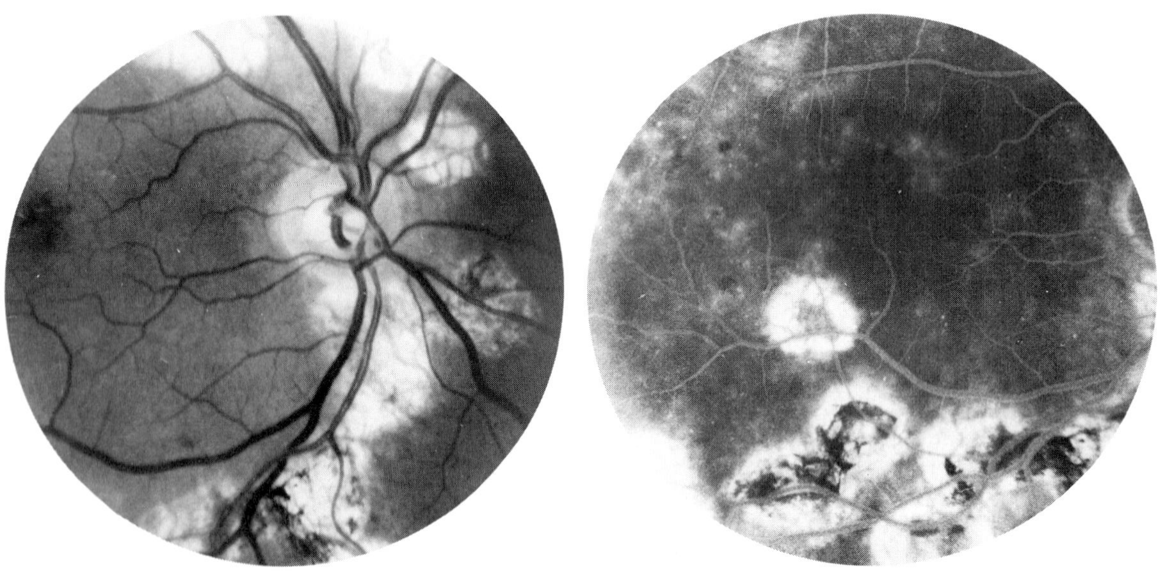 B

Fig. 15-13. A, Pigment proliferation and glial hypertrophy around the border of photocoagulation scars 3 months after xenon-arc photocoagulation in a 52-year-old man with diabetic retinopathy. **B,** Early pseudofluorescence demonstrated by the reflection of the blue exciting light from the glial scars back through an imperfect barrier filter onto the photographic film.

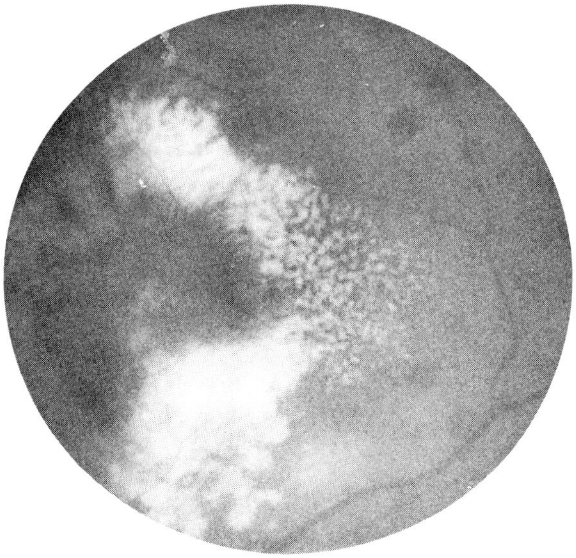

Fig. 15-14. Late pseudofluorescence illustrated by the recording of a large exudate patch on the photographic film following leakage and fluorescence of the fluorescein dye in the vitreous cavity.

camera filters to be recorded on the film. This situation occurs before the injection of fluorescein and is simply related to the problem of the blue excitation light reflected from the optic disc, areas of chorioretinal atrophy, exudates, and zones of gliotic tissue being able to pass through the barrier filter and therefore being recorded on the film of the camera. The use of filters with mutually exclusive transmission spectra eliminates the problem of early pseudofluorescence (Fig. 15-13).

Late pseudofluorescence. Late pseudofluorescence can be seen during the later phases of the fluorescein angiography and is caused by the stimulation and excitation of the fluorescein in the anterior vitreous and aqueous to produce fluorescence. The green fluorescence is then reflected from whitish surfaces, such as mentioned previously, and passes through the barrier filter onto the camera film (Fig. 15-14).

General discussion

Fluorescein angiography is tremendously valuable in the evaluation and diagnostic interpretation of disease states and as an indicator and guide for photocoagulation treatment. Color fluorescein angiography can be useful in documenting the relationship of areas of pigment, hemorrhage, and exudates to the angiographic defect. Stereoscopic fluorescein angiography can add another dimension to the analysis of these problems and should be employed whenever possible. Stereo Kodachrome fundus photography of the diseased area, the use of slit lamp biomicroscopy with a contact lens, and indirect ophthalmoscopy are extremely helpful in interpreting the fluorescein angiogram correctly.

Fluorescein ophthalmoscopy should be conducted in those instances where a photographic fluorescein angiographic system is not available. The influx of fluorescein into the posterior polar defect can be seen precisely in many patients and serves to delineate the disease process. Fluorescein angiography, combined with the other ophthalmoscopic and subjective ancillary tests, can provide increased accuracy in the diagnostic and therapeutic approach to the disease.

HEMOBAROMETRY AND HEMOTOPOGRAPHY

Hemobarometry is a technique that makes possible the measurement of the blood pressure in the various branches of the choroidal and retinal vasculature. Relative and near-absolute pressures in the central retinal artery, main arterioles, terminal arterioles, venules, and veins can be calculated accurately by this method, and results are reproducible. The basic principle of hemobarometry involves the measurement of the blood pressure within a vessel by raising the intraocular pressure by the suction ophthalmodynamometry method to a level sufficient to overcome the internal pressure and thereby collapse the vessel or restrict its blood flow. The intraocular pressure necessary to collapse a vessel or prevent forward movement of the blood can be determined by photographing simultaneously the suction ophthalmodynamometer vacuum reading and the fundus angiography phase, thus recording precisely the pressure and moment that the fluorescent blood column reaches the particular vessel in which the pressure is being measured (Fig. 15-15). The superimposition of external pressure on the tissue and vessels along the vascular channels makes it more dificult for blood to flow either into the tissue or the vessels themselves; therefore, the fluorescein-blood mixture can be used as an indicator of the pressure within the individual vascular complexes.

High intraocular pressures work in a manner similar to hemobarometry to prevent the easy passage of blood into the vessels of the retina. Localized patches of retinal edema, exudate formation, or intraretinal hemorrhages in any region of the posterior segment or, more commonly, in the macular area can lead to increased tissue resistance to blood flow. The pressure required for macular perfusion is thereby increased, and the actual perfusion gradients are decreased.

These relationships might be summed up in the following equation:

$$\text{HBM} + \text{TR} + \text{VR} = \text{RVP}$$

In this equation HBM represents the pressure applied to the globe to increase the pressure on the retinal and choroidal vasculature; TR represents the tissue resistance, which may be increased in pathologic states affecting retinal tissue pressure, such as senile exudative maculopathy, diabetic maculopathy, hypertensive retinopathy, and other vascular conditions; VR represents the resistance to vascular blood flow in the larger vessels that can considerably alter the perfusion pressure at right angles to this larger vessel. Increased

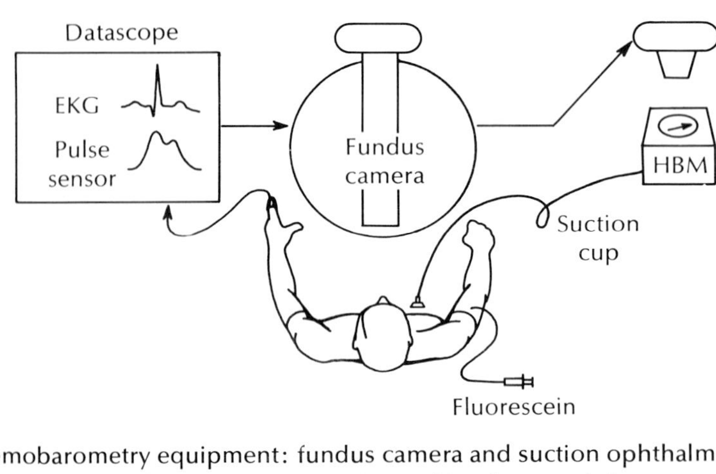

Fig. 15-15. Hemobarometry equipment: fundus camera and suction ophthalmodynamometer camera to record the fundus fluorescein angiographic phase and the pressure dial reading when the cameras are triggered by the finger pulse sensor.

resistance (gliotic, edematous, or photocoagulated areas) or decreased resistance (higher velocity systems, such as the extramacular shunting disease states) to vascular flow becomes important and significantly affects nearby pressure and perfusion relationships. The retinovascular pressure, RVP, is the pressure that is documented hemobarometrically; it is the pressure that is sufficient to overcome the factors on the left side of the equation. If two of the factors on the left side of the equation are known and remain constant, the third can be calculated, interpreted, and compared with normal levels.

A second diagnostic technique, hemotopography, uses a wide-angle fundus photographic system connected to video recording equipment, so that the blood flow rates through the individual vascular systems can be determined, and the fluorescent density in

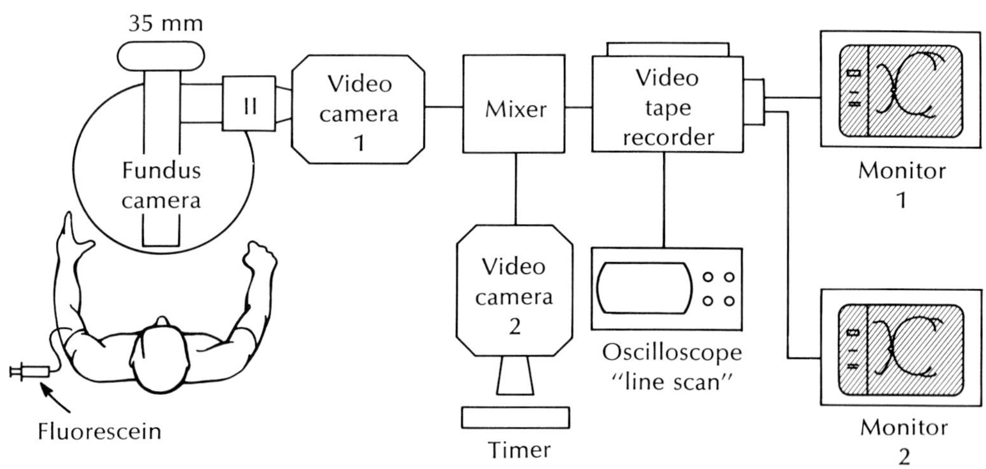

Fig. 15-16. Video retinal hemotopography equipment: line-scanning oscilloscope, fundus camera, tape recorder, and video monitors.

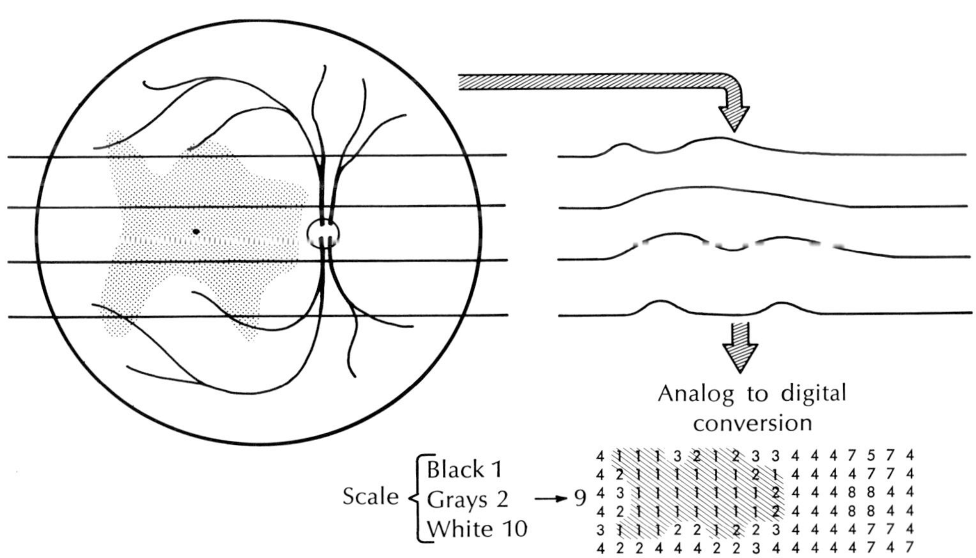

Fig. 15-17. Conversion of fluorescein angiographic or hemobarometric photographs to analog symbols that can be digitalized by computer techniques to form a densitometric pattern of the foveal and macular region.

the various portions of the macular region can be analyzed by line selection techniques (Fig. 15-16). Photographs taken during hemobarometry are converted to analog symbols by line selection analysis and are digitized by computer techniques (Fig. 15-17) or are scanned directly by a specialized microscope for a densitometric analysis of the fluorescein content in the macular region.

The data generated by the diagnostic techniques of hemobarometry and hemotopography are compared by multidimensional evaluation computer techniques to determine perfusion patterns, pressure gradients, and overall competency of the circulation in the macular and paramacular regions. Recommendations are then made for photocoagulation or other therapeutic measures that might be beneficial.

MACULAR TESTING

Amsler grid

The Amsler grid is most important for evaluation of the patient with a macular lesion causing visual field distortion. The distortion can be monitored in the office or at home if the patient is given a copy of the Amsler grid. With the grid the patient can measure the change in distortion and relay this information to the physician.

Modified Amsler grid

The modified Amsler grid consists of dense photographic film placed over an x-ray viewing box. Clear lines on the film represent the grid. The patient is asked to fixate for approximately 30 sec at the center of the viewing box, which is covered with a blue or red filter. At the end of this time the grid is placed over the filter and viewing box, and following the photic stress with light from the long (red) or short (blue) end of the visible spectrum, the patient draws the distortions as he sees them. Various defects in the layers of the retina can be elicited more easily with this method, particularly when an equivocal response is obtained with the conventional Amsler grid testing technique.

Visual fields

Tangent screen campimetry should be performed on all patients with macular lesions so that the proper course of treatment can be decided and the lesion can be evaluated at a future date. The 1- and 2-mm white, red, and green testing objects should be used in the foveal and perifoveal regions if macular disease is suspected. The integration of the results of visual field testing with the Amsler grid examinations can provide a thorough evaluation of the macular function.

Color vision

The AO-HRR pseudoisochromatic charts or the Ishihara color vision booklet can be of some importance in differentiating a treatable lesion from a heredodegenerative dystrophy. All patients should be examined for color vision defects before they are tested with the modified Amsler grid apparatus. Defects in color vision can be important in the characterization of the particular macular defect.

Chapter 16

Future photocoagulation developments

KRYPTON LASER

The krypton laser has the ability to produce laser beams at various portions of the visible spectrum. Laser beams in the blue (488.0 nm), green (514.5 nm), pea green (530.8 nm), yellow (568.2 nm), and red (647.1 nm) portions of the visible radiations are prominent with this particular energy source. Most of these outputs have sufficient power to produce coagulations in the majority of patients, but their power is somewhat limited for those patients with extensive lenticular or vitreous opacities. The great advantage of the krypton laser is that the pea green and yellow wavelengths are more highly absorbed by hemoglobin and lipofuscin than are the argon wavelengths, and one would therefore expect a more efficient conversion of light energy to heat energy. Furthermore, the 647.1-nm radiation in the red part of the visible spectrum could be used for the coagulation of the pigment epithelium when blood is present in the vitreous or in the preretinal space. The greatest disadvantage of the krypton laser is the large amount of input electrical power necessary to produce laser beam power adequate for photocoagulation. At this time the krypton laser is too unwieldy to be considered as a photocoagulation tool, although this difficulty may be overcome with advanced technology in the near future.

YAG LASER

The frequency-doubled neodymium yttrium-aluminum-garnet (YAG) laser has the great potential for providing a laser photocoagulation system that would fit within a small suitcase and be entirely portable. The beam that is generated by the basic laser system is produced in the infrared portion of the spectrum (1,064.0 nm) and is then passed through a nonlinear crystal (barium sodium lithium niobate) that doubles the frequency of the incoming beam while it halves the wavelength, producing a pea green beam (532.0 nm). This beam is also more highly absorbed by hemoglobin and the pigment epithelium than is the argon laser beam, and there is a greater potential for absorption and conversion to heat energy by these pigments.

At present this laser can generate sufficient energy for photocoagulation of most cases but is restricted by the stability and technical production problems of the nonlinear crystal. It is therefore difficult to mass-produce these lasers with any degree of reliability of the nonlinear crystal and the resulting laser beam power. If these technologic difficulties can be overcome, this laser will certainly be one of the more useful devices.

GLAUCOMA SURGERY

During the past 6 years there has been interest in the use of lasers for the treatment of glaucoma. There are basically three techniques: peripheral iridotomy, alteration of the trabecular meshwork, and destruction of the ciliary body. All three have their counterpart in established surgical techniques, including cryocyclotherapy. At the present time there is inadequate information and experience to consider these three modalities safe or effective enough to replace existing techniques.

Peripheral ruby laser iridotomy has recently been reported to have an overall 76% success rate. It failed to relieve the glaucoma in 24% of the patients with angle-closure glaucoma (Perkins, 1973).

Laser treatment of the angle has variously been termed "laseropuncture" (Krasnov, 1973), "laser trabecular puncture" (Hager, 1973), and "laser trabeculotomy" (Worthen, 1973, 1974). With all of these terms it is assumed that an opening is made in the trabecular meshwork. Both the Q-switched ruby laser and the argon laser have been utilized in these patients, and it has been found that the effect of the treatment is transitory, lasting 1 to 3 months (Krasnov, 1973; Hager, 1973). It has been observed that laser treatments to the iris and trabecular meshwork could be more effectively produced with faster pulses and higher-intensity laser bursts because of the greater vaporization and hole creation with minimal thermal or burning effects. It has appeared that an argon laser, when pulsed rapidly with high-intensity bursts, would be considered appropriate for this task, although the Q-switched ruby laser with a pulse duration of nanoseconds, could possibly have the theoretical advantage of a minimal thermal effect and a high vaporization potential.

The treatment of the ciliary body has been approached from two standpoints. The ruby and argon lasers have been used to photocoagulate the ciliary body of rabbits and man transcorneally, but success has been limited (Lee, 1971; Zimmerman, 1973). Because of the regenerative capacity of the ciliary epithelium, this approach has not been effective over a long period of time. The other approach has utilized both ruby and neodymium lasers through the sclera to affect the ciliary body in a manner analogous to that of cryocautery destruction (Beckman, 1972). Reportedly, with this procedure a decrease in intraocular pressure has been obtained for a period of about 6 months.

The carbon dioxide laser has been used in animal studies to produce a trephination hole at the limbus through the sclera into the anterior chamber (Beckman, 1971). This procedure could be refined and might have some advantages over conventional trephination because of the hemostatic effect of this laser beam.

Several years ago my laboratory attempted to produce a filtering cicatrix by directing an argon laser beam across the anterior chamber with a three-mirror lens in such a way that the argon beam would burn its way through the trabecular meshwork outward into the subconjunctival space. In three patients success over a several-week to 2-month period was only partial. Theoretically, additional research in this area could provide a workable method of nonoperative creation of a filtering bleb.

Although initial results have been encouraging, it is mandatory that these new techniques be compared with those already established, and it must be clearly demonstrated that the newer techniques are either safer, more effective, or longer lasting before they are put into use. Further careful study will place these new techniques in their proper perspective in the field of glaucoma surgery.

Several interesting techniques concerning the application of laser energy in the surgical approach to cataracts have been attempted in my laboratory. The rupture, splitting, and hydration of the anterior capsule and cortical material have been accomplished in animals and humans with the ruby and argon lasers. The introduction of fluorescein dye and carbon particles into these areas has been attempted to increase the absorption of the laser beam and its effectiveness. These procedures have been employed to soften the cortical and nuclear material sufficiently for aspiration of the intracapsular material through an extremely small cannula. These studies are purely investigative at the present time and must be regarded as highly experimental.

During the past 2 years I have also designed and constructed a delivery system to conduct the carbon dioxide laser beam from its energy source to the lens body (L'Esperance, 1975). This delivery system incorporates an infusion and exhaust system from the anterior chamber to keep the eye at constant pressure, an internal pressure system to clear a small cannula to the surface of the lens so that the carbon dioxide laser beam can vaporize the surface of the lens at the point of impact, and a small aeration system to remove the vaporized debris from the eye. An energy-sampling device, an articulated arm delivery system, and methods to precisely vary the level of the carbon dioxide laser power have been built into the phaco-vaporization instrument (Fig. 16-1). With this procedure the carbon dioxide laser beam, operating at 10.6μ wavelength in the far infrared portion of the spectrum, is completely absorbed and converted to heat at an astonishingly shallow depth of 200μ of tissue. Only the surface of the lens, iris, or vitreous

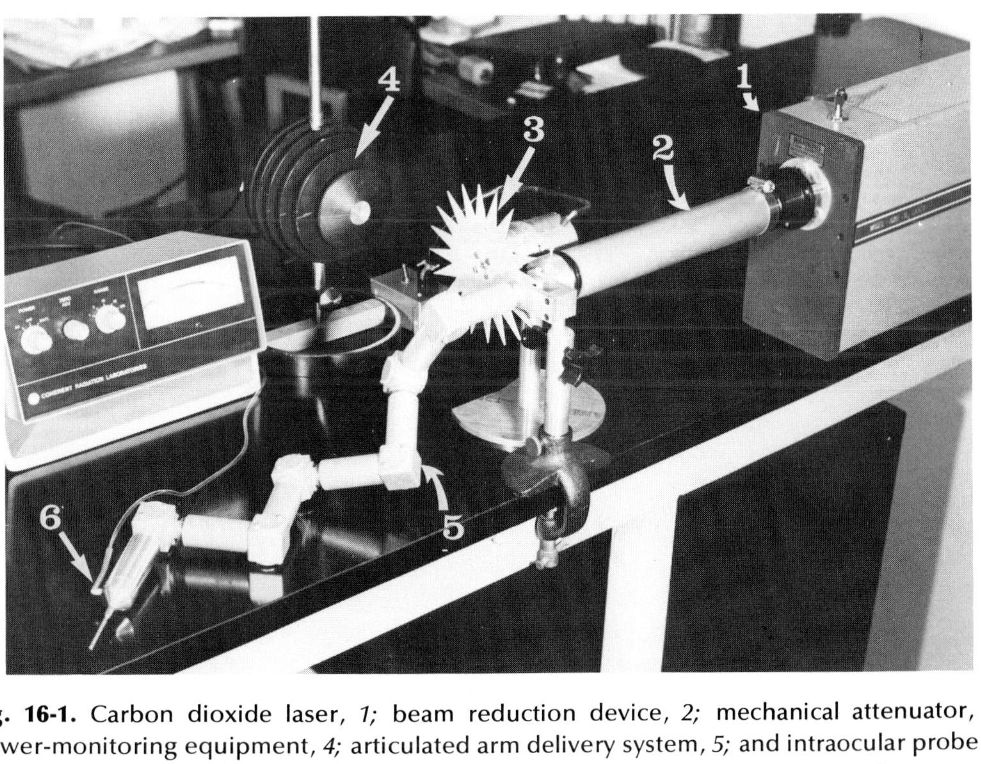

Fig. 16-1. Carbon dioxide laser, *1;* beam reduction device, *2;* mechanical attenuator, *3;* power-monitoring equipment, *4;* articulated arm delivery system, *5;* and intraocular probe to channel the laser beam to the lens for phaco-vaporization of the cataract, *6.* Vitreous and iris tissue can also be removed through the probe by vaporization with the CO_2 laser beam.

body on which the carbon dioxide laser beam impinges absorbs the beam and is vaporized. No char or residue remains, and the lens can be virtually vaporized from the center of the eye. This system has been used successfully in animals and clinically on human eyes, but the instrumentation and technique require further evaluation and refinement before a definite degree of effectiveness can be ascertained.

CORNEAL SURGERY

The carbon dioxide laser with a special lens to produce a cone of laser energy has been used to cut corneal buttons from eyes. Although the laser does not damage tissue beyond the point of contact, the technique was not practical for widespread use. Superficial corneal blood vessels can be eradicated with either the argon or carbon dioxide laser, but vessels recur several weeks after photocoagulation. It is very difficult to restrict the growth of blood vessels from the limbus into the cornea for any period of time.

Pseudomonas aeruginosa and *Candida albicans* corneal ulcers have been treated in animals by unfocused argon laser radiation after the ulcers had been conjugated with fluorescein-tagged antibodies that had attached to each particular organism. The destructive action of the ulcers was stopped immediately, and they healed rapidly thereafter. It is apparent that the fluorescein component of the antibody complex that was attached to the individual organism absorbs sufficient argon laser radiation to raise the fluorescein particle and the organism above the organism's thermal death point. This phototherapy research is being continued in my laboratory and may have more widespread application.

References

Aiello, L. M., Beetham, W. P., Balodimos, M. C., and others: Ruby laser photocoagulation in treatment of diabetic proliferating retinopathy: preliminary report. In Goldberg, M. F., and Fine, S. L., editors: Symposium on the Treatment of Diabetic Retinopathy, Arlington, Va., 1968, U.S. Department of Health, Education, and Welfare.

Annesley, Jr., W. H., Tasman, W. S., LeWin, D. P., and Tomer, T. L.: Retrospective evaluation of photocoagulation for idiopathic central serous chorioretinopathy: limitations and prospects for retinal surgery, Mod. Probl. Ophthalmol. **12**:234-238, 1974.

Beckman, H., Barraco, R., Sugar, H. S., Gaynes, E., and Blau, R.: Laser iridectomies, Am. J. Ophthalmol. **72**:393, 1971.

Beckman, H., Kinoshita, A., Rota, A. N., and others: Transcleral ruby laser irradiation of the ciliary body in the treatment of intractable glaucoma, Trans. Am. Acad. Ophthalmol. Otolaryngol. **76**:423, 1972.

Beckman, H., Rota, A., Barraco, R., Sugar, H. S., and Gaynes, E.: Limbectomies, keratectomies, and keratostomies performed with a rapid-pulsed carbon dioxide laser, Am. J. Ophthalmol. **71**:1277-1283, 1971.

Beetham, W. P., Aiello, L. M., Balodimos, M. C., and others: Ruby laser photocoagulation of early diabetic neovascular retinopathy: preliminary report of a long-term controlled study, Arch. Ophthalmol. **83**:261-272, 1970.

Behrendt, T.: Multiline argon laser, Arch. Ophthalmol. **85**:355-358, 1971.

Bessis, M., Gires, F., Mayer, G., and Nomarski, G.: Irradiation des organites cellulaires a l'aide d'un laser a rubis, Compt. Rend. Acad. Sci. **255**:1010-1012, 1962.

Birch-Hirschfeld, A.: Zum kapitel der Sonnenblendung des Auges, Ztschr. Augenh. **28**:444, 1912.

Blessing: Petersbrg. Med. Ztschr. **37**:365, 1912.

Bonetus, T.: Cited by Hamm, H.: Zentralskotom nach sonnenblendung, dissertation, Hamburg, 1947.

Boniuk, I., Okun, E., Johnston, G. P., and Arribas, N.: Xenon photocoagulation vs. cryotheraphy in the prevention of retinal detachment: limitations and prospects for retinal surgery, Mod. Probl. Ophthalmol., **12**:81-92, 1974.

Brockhurst, R. J.: Photocoagulation in congenital retinoschisis, Arch. Ophthalmol. **84**:158-165, 1970.

Burton, T. C.: Central serous retinopathy. In Blodi, F. C., editor: Current concepts in ophthalmology, vol. 3, St. Louis, 1972, The C. V. Mosby Co.

Campbell, C. J., Rittler, M. C., and Koester, C. J.: The optical maser as a retinal coagulator: an evaluation, Trans. Am. Acad. Ophthalmol. **67**:58-67, 1963.

Campbell, C. J., and others: Clinical studies in laser photocoagulation, Arch. Ophthalmol. **74**:57-65, 1965.

Campbell, C. J., Rittler, M. C., Noyori, K. S., and others: The threshold of the retina to damage by laser energy, Arch. Ophthalmol. **76**:437-442, 1966.

Campbell, C. J., and others: Ocular effects produced by experimental lasers. I. Q-switched ruby laser, Am. J. Ophthalmol. **66**:459-470, 1968.

Campbell, C. J., and others: Ocular effects produced by experimental lasers. II. Carbon dioxide laser. Am. J. Ophthalmol. **66**:604-614, 1968.

Campbell, C. J., and others: Ocular effects produced by experimental lasers. III. Neodymium laser, Am. J. Ophthalmol. **66**:614-632, 1968.

Campbell, C. J., Rittler, M. C., Swope, C. H., and others: The ocular effects produced by experimental lasers. IV. The argon laser, Amer. J. Ophthalmol. **67**:671-681, 1969.

Cleasby, G. W., Hall, D. L., Fung, W. E., and Webster, R. G., Jr.: Retinal branch vein occlusion: treatment by photocoagulation: limitations and prospects for retinal surgery, Mod. Probl. Ophthalmol. **12**:254-260, 1974.

Colyear, B. H., Jr.: Retinal vascular lesions treated by photocoagulation, Am. J. Ophthalmol. **63**:262-270, 1967.

Cords, Z.: Sonnenblendung Ztschr. Augenh. **27**:511, 1912.

Curtin, V. T., and Norton, E. W. D.: Early pathological changes of photocoagulation in the human retina, Arch. Ophthalmol. **69**:744, 1963.

Czerny: Ber. Wien. Acad. Wiss. **2**:56, 1867.

Dellaporta, A., and Declercq, S. D.: Xenon photocoagulation in diabetic retinopathy, Trans. Am. Acad. Ophthalmol. Otolaryngol. **77**:27-33, 1973.

Deutschmann, R.: Ein Experimenteller Beitrag zur Pathogense der Sympathischen Augen-Entzündung, von Graefes Arch. Ophthalmol. **28**:291, 1882.

Dobree, J.: Simple diabetic retinopathy, Br. J. Ophthalmol. **54**:1-10, 1970.
Gass, J. D. M.: Pathogenesis of disciform detachment of the neuroepithelium. I. General concepts and classification, Am. J. Ophthalmol. **63**:573-585, 1967.
Gass, J. D. M.: Pathogenesis of disciform detachment of the neuroepithelium. II. Idiopathic central serous choroidopathy, Am. J. Ophthalmol. **63**:587-615, 1967.
Gass, J. D. M.: Pathogenesis of disciform detachment of the neuroepithelium. III. Senile disciform macular degeneration, Am. J. Ophthalmol. **63**:617-644, 1967.
Gass, J. D. M.: Pathogenesis of disciform detachment of the neuroepithelium. IV. Fluorescein angiographic study of senile disciform macular degeneration, Am. J. Ophthalmol. **63**:645-659, 1967.
Gass, J. D. M.: Pathogenesis of disciform detachment of the neuroepithelium. V. Disciform macular degeneration secondary to focal choroiditis, Am. J. Ophthalmol. **63**:661-687, 1967.
Gass, J. D. M.: Pathogenesis of disciform detachment of the neuroepithelium. VI. Disciform detachment secondary to heredodegenerative, neoplastic and traumatic lesions of the choroid, Am. J. Ophthalmol. **63**:689-711, 1967.
Gass, J. D. M.: Laser grid photocoagulation of the macula. Presented at a meeting of the Association for Residents in Ophthalmology, Miami, Fla., 1970.
Gass, J. D. M.: Stereoscopic atlas of macular diseases, St. Louis, 1970, The C. V. Mosby Co.
Gass, J. D. M., Sever, R. J., Sparks, D., and others: A combined technique of fluorescein funduscopy and angiography of the eye, Arch. Ophthalmol. **78**:455-461, 1967.
Geeraets, W. J.: Some aspects of laser coagulation, Int. Ophthalmol. Clin. **6**:263-273, 1966
Geeraets, W. J., Williams, R. C., Chan, G., Ham, W. T., Guerry, D. III and Schmidt, F. H.: The relative absorption of thermal energy in retina and choroid, Invest. Ophthalmol. **1**:340-348, 1962.
Geeraets, W. J., and others: The relative absorption of thermal energy in retina and choroid, Invest. Ophthalmol. **1**:340-348, 1962.
Geeraets, W. J., and others: Laser versus light coagulator: a funduscopic and histologic study of chorioretinal injury as a function of exposure time, Fed. Proc. **24** (Suppl. 14):S-48-61, 1965.
Gifford, S. R., and Marquardt, G.: Central angiospastic retinopathy, Arch. Ophthalmol. **21**: 211-228, 1939.
Goldberg, M. F., and Fine, S. L., editors: Symposium on the Treatment of Diabetic Retinopathy, Arlington, Va., 1968, U.S. Department of Health, Education, and Welfare.
Guerry, D., and Wiesinger, H.: Light coagulation, Am. J. Ophthalmol. **49**:87-96, 1960.
Hager, H.: Besondere mikrochirurgische Eingriffe. II. Erste Erfahrugen mit dere Argon-Laser Gerät 800, klin. Monat. Augenh. **172**:437, 1973.
Ham, W. T., Jr., Wiesinger, H., Schmidt, F. H., and others: Flash burns in the rabbit retina: as a means of evaluating the retinal hazard from nuclear weapons, Am. J. Ophthalmol. **46**:700-723, 1958.
Hamm, H.: Zentralskotom nach sonnenblendung, dissertation, Hamburg, 1947.
Harris, G. S.: Photocoagulation of macular lesions following fluorescein angiography, Can. J. Ophthalmol. **4**:16-19, 1969.
Hepler, R. S., and others: Photocoagulation of choroidal melanomas, Arch. Ophthalmol. **79**:177-181, 1968.
Hudson, J. R.: Functional results of retinal detachment surgery. In McPherson, A., editor: New and controversial aspects of retinal detachment, New York, 1968, Harper & Row, Publishers.
Irvine, A. R., and Norton, E. W. D.: Photocoagulation for diabetic retinopathy, Am. J. Ophthalmol. **71**:437-445, 1971.
Jack, M. K.: Central serous retinopathy with optic pit treated with photocoagulation, Am. J. Ophthalmol. **67**:519-521, 1969.
Jenkins, F. A., and White, H. E.: Fundamentals of optics, ed. 3, New York, 1957, McGraw-Hill Book Co.
Jepson, C. N., and Wetzig, P. C.: Photocoagulation in disciform macular degeneration, Am. J. Ophthalmol. **67**:920-930, 1969.
Klien, B. A.: Clinical manifestations. In Symposium on Macular Diseases, Trans. Am. Acad. Ophthalmol. Otolaryngol. **69**:614-620, 1965.
Krasnov, M. M.: Laseropuncture of anterior chamber angle in glaucoma, Am. J. Ophthalmol. **75**:674, 1973.
Krill, A. E., and Archer, D. B.: Choroidal neovascularization in multifocal (presumed histoplasmin) choroiditis, Arch. Ophthalmol. **84**:595-604, 1970.
Krill, A. E., Archer, D. B., and Newell, F. W.: Photocoagulation in complications secondary to branch vein occlusion, Arch. Ophthalmol. **85**:48-60, 1971.
Krill, A. E., Archer, D. B., Newell, F. W., and others: Photocoagulation in diabetic retinopathy, Am. J. Ophthalmol. **72**:299-321, 1971.
Krill, A. E., Chishti, M. I., Klien, B. A., and others: Multifocal inner choroiditis, Trans. Am. Acad. Ophthalmol. Otolaryngol. **73**:222-245, 1969.
Kuwabara, T., and Aiello, L. M.: Effect of the ruby laser on the monkey retina: an electron microscopic study. In Goldberg, M. F., and Fine, S. L., editors: Symposium on Treatment of Diabetic Retinopathy, Arlington, Va., 1968, U.S. Department of Health, Education, and Welfare.
Lappin, P. W., and Coogan, P. S.: Histologic evaluation of ophthalmoscopically subvisible retinal laser exposures, Invest. Ophthalmol. **9**:537-542, 1970.
Lappin, P. W., and Coogan, P. S.: Relative sensitivity of various areas of the retina to laser radiation, Arch. Ophthalmol. **84**:350-354, 1970.
Lee, P., and Pomerantzeff, O.: Transpupillary cyclophotocoagulation of rabbit eyes, Am. J. Ophthalmol. **71**:911-920, 1971.
L'Esperance, F. A., Jr.: The effect of laser radiation on the retinal vasculature, Arch. Ophthalmol. **74**:752-759, 1965.
L'Esperance, F. A., Jr.: Clinical comparison of xenon-arc and ruby laser photocoagulation of retinal lesions, Arch. Ophthalmol. **75**:61-67, 1966.
L'Esperance, F. A., Jr.: An ophthalmic argon laser photocoagulation system: design, construction, and laboratory investigations, Trans. Am. Ophthalmol. Soc. **66**:827-904, 1968.
L'Esperance, F. A., Jr.: The treatment of ophthalmic vascular disease by argon laser photocoagulation, Trans.

Am. Acad. Ophthalmol. Otolarngol. 73:1077-1096, 1969.
L'Esperance, F. A., Jr.: Clinical applications of argon laser photocoagulation, Trans. Ophthal Soc. U.K. 89:557-573, 1969.
L'Esperance, F. A., Jr.: The ocular histopathologic effect of krypton and argon laser radiation, Am. J. Ophthalmol. 68:263-273, 1969.
L'Esperance, F. A., Jr.: Argon laser photocoagulation of diabetic retinal neovascularization (a five-year appraisal), Trans. Am. Acad. Ophthalmol. Otolaryngol. 77:6-24, 1973.
L'Esperance, F. A., Jr.: Carbon dioxide laser phacovaporization, Arch. Ophthalmol. In press.
L'Esperance, F. A., Jr., and Kelly, G. R.: The threshold of the retina to damage by argon laser radiation, Arch. Ophthalmol. 81:583-588, 1969.
L'Esperance, F. A., Jr., Labuda, E. F., and Johnson, A. M.: Photocoagulation delivery systems for continuous-wave lasers, Br. J. Ophthalmol. 53:310-322, 1969.
Little, H. L.: Preventing complications in argon laser retinal photocoagulation. In Francois, J., editor: Symposium on Light Coagulation, Argon and Xenon, Vol. 1, Dr. W. Junk, B. V., Publishers, The Hague, 1973.
Little, H. L., and Zweng, H. C.: Complications of argon laser retinal photocoagulation, Trans. Pac. Coast Otoophthalmol. Soc. 52:115-129, 1971.
Little, H. L., Zweng, H. C., and Peabody, R. R.: Argon laser slit-lamp retinal photocoagulation, Trans. Am. Acad. Ophthalmol. Otolaryngol. 74:85-97, 1970.
Maggiore, L.: Soc. Ital. Oftal, 1927.
Maiman, T. H.: Stimulated optical radiation in ruby, Nature 187:493-494, 1960.
Marshall, J.: Thermal and mechanical mechanisms in laser damage to the retina, Invest. Ophthalmol. 9:97-115, 1970.
Marshall, J., and Mellerio, J.: Histology of retinal lesions produced with Q-switched lasers, Exp. Eye Res. 7:225-230, 1968.
Maumenee, A. E.: Serous and hemorrhagic disciform detachment of the macula, Trans. Pac. Coast Otoophthalmol. Soc. 40:139-160, 1959.
Maumenee, A. E.: Clinical manifestations. In Symposium on Macular Diseases, Trans. Am. Acad. Ophthalmol. Otolaryngol. 69:605-613, 1965.
Maumenee, A. E.: Pathogenesis. In Symposium on Macular Diseases, Trans. Am. Acad. Ophthalmol. Otolaryngol. 69:691-699, 1965.
Maumenee, A. E.: Pathogenesis. In Symposium on Macular Diseases, Trans. Am. Acad. Ophthalmol. Otolaryngol. 72:389-395, 1968.
Meyer-Schwickerath, G.: Indications and limitations of light coagulation of the retina, Trans. Am. Acad. Ophthalmol. Otolaryngol. 63:725-738, 1959.
Meyer-Schwickerath, G.: Light coagulation, translated by S. M. Drance, St. Louis, 1960, The C. V. Mosby Co.
Meyer-Schwickerath, G., and Schott, K.: Diabetic retinopathy and photocoagulation, Am. J. Ophthalmol. 66:597-603, 1968.
Moran-Salas, J.: Arch. Soc. Oftal. Hispano-Am. 10:566, 1950.
Norton, E. W. D., and Gutman, F.: Fluorescein angiography and hemangiomas of the choroid, Arch. Ophthalmol. 78:121-125, 1967.
Noyori, K. S., Campbell, C. J., Rittler, C., and others: The characteristics of experimental laser coagulations of the retina, Arch. Ophthalmol. 72:254-263, 1964.
Okun, E.: The effectiveness of photocoagulation in the therapy of proliferative diabetic retinopathy (PDR). In Symposium on Diabetic Retinopathy, Trans. Am. Acad. Ophthalmol. Otolaryngol. 72:246-252, 1968.
Okun, E., Boniuk, I., Johnston, G. P., and Arribas, N. P.: Xenon photocoagulation of presumed histoplasmic maculopathy: limitations and prospects for retinal surgery, Mod. Probl. Ophthalmol. 12:295-314, 1974.
Okun, E., and Cibis, P. A.: The role of photocoagulation in the therapy of proliferative diabetic retinopathy, Arch. Ophthalmol. 75:337-352, 1966.
Okun, E., and Cibis, P. A.: Photocoagulation in "limited" retinal detachment and breaks without detachment. In McPherson, A., editor: New and controversial aspects of retinal detachment, New York, 1968, Harper & Row, Publishers.
Okun, E., and Collins, E. M.: Histopathology of experimental photocoagulation in the dog eye. III. Microaneurysmlike formations following branch vein occlusion, Am. J. Ophthalmol. 56:40-45, 1963.
Okun, E., Johnston, G., and Boniuk, I.: Management of Diabetic Retinopathy, St. Louis, 1973, The C. V. Mosby Co.
Patz, A., and Berkow, J. W.: Visual and systemic prognosis in diabetic retinopathy. In Symposium on Diabetic Retinopathy, Trans. Am. Acad. Ophthalmol. Otolaryngol. 72:253-258, 1968.
Patz, A., Maumenee, A. E., and Ryan, S. J.: Argon laser photocoagulation, Trans. Am. Acad. Ophthalmol. Otolaryngol. 75:569-579, 1971.
Patz, A., Schatz, H., Berkow, J. W., Gittelsohn, A. M., and Ticho, U.: Macular edema—an overlooked complication of diabetic retinopathy, Trans. Am. Acad. Ophthalmol. Otolaryngol. 77:34-42, 1973.
Patz, A., Schatz, H., Ryan, S. J., and others: Argon laser photocoagulation for treatment of advanced diabetic retinopathy, Trans. Am. Acad. Ophthalmol. Otolaryngol. 76:981-989, 1972.
Peabody, R. R., Zweng, H. D., and Little, H. L.: Treatment of persistent central serous retinopathy, Arch. Ophthalmol. 79:166-169, 1968.
Peabody, R. R., Zweng, H. C., and Little, H. L.: Treatment of retinal vascular disease with argon laser slit lamp photocoagulation, Trans. Pac. Coast Otoophthalmol. Soc. 51:307-326, 1970.
Perkins, E. S., and Brown, N. A. P.: Iridotomy with a ruby laser, Br. J. Ophthalmol. 57:487, 1973.
Pischel, D. K., Clark, G., and Cibis, P. A.: Symposium: photocoagulation, Trans. Am. Acad. Ophthalmol. Otolaryngol. 66:57-87, 1962.
Pischel, D. K., and Colycar,B. H., Jr., Light coagulation therapy, Am. J. Ophthalmol. 50:590-595, 1960.
Reese, A. B.: Telangiectasis of the retina and Coats' disease, Am. J. Ophthalmol. 42:1-8, 1956.
Rosan, R. C., Flocks, M., Vassiliadis, A., and others: Pathology of monkey retina following irradiation with an argon laser, Arch. Ophthalmol. 81:84-88, 1969.

Rose, H. W., and others: Human chorioretinal burns from atomic fireballs, Arch. Ophthalmol. **55**:205-210, 1956.

Rubinstein, K., and Myska, V.: Treatment of diabetic maculopathy with photocoagulation: limitations and prospects for retinal surgery, Mod. Probl. Ophthalmol. **12**:271-274, 1974.

Schlaegel, T. F., Jr., Cofield, D. D., Clark, G., and others: Photocoagulation and other therapy for histoplasmic choroiditis, Trans. Am. Acad. Ophthalmol. Otolaryngol. **72**:355-363, 1968.

Schneider, R. J.: Serous detachment of the macula, Can. J. Ophthalmol. **5**:117-126, 1970.

Schott, K.: Weitere Erfahrungen mit der Lichtocoagulation bei Retinopathia diabetica, Dtsch. Ophthal. Ges. **66**:349-355, 1964.

Shikano, S., and Shimizu, K.: Atlas of fluorescence fundus angiography, ed. 1, Philadelphia, 1968, W. B. Saunders Co.

Smith, R. S., and Stein, M. N.: Transcleral laser radiation, Am. J. Ophthalmol. **67**:100-109, 1969.

Solon, L. R., and others: Physiological implications of laser beams, Science **134**:1506-1508, 1961.

Spalter, H. F.: Photocoagulation of central serous retinopathy: a preliminary report, Arch. Ophthalmol. **79**: 247-253, 1968.

Straatsma, B. R., Allan, R. A., and Petit, T. H.: Central serous retinopathy, Trans. Pac. Coast Otoophthalmol. Soc. **47**:107-127, 1966.

Taleff, M., Ritter, E. J., Rockwell, R. J., and others: Laser coagulation of the retina using the argon laser, Am. J. Ophthalmol. **67**:666-670, 1969.

Taylor, E.: Proliferative diabetic retinopathy, Br. J. Ophthalmol. **54**:535-539, 1970.

Townes, C. H.: Optical masers and their possible application in biology, Biophys. J. **2**: 325-329, 1962.

Vedmedenko, L. A.: Photocoagulation of the iris, Ophthalmol. J. (Odessa) 3:182, 1969.

Verhoeff, F. H., Bell, L., and Walker, C. B.: The pathological effects of radiant energy on the eye, Proc. Am. Acad. Arts. Sci. **51**:630-818, 1916.

von Graefe, A.: Neber centrale recidivirende retinitis, von Graefes Arch. Ophthalmol. **12**:211-215, 1866.

Vos, J. J.: A theory of retinal burns, Bull. Math. Biophys. **24**:115-128, 1962.

Wallow, I. H. L., and Tso, M. O. M.: Failure of formation of chorioretinal adhesions following xenon arc photocoagulation: limitations and prospects for retinal surgery, Mod. Probl. Ophthalmol. **12**:189-201, 1974.

Watzke, R. C., and Snyder, W. B.: Light coagulation for hemorrhagic disciform degeneration of the macula, Trans. Am. Acad. Ophthalmol. Otolaryngol. **72**:389-395, 1968.

Wessing, A.: Central serous retinopathy and related lesions, Mod. Probl. Ophthalmol. **9**:148-151, 1971.

Wetzig, P. C., and Worlton, J. T.: Treatment of diabetic retinopathy by light-coagulation, Br. J. Ophthalmol. **47**:539-541, 1963.

Widmark: Skand. Arch. **4**:281, 1893 (also cited by Birch-Hirschfeld).

Wise, G. N.: Retinal neovascularization, Trans. Am. Ophthalmol. Soc. **54**:729-826, 1956.

Wise, G. N., Campbell, C. J., Wendler, P. F., and others: Photocoagulation of vascular lesions of the macula, Am. J. Ophthalmol. **66**:452-459, 1968.

Wise, G. N., Dollery, C. T., and Henkind, P.: The retinal circulation, New York, 1971, Harper & Row, Publishers.

Woods, A. C., and Wahlen, H. E.: The probable role of benign histoplasmosis in the etiology of granulomatous uveitis, Am. J. Ophthalmol. **49**:205-220, 1960.

Worthen, D. M., and Wickham, M. G.: Laser trabeculotomy in monkeys, Invest. Ophthalmol. **12**: 707-711, 1973.

Worthen, D. M., and Wickham, M. G.: Argon laser trabeculotomy, Trans. Am. Acad. Ophthalmol. Otolaryngol. **78**:371-375, 1974.

Yannuzzi, L.: A classification of abnormal fundus fluorescence, Ann. Ophthalmol. **3**:711-718, 1971.

Zaret, M. M., and others: Ocular lesions produced by an optical maser (laser), Science **134**:1525-1526, 1961.

Zimmerman, T. J., Worthen, D. M., and Wickham, M. G.: Argon laser photocoagulation of ciliary processes and pigmented pupillary membranes in man, Invest. Ophthalmol. **12**:622-623, 1973.

Zweng, H. C.: Further observations on argon laser photocoagulation of diabetic retinopathy, Trans. Am. Acad. Ophthalmol. Otolaryngol. **76**:990-1004, 1972.

Zweng, H. C., Flocks, M., Kapany, N. S., Silbertrust, N., and Peppers, N. A.: Experimental laser photocoagulation, Am. J. Ophthalmol. **58**:353-362, 1964.

Zweng, H. C., Little, H. L., and Peabody, R. R.: Laser photocoagulation of macular lesions, Trans. Am. Acad. Ophthalmol. Otolaryngol. **72**:377-388, 1968.

Zweng, H. C., Little, H. L., and Peabody, R. R.: Laser photocoagulation and retinal angiography, St. Louis, 1969, The C. V. Mosby Co.

Zweng, H. C., Little, H. L., and Peabody, R. R.: Argon laser photocoagulation of diabetic retinopathy, Arch. Ophthalmol. **86**:395-400, 1971.

Zweng, H. C., Paus, G. L., Vassiliadis, A., and Rose, H.: Laser photocoagulation of the iris, Arch. Ophthalmol. **84**:193-199, 1970.

Index

I

K

L

M

N

O

Q

R

Peripheral retinal structural abnormalities

Reel I-1. Retinal tear with operculum
Reel I-2. Retinal tear after photocoagulation
Reel I-3. Healed retinal tear
Reel I-4. Peripheral retinal degeneration after photocoagulation
Reel I-5. Peripheral retinal degeneration after photocoagulation
Reel I-6. Retinal detachment after barrier photocoagulation
Reel I-7. Healed retinal detachment
Reel II-1. Retinal detachment after barrier photocoagulation
Reel II-2. Retinoschisis after barrier photocoagulation
Reel II-3. Retinoschisis, healed, after barrier photocoagulation

Peripheral retinal vascular abnormalities

Reel II-4. Fluorescein angiography, Eales' disease
Reel II-5. Leber's miliary aneurysms before photocoagulation
Reel II-6. Leber's miliary aneurysms after photocoagulation
Reel II-7. Leber's miliary aneurysms after photocoagulation
Reel III-1. Leber's miliary aneurysms, healed
Reel III-2. Coats' disease before photocoagulation
Reel III-3. Coats' disease after photocoagulation
Reel III-4. Coats' disease, healed
Reel III-5. Proliferative sickle retinopathy before photocoagulation
Reel III-6. Proliferative sickle retinopathy after photocoagulation
Reel III-7. Proliferative sickle retinopathy, healed
Reel IV-1. Proliferative sickle retinopathy, healed
Reel IV-2. Nonproliferative diabetic retinopathy before photocoagulation
Reel IV-3. Nonproliferative diabetic retinopathy after photocoagulation
Reel IV-4. Nonproliferative diabetic retinopathy, healed
Reel IV-5. Epipapillary neovascularization before photocoagulation
Reel IV-6. Epipapillary neovascularization after photocoagulation
Reel IV-7. Epipapillary neovascularization, healed
Reel V-1. Epipapillary neovascularization after photocoagulation
Reel V-2. Peripapillary neovascularization
Reel V-3. Peripapillary neovascularization after photocoagulation
Reel V-4. Peripapillary neovascularization after photocoagulation
Reel V-5. Peripapillary neovascularization, healed
Reel V-6. Peripapillary neovascularization, healed
Reel V-7. Peripapillary neovascularization after photocoagulation
Reel VI-1. Papillovitreal neovascularization
Reel VI-2. Papillovitreal neovascularization after photocoagulation
Reel VI-3. Papillovitreal neovascularization, healed
Reel VI-4. Retinovitreal neovascularization
Reel VI-5. Retinovitreal neovascularization after photocoagulation
Reel VI-6. Retinovitreal neovascularization, healed
Reel VI-7. Preretinal neovascularization
Reel VII-1. Preretinal neovascularization after photocoagulation
Reel VII-2. Preretinal neovascularization, healed
Reel VII-3. Preretinal neovascularization, healed
Reel VII-4. Papillovitreal neovascularization
Reel VII-5. Papillovitreal neovascularization, obliterated
Reel VII-6. Papillovitreal neovascularization
Reel VII-7. Papillovitreal neovascularization, obliterated

Peripheral chorioretinal tumors

Reel VIII-1. Malignant melanoma
Reel VIII-2. Malignant melanoma after photocoagulation
Reel VIII-3. Malignant melanoma, early healed stage
Reel VIII-4. Angiomatosis retinae
Reel VIII-5. Angiomatosis retinae after photocoagulation
Reel VIII-6. Angiomatosis retinae, obliterated
Reel VIII-7. Choroidal hemangioma
Reel IX-1. Choroidal hemangioma, obliterated

Macular intraretinal abnormalities

Reel IX-2. Pigment epithelial detachment after photocoagulation
Reel IX-3. Pigment epithelial detachment
Reel IX-4. Pigment epithelial detachment after photocoagulation
Reel IX-5. Pigment epithelial detachment, healed
Reel IX-6. Central serous choroidopathy (SDSR)
Reel IX-7. Central serous choroidopathy after photocoagulation
Reel X-1. Central serous choroidopathy (SDSR), healed
Reel X-2. Central serous choroidopathy after photocoagulation
Reel X-3. Hemorrhagic detachment of pigment epithelium
Reel X-4. Hemorrhagic detachment after barrier photocoagulation
Reel X-5. Hemorrhagic detachment after photocoagulation
Reel X-6. Hemorrhagic detachment, healed

Macular interretinal abnormalities

Reel X-7. Branch retinal artery occlusion
Reel XI-1. Branch retinal artery occlusion
Reel XI-2. Branch retinal artery occlusion after photocoagulation
Reel XI-3. Branch retinal vein occlusion after photocoagulation
Reel XI-4. Branch retinal vein occlusion, healed
Reel XI-5. Branch retinal vein occlusion after photocoagulation
Reel XI-6. Branch retinal vein occlusion after photocoagulation
Reel XI-7. Branch retinal vein occlusion, early healed
Reel XII-1. Central retinal vein occlusion
Reel XII-2. Central retinal vein occlusion after PRP
Reel XII-3. Central retinal vein occlusion, early healed
Reel XII-4. Irvine-Gass maculopathy, healed

Miscellaneous macular diseases

Reel XII-5. Macular hole after photocoagulation
Reel XII-6. Macular hole after photocoagulation
Reel XII-7. Preretinal fibrosis after photocoagulation
Reel XIII-1. Toxoplasmic retinochoroiditis
Reel XIII-2. Toxoplasmic retinochoroiditis after photocoagulation
Reel XIII-3. Toxoplasmic retinochoroiditis, healed
Reel XIII-4. Toxoplasmic retinochoroiditis after photocoagulation
Reel XIII-5. Toxoplasmic retinochoroiditis
Reel XIII-6. Toxoplasmic retinochoroiditis after photocoagulation
Reel XIII-7. Toxoplasmic retinochoroiditis, early healed
Reel XIV-1. *T. canis* granuloma after photocoagulation
Reel XIV-2. *T. canis* granuloma, early healed
Reel XIV-3. Retinal pigment epitheliopathy
Reel XIV-4. Retinal pigment epitheliopathy after photocoagulation
Reel XIV-5. Retinal pigment epitheliopathy, healed
Reel XIV-6. Angioid streaks, early healed stage
Reel XIV-7. Angioid streaks, late healed stage
Reel XV-1. Subretinal neovascularization after photocoagulation
Reel XV-2. Subretinal neovascularization after photocoagulation
Reel XV-3. Subretinal neovascularization, healed

Iris abnormalities

Reel XV-4. Miotic pupil
Reel XV-5. Miotic pupil after photomydriasis
Reel XV-6. Photomydriatic iris after miotics
Reel XV-7. Iris after photoiridotomy
Reel XVI-1. Photoiridotomy, early healed stage
Reel XVI-2. Photoiridotomy, late healed stage
Reel XVI-3. Implantation iris cyst
Reel XVI-4. Implantation iris cyst after photocoagulation
Reel XVI-5. Implantation iris cyst, obliterated
Reel XVI-6. Iridocyclitic membrane after photocoagulation
Reel XVI-7. Iridocyclitic membrane after discission